The Fundamentals of Clinical Research

The Fundamentals of Clinical Research

A Universal Guide for Implementing Good Clinical Practice

P. Michael Dubinsky
Spartansburg, PA, USA

Karen A. Henry
University of California, Berkeley
Richmond, CA, USA

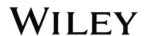

Registered Office
John Wiley & Sons, Inc., 111 River Street, Hoboken, NJ 07030, USA

Editorial Office
111 River Street, Hoboken, NJ 07030, USA

For details of our global editorial offices, customer services, and more information about Wiley products visit us at www.wiley.com.

Wiley also publishes its books in a variety of electronic formats and by print-on-demand. Some content that appears in standard print versions of this book may not be available in other formats.

Library of Congress Cataloging-in-Publication Data

Names: Dubinsky, P. Michael, author. | Henry, Karen A., author.
Title: The fundamentals of clinical research : a universal guide for
    implementing good clinical practice / P. Michael Dubinsky, Spartansburg,
    PA, USA, Karen A. Henry, University of California, Berkeley Richmond,
    CA, USA.
Description: Hoboken, NJ : Wiley, 2022. | Includes index.
Identifiers: LCCN 2021033034 (print) | LCCN 2021033035 (ebook) | ISBN
    9781118949597 (hardback) | ISBN 9781118949603 (adobe pdf) | ISBN
    9781118949610 (epub)
Subjects: LCSH: Medicine–Research.
Classification: LCC R850 .D83 2021 (print) | LCC R850 (ebook) | DDC
    610.72–dc23
LC record available at https://lccn.loc.gov/2021033034
LC ebook record available at https://lccn.loc.gov/2021033035

Cover Design: Wiley
Cover Image: © Mira N. Henry

Set in 9.5/12.5pt STIXTwoText by Straive, Pondicherry, India

10   9   8   7   6   5   4   3   2   1

Contents

Preface

Goal

Since 1996 the emergence of the good clinical practice (GCP) framework for the conduct of clinical trials, more than any other requirement or guidance, has served as a singular reference point for performing trials in humans in conformance with ethical and regulatory expectations. Certainly GCP is mentioned and described in all clinical trial texts, manuscripts, papers, and presentations, and it has moved beyond the role of guidance and become law in a number of global regions and countries: the GCP guidance document developed and published by the International Council for Harmonization of Technical Requirements for Registration of Pharmaceuticals for Human Use (ICH) has been adopted into law in both the European Union (EU) and Canada, and the World Health Organization has developed a set of GCPs for its constituency. For medical device products, the ISO standard 14155 was revised in 2011 and now serves as the GCP reference point for device-related clinical research. That step eliminated the need for clinical investigators studying medical devices to debate whether they should be following the ICH-GCP that was targeted at pharmaceutical drug studies. As a result, GCP has become the universal language of trials that involve human subjects.

GCP provides a framework for clinical trial professionals to work within and guidance in how to abide by their local, national, and/or regional regulatory requirements. In turn, regional and national regulatory authorities integrate GCP into their clinical trial regulations, adopt it to their existing regulations, or call their regulations GCP. The regulatory authorities have established requirements that govern the conduct of trials, and these requirements represent the baseline for compliance. That said, much of the interpretation of the requirements is left to the trial sponsor, investigator, and clinical teams.

The authors, based on their experience both on the job and as teachers, recognize that a comprehensive and integrated understanding of the clinical trial process, with a firm grasp of the fundamental concepts, is vital to improving the quality and outcomes of clinical trials. Both seasoned and novice clinical research professionals wish to obtain a complete overview of the industry and would benefit from learning the fundamentals of clinical research. The comprehensive overview we present in this text will give professionals insight into why they do what they do and provide an integrated understanding of the various disciplines and stages of clinical research. This vantage point allows for judicious application of GCP in practice.

We have designed this text to be used as source material in educational settings such as university courses and as a training aid for the clinical research industry. Our goal is to provide a universal working reference for all of the players in clinical trials: an educational resource that integrates the fundamentals of clinical research for working individuals, clinical research students, or any curious person. By "working individual," we mean everyone from the novice to the seasoned clinical research professional in academia, industry, or a regulatory environment. From a practical viewpoint, this text has been written to address the regulatory, scientific, administrative, business, and ethical considerations of clinical research trials within a GCP framework. It describes how to implement clinical research to meet research, regulatory, and ethical objectives, such that the process succeeds the first time and does not need to be repeated.

Scope of this Book

Clinical research has reached global proportions. This text will not attempt to touch on each individual country, but rather will look at global regions and nations, such as the EU and the United States, which set the pace for the implementation of GCP worldwide. We have aimed to give perspective to each element of GCP from as many vantage points as we can, and have expanded our discussion of the elements of GCP to include regulatory, scientific, technological, site investigator, sponsor, quality, and IRB viewpoints, as appropriate.

We have focused the scope of our clinical research discussion on trials involving humans in a biomedical context. From an investigative product/test article perspective, the text favors pharmaceutical drugs since they are associated with the majority of clinical trials. Biological products fit into the same niche. We have also addressed medical devices, though we recognize that despite the similarities in areas such as regulatory controls in the United States, there is a plethora of differences. While we cannot discuss all of these differences, we have highlighted some of the most significant ones.

How to Use this Book

This text is divided into sections that contain relevant chapters on the history of GCP, drug development in the regulatory environment, the GCP framework, GCP for the individual clinical trial, and quality in clinical trials. Each chapter builds on a key GCP concept and contains chapter objectives, content, a summary, and a set of knowledge check questions so that the reader can self-check their learning and comprehension. The ICH-GCP Guidelines serve as the glossary of terms and definitions. Plates visually summarize the content for certain chapters, and the reader is also able to cross-reference details in pertinent chapters from the plates. Figures, tables, and other illustrations also enhance the text materials.

Opinion of the Authors

The authors of this text have a combined approximately 76 years of experience working in various areas of clinical research, as well as approximately 25 years of experience as part-time instructors in university-sponsored classrooms and online courses of study designed to introduce students to the clinical research industry. They have also developed some of the educational and learning materials that make up these university-sponsored courses. This text is written from their individual viewpoints as they have interpreted and applied the GCP Guidelines. Except for direct references to the ICH E6 (R2) Guideline or other sources, all statements are the opinions of the authors.

The authors would like to thank Kay Ranganathan for introducing them to the instructional arena for clinical research; their esteemed colleagues for their review of the manuscript; and their families for their patience and support through the times when writing this book got in the way of family life.

About the Authors

P. Michael Dubinsky has more than 40 years of experience in the field of GxP quality and compliance in government and industry. He has worked with the FDA and as a regulatory consultant for private corporations. He was also an Instructor in the areas of clinical trial compliance, regulatory audits, and quality at the University of California Berkeley Extension Programs.

Karen A. Henry has worked as a clinical research professional since 1990. She has expertise in regulatory medical writing, standards and processes, trial management and monitoring, biostatistics, and data management. She is also a Lead Instructor for the Certificate Program in Clinical Research Conduct Management at the University of California Berkeley Extension Programs.

About the Companion Website

This book is accompanied by a companion website.

www.wiley.com/go/dubinsky/clinicalresearch

This website includes:

- Solutions to the Problems
- Further References Section

Protocol Synopsis and Schedule of Trial Activities Template

Part I

Good Clinical Practice History

1

History

P. Michael Dubinsky

> **GCP Key Point**
>
> *Good Clinical Practice might be termed a cultural approach to applying ethics and integrity to human biomedical clinical trials with investigational products.*

1.1 Introduction

This chapter will briefly outline the history of biomedical clinical trials from the standpoints of regulatory oversight and ethical expectations and the emergence of good clinical practice (GCP).

1.2 Objectives

The objectives of this chapter are to:

- Provide an outline of legislation, events, and circumstances which provide the background and history for the development of the ICH GCP Guideline E6 R2.
- Offer thoughts and points of view on why the GCP mindset emerged among the global regions most involved in pharmaceutical drug development occurred.

1.3 Chronology

If you research the history of GCP, you will find that it is aligned with the events which form the stepping stones on the pathway of clinical trial regulation. The best known events involve abuses of humans during medical experimentation

The Fundamentals of Clinical Research: A Universal Guide for Implementing Good Clinical Practice,
First Edition. P. Michael Dubinsky and Karen A. Henry.
© 2022 John Wiley & Sons, Inc. Published 2022 by John Wiley & Sons, Inc.
Companion website: www.wiley.com/go/dubinsky/clinicalresearch

and the subsequent legislative and regulatory initiatives to prevent the recurrence of those abuses. The following events, policies, and legislation stand out.

- 1902 – The Biologics Control Act [1] is enacted by the US Congress requiring licensing of vaccines, serums, and similar products. The legislation was prompted by the distribution of a contaminated batch of diphtheria antitoxin contaminated with tetanus which killed 13 children. This legislation eventually became part of the Public Health Service Act and serves as the primary regulatory control for the same group of products which now includes cell therapies and many biotechnology-derived products.
- 1906 – The Food and Drugs Act [2] is passed by the US Congress and gives the Federal Government control over misbranded or adulterated drugs.
- 1938 – The US Congress enacts the Federal Food, Drug and Cosmetic Act (FFDCA) [3] in part due to the Elixir of Sulfanilamide [3] episode in which 107 deaths occurred. The new law required proof of safety prior to marketing and drew cosmetics and therapeutic devices into the regulatory scheme.
- 1949 – The Nuremburg Code [4] is born out of the criminal trials of Nazi researchers who conducted unethical experiments on humans during WWII. The Code is a set of 10 points that establishes a foundation for voluntary consent of research subjects as well as most of the key ethical principles which emerge in subsequent documents.
- 1962 – The Kefauver–Harris Drug Amendments to the FFDCA [5] required that drugs must demonstrate efficacy as well as safety and the investigational new drug (IND) application as we know it today is launched in the regulations. One of the driving forces behind these legislative amendments to the FFDCA was the thalidomide tragedy of 1961 when newborns suffered severe birth defects. The FDA's IND regulations followed circa 1963.
- 1964 – The Declaration of Helsinki [6] takes the ethical principles for conducting research on humans to a new level through the efforts of the World Medical Association.
- 1965 – The US National Institutes of Health proposed that their research involving humans be examined by an impartial panel of peers to ensure ethical integrity. By 1971 the Public health Services' policy of ethical review for human research was expanded to include Department of Health Education and Welfare research however the policy was not well enforced. In 1974. Regulations requiring group ethics review were published and the term institutional review board was born [7].
- 1972 – The US Public Health Service's Tuskegee Syphilis Study [8], which began circa 1932, is publically exposed for its deficiencies and ethical failures.
- 1974 – The US Congress reacts to the Tuskegee study episode by enacting the National Research Act [9] (National Research Act 1974) which establishes the

National Commission for the Protection of Human Subjects of Biomedical and Behavioral Research (National Commission).

- 1976 – the US Congress is provided a report [10] from the General Accounting Office which reported that based on a special survey of sponsor and investigator inspections 74% failed to comply with legal requirements pertaining to informed consent, drug accountability, adherence to protocol, record accuracy, and availability as well as the appropriate supervision by the clinical investigator. This report prompts Congress to recommend that FDA undertake adequate monitoring / inspection programs of clinical trial sponsors, investigators, and institutional review boards.

> "the Food and Drug Administration (FDA) is not adequately regulating new drug testing to insure that human subjects are protected and the test data is accurate and reliable."

- In 1979 the Belmont Report [11] is published by the National Commission and joins the Nuremburg Code and Declaration of Helsinki as a fundamental policy document describing the application of ethical principles such as respect for persons, beneficence, and justice in the conduct of behavioral and biomedical research involving humans.

- 1980s – Global regions, countries with mature drug regulatory systems such as Japan, the European Union (EU), and the United States, as well as global health authorities, e.g. World Health Association, independently establish or enhance regulations and guidelines governing the conduct of human clinical trials. Harmonization of requirements for drug approval is championed by many.
- 1990 – The International Conference on Harmonization of Technical Requirements for Registration of Pharmaceuticals for Human Use (ICH) [12] is founded by the regulatory authorities and pharmaceutical associations of Japan, the United States and the European Union.
- 1996 – The ICH guidance GUIDELINE FOR GOOD CLINICAL PRACTICE E6 (R1) [13] (ICH E6(R2) is finalized. It remains the gold standard for the design, conduct, recording, and reporting of clinical trials involving human subjects. Note – It was revised in 2016 to (R2).
- 2004 – The EU Clinical Trial Directive 2001/20/EC [14] becomes effective and EU member states must move to adopt it into their legal requirements. The Directive sets universal requirements for clinical trials including approval by an

ethics committee, harmonization of technical requirements through participation in the ICH, and application of GCPs in the conduct of human trials.

> The verification of compliance with the standards of GCP and the need to subject data, information, and documents to inspection in order to confirm that they have been properly generated, recorded, and reported are essential in order to justify the involvement of human subjects in clinical trials.

- 2011 – The International Standards Organization (ISO) in conjunction with its standard setting partners publishes the medical device version of the GCP requirements in the form of the standard ANSI/AAMI/ISO 14155 Clinical investigation of medical devices for human subjects – GCP [15] (ISO 14155-2011). 14155 Represents the medical device version of the ICH GCP standard for pharmaceuticals. This publication solidified the application of GCP expectations for human clinical trials in essentially all investigative (unapproved) articles intended for the cure, mitigation, or treatment of disease and injury in man.

This chronology does not however speak directly to the driving forces that were in play as the events unfolded and the progress towards an international acceptance of GCP as a standard was underway.

1.4   The Emergence of the ICH and Its Guidelines

GCP as we know it today was born not just out of tragic episodes in human experimentation such as the Tuskegee Syphilis Study and the abuses of Nazi researchers in the WWII concentration camps. It was very much a work-product of the for-profit drug industry which needed harmonized standards to facilitate the marketing application process among the world's primary producers and consumers of pharmaceuticals. An additional motivation for the ICH concept was to remove duplicative testing which would reduce the exposure of humans to investigational medicinal products, unnecessarily. Viola!, the emergence of the ICH. The ICH was born out of collaboration between the regulatory authorities and industry trade associations. It therefore had the best of both regulatory thinking and for-profit science. The newly born organization moved quickly to develop and propose a number of key guidelines which would benefit the entire pharmaceutical industry. GCP was one of the efficacy guidelines defining approaches to clinical trial activities. Others included clinical safety for Drugs Used in Long Term Treatment (E1) and general considerations in clinical trials (E8).

It is important to note that in establishing the ICH approach the industry and regulators did not attempt to cut corners or somehow create a shortcut bypassing a structured process. Instead the ICH framework has become a model for sound business accomplishment while operating in a transparent and efficient manner. Inclusion of interested parties was encouraged and while the founding members remain in place as the governing entity, participation by other global regions and countries has been fostered and encouraged as observers and as part of global cooperation. Canada, Brazil, China and Australia to name a few participate in ICH meetings and workgroups.

In 2015 the ICH took several steps to solidify its organizational presence and expand its influence. It established itself as an association under Swiss law and it invited regulators and industry counterparts from Switzerland, and Canada to join as full members. It also adopted a name change – The International Council for Harmonization – and continues to grow and prosper today.

Notwithstanding the harmonization mission of the ICH, implementation of guidelines such as GCP even among the founding members of the ICH has not been identical. The European Union and Japan have adopted the GCP guideline into their legal requirements for the conduct of clinical trials. The United States has not, however, done so. The reasons for this difference in adoption of the GCP, as well as other ICH guidelines, lie primarily in the legal system supporting the regulatory framework. For example the United States has had in place regulations governing new drug studies since the early 1960s including requirements associated with informed consent. Modifying those regulations to integrate or adopt the GCP guideline would have been a monumental task. In addition, the system in place to modify/change regulations is a cumbersome one which would encounter difficulties and complexities in keeping up with the technology changes that can more efficiently be processed by a nongovernmental entity such as the ICH.

Without doubt, the US FDA agrees with the ICH GCP guidance, they helped write it! The manner in which the FDA has integrated GCP into its regulatory scheme provides a good example of harmonization with its ICH counterparts as well as demonstrating its support and approval for the application of GCP for human clinical trials.

FDA in a 2004 Federal Register Notice of Proposed Rulemaking (NOPR) [16] to adopt GCP in 21 Code of Federal Regulations (CFR) 312.120 as a reference point for the acceptance of foreign clinical studies not conducted under an IND. At the time, the criteria in 21 CFR 312.120 called for foreign clinical studies to be conducted in accordance with the ethical principles in the Declaration of Helsinki. In reviewing the Preambles to both the NOPR and the 2008 Final Rule [17] it is apparent that the FDA wanted to demonstrate its support and agreement with GCP but was grappling with adopting GCP as a document into law because it would pose administrative difficulties from a procedural and regulatory standpoint. The end product is that FDA removed the reference to the Declaration of Helsinki, which itself had become problematic from several policy standpoints and substituted GCP as the criteria for acceptance of data generated in studies not conducted under an IND. They even devised a set of 11 specific pieces of information that should be described as evidence that GCP was followed during the course of the human clinical trial. It was a win for the FDA and a win for GCP.

Contemporaneous with the development of the ICH GCP was the development of a set of GCP expectations by the World Health Organization [18]. Subsequent to the publication of the ICH GCP, a number of countries has published its own version by modifying the standard to include requirements that fit their regulatory model.

In the next Chapters we will outline the regulatory environment within which GCP is enabled.

1.5 Summary

The advent of the GCP Guideline and its adoption as a global reference for the conduct of human biomedical clinical trials is a story that emerges from a number of business and regulatory objectives that came together in the early 1990s. The chronology of regulatory legislation, historical incidents, and ethical policy development listed earlier formed the backdrop for the success of the ICH organization. It is noteworthy that GCP stood out as a key early guideline development project. Protection of trial subjects and the assurance that data can be trusted were central themes for regulators and the pharmaceutical drug manufacturers were keen to find the protocols which would have a universal appeal. The story of the ICH in general and the development of GCP in particular is one where everyone was a winner.

Knowledge Check Questions

1) The emergence of legislative regulatory controls over pharmaceutical drug development and clinical trials was often prompted by:
    a) Protests from university medical students _____
    b) Tragic outcomes from administration of unsafe and/or ineffective drug products_____
    c) Promises made to voters by candidates for political office_____
2) Failure of medical researchers to apply ethical principles has never been a problem that needed solving? True ____ False _____
3) The Belmont Report was authorized by the National Research Act of 1974. True ____ False _____
4) The ICH Efficacy Guideline – GCP – is considered the industry standard for the conduct of human biomedical clinical trials with drug products. It was developed because:

a) Of continuing abuses against study subjects by drug researchers
_____

b) The United States, Japan, and the European Union wanted manufacturers in their countries to have a monopoly on drug marketing _____

c) Manufactures and regulatory authorities wanted to establish harmonized standards to facilitate the mutual acceptance of clinical data supporting drug approval_____

5) The ICH headquarters are located in the United States and the organization is under the US FDA. True _____ False _____

References

1 NIH1908. A short History of the National Institutes of Health, p. 3 http://history.
nih.gov/exhibits/history/docs/page_03.html (accessed 11 November 2019)

2 Janssen, W.F. (1981). Story of the laws lehind the labels, Part 1. The 1906 Food and
Drugs Act. https://wayback.archive-it.org/7993/20170111191530/http://www.fda.
gov/AboutFDA/WhatWeDo/History/Overviews/ucm056044.htm (accessed
27 November 2019)

3 FDA (2012). History of drug regulation in the United States, 1906–2006, p6,
wayback.archive-it.org/7993/20170114041745/http://www.fda.gov/downloads/
AboutFDA/WhatWeDo/History/ProductRegulation/PromotingSafeandEffectiveDr
ugsfor100Years/UCM114468.pdf (accessed 27 November 2019)

4 United States Holocaust Memorial Museum. United States Holocaust Memorial
Museum Note https://www.ushmm.org/information/exhibitions/online-
exhibitions/special-focus/doctors-trial/nuremberg-code (assessed
27 November 2019)

5 FDA (2012). Consumer updates, Kefauver-Harris Amendments Revolutionized
Drug Development http://www.fda.gov/ForConsumers/ConsumerUpdates/
ucm322856.htm (accessed 27 November 2019)

6 World Medical Association (2018). WMA Declaration of Helsinki – Ethical
Principles for Medical Research Involving Human Subjects. https://www.wma.net/
policies-post/wma-declaration-of-helsinki-ethical-principles-for-medical-research-
involving-human-subjects/ (accessed 27 November 2019)

7 Grady, C. Institutional review boards, purpose and challenges, commentary, chest,
November 2015 (1148–1155) https://www.ncbi.nlm.nih.gov/pmc/articles/
PMC4631034/pdf/chest_148_5_1148.pdf (accessed 28 May 2020)

8 Centers for Disease Control and Prevention. U.S. Public Health Service Syphilis
Study at Tuskegee. http://www.cdc.gov/tuskegee/timeline.htm (accessed
27 November 2019)

9 NIH (1908). National Research Act – Office of NIH History. https://history.nih. gov/research/downloads/PL93-348.pdf (accessed 27 November 2019)

10 US Government Accountability Office. Federal control of new drug testing is not adequately protecting human test subjects and the public HRD-76–96: published: Jul 15, 1976. publicly released: July 15, 1976. http://www.gao.gov/products/ HRD-76-96. (accessed 27 November 2019)

11 US Department of Health and Human Services. Office of human research protections, the belmont report. http://www.hhs.gov/ohrp/humansubjects/ guidance/belmont.html (accessed 27 November 2019)

12 ICH. The international council for harmonisation of technical requirements for pharmaceuticals for human use (ICH), http://www.ich.org/ (accessed 27 November 2019)

13 *ICH E6 (R2). ICH E6 (R2) (2016) INTEGRATED ADDENDUM TO ICH E6(R1):GUIDELINE FOR GOOD CLINICAL PRACTICE*: International Council on Harmonization https://database.ich.org/sites/default/files/E6_R2_Addendum. pdf (accessed 27 November 2019)

14 European Commission European commission directive 2001/20/EC, clinical trials. https://ec.europa.eu/health/human-use/clinical-trials/directive_en (accessed 27 November 2019)

15 ANSI WEBSTORE. *Clinical Investigation of Medical Devices for Human Subjects - Good Clinical Practice*. International Standards Organization http://webstore. ansi.org/RecordDetail.aspx?sku=ISO%2014155:2011&source=google&adgro up=iso11&gclid=CO6fhuXkx70CFU5rfgodQGwA9Q (accessed 27 November 27, 2019).ISO 14155:2011

16 GPO. Federal register, 32467, Vol. 69, No. 112, Thursday, June 10, 2004 human subject protection; foreign clinical studies not conducted under an investigational new drug application – proposed rule http://www.gpo.gov/fdsys/pkg/ FR-2004-06-10/pdf/04-13063.pdf (accessed 27 November 2019)

17 Authenticated U.S. Government Information. Federal register/Vol. 73, No. 82/ Monday, April 28, 2008/Rules and regulations, human subject protection; foreign clinical studies not conducted under an investigational new drug application, final rule https://www.govinfo.gov/content/pkg/FR-2008-04-28/pdf/E8-9200.pdf (accessed 27 November 2019)

18 World Health Organization. *Handbook for Good Clinical Research Practice*. ISBN: ISBN 92 4 159392 X https://www.who.int/medicines/areas/quality_safety/ safety_efficacy/gcp1.pdf.

Part II

Drug Development in the Regulatory Environment

2

Regulatory Environment

P. Michael Dubinsky

GCP Key Point

Regulatory authorities along with medical institutions and professional groups form a network of controls which set the boundaries for human biomedical clinical trials thereby ensuring that GCP is followed.

2.1   Introduction

Is it idealistic to think that all clinical research whether commercial, academic, governmental or otherwise will be conducted under ethical guidelines and according to best scientific and professional practices such as GCP? Unfortunately idealism has not always been the guiding force in human biomedical research and along the way governmental and professional oversight has been implemented to ensure that abuses are avoided. This chapter explores the regulatory environment that has evolved to oversee human biomedical clinical trials.

2.2   Objective

To describe the nature and scope of controls that are in place to ensure that human biomedical clinical trials are conducted in a manner which ensures the protection of human subjects participating in them and the scientific integrity of the trial plan. Understanding the nature, scope and reach of the regulatory controls as well as their enforceability is essential to applying the GCP principles.

The Fundamentals of Clinical Research: A Universal Guide for Implementing Good Clinical Practice, First Edition. P. Michael Dubinsky and Karen A. Henry.
© 2022 John Wiley & Sons, Inc. Published 2022 by John Wiley & Sons, Inc.
Companion website: www.wiley.com/go/dubinsky/clinicalresearch

2.3 Regulatory Matrix

The regulatory environment within which human biomedical clinical trials are conducted is a matrix composed of: (i) the policies, laws, and regulations which describe the requirements and guidance; (ii) the governmental jurisdictions (Federal, State, Country, Region e.g. EU) which are responsible for implementing the requirements through regulatory authorities; (iii) nongovernmental organizations, e.g. Academic Medical Centers (AMCs), which both sponsor clinical trials and set their own internal standards for how clinical trials will be conducted; and (iv) the professional organizations (e.g. WHO, WMA) which support, define, and interpret the requirements, standards, and guidelines for their professional members.

It is not always clear whether this matrix works together under a planned scenario but the end result is that if a commercial sponsor, medical establishment, or individual practitioner wishes to conduct experimental biomedical studies in humans, that activity receives considerable oversight and review. There are complexities which the regulatory environment matrix introduces to the conduct of clinical trials; therefore it is important to understand the makeup of the regulatory environment. For example conducting trials in conformance with ICH E6(R2) does not guarantee that a trial meets all of the applicable regulatory standards called for by the country or region where the study is performed but it is probable that the use of the those guidelines would ensure that 90% or more of applicable requirements will be met.

Let us begin the examination of the regulatory environment by reviewing each of the four part matrix as depicted in Figure 2.1.

2.4 Laws, Regulations, and Policies

The enforceable requirements governing human biomedical clinical trials are found in the written laws (statutes) and implementing regulations. These laws and regulations, which are based on governmental policies provide the societal backbone for the authorities to regulate and affect control over human biomedical clinical trial activities. The laws are written by the elected legislatures which in the United States is the Congress. Congress is composed of the Senate and House of Representatives. The laws are passed by the Legislature, i.e. Congress and approved by the President and as needed interpreted by the US Supreme Court. Laws however are very high level statements and call for implementing details. Once in place, USA laws are implemented by the executive departments who report to the President. In the United States, the Federal Food Drug and Cosmetic Act (FFDCA) is a primary governing statute and the implementing regulations

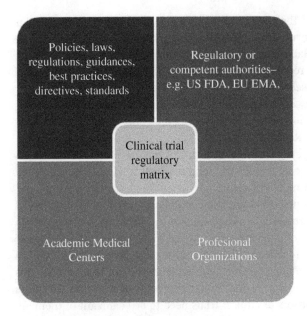

Figure 2.1 The clinical trial regulatory matrix.

are developed/written by staff in the Food and Drug Administration (FDA) which is part of the Department of Health and Human Services (DHHS). The regulations are memorialized in the US Code of Federal Regulations (CFR). Regulations are developed according to the Administrative Procedures Act of 1946 (APA) which calls for agencies such as the FDA/DHHS to (i) keep the public informed of their organization, procedures and rules; (ii) provide for public participation in the rulemaking process; (iii) to establish uniform standards for the conduct of formal rulemaking and adjudication; (iv) to define the scope of judicial review. The rules developed pursuant to the APA have the force and effect of law, i.e. they are enforceable. There are sanctions and penalties if the rules are not followed.

The rules applicable to the conduct of clinical trials in the USA are found in Title 21 of the Code of Federal Regulations. The FDA considers the following Parts to be GCP:

- 21 CFR Part 50 – Protection of Human Subjects
- 21 CFR Part 54 – Financial Disclosure by Clinical Investigators
- 21 CFR Part 56 – Institutional Review Boards (IRBs)
- 21 CFR Part 312 – Investigational New Drug Application (prescription drugs)
- 21 CFR Part 812 – Investigational Device Exemptions (medical devices)

These regulations define the must do ground rules that apply to regulated biomedical research from informed consent to the content of an application for authorization to conduct the trial in humans. There are additional regulations which have impact on drug development and clinical trials activities such as electronic records, good laboratory practices, and marketing applications.

In addition to the FDA regulations the DHHS has an organizational group titled the Office of Human Research Protections (OHRP) which has responsibility for regulations governing research funded or performed by the federal government. Specifically: 45 CFR Part 46 – Federal Policy for the Protection of Human Research Subjects – "the Common Rule."

The title of the rule speaks for itself in terms of content. It applies to all US Federal government biomedical and behavioral research conducted or sponsored by over 15 Federal department and agencies.

Federal regulations do not stand completely alone in terms of governmental oversight of clinical trial requirements and each of the 50 States has rules which affect one or more aspects of the conduct of clinical trials. For example the age of consent for trial subjects is reflected in State rather than Federal laws. The full nature and scope of the Federal and State requirements will not be covered in this text. The important point is that regulatory requirements may be found in more than one source and sponsors of clinical trials need to be cognizant of them all. ICH E6(R2) 5.1.1 speaks to that expectation.

Another well-known example of the law and regulation framework is that of the European Union. The European Union's approach is a bit different than the USA due to its regional construct but the legal arrangement resembles that of the USA. The European Union currently comprises 28 Member States. There is a central government organization, the European Council (EC) located in Brussels, Belgium. The EC, in conjunction with the European Parliament issues Directives which each of the member states are expected to implement or place into law and regulation within their own country's legislative/governmental system. With regard to GCP the EC issued Directive 20/2001/EC – The Clinical Trial Directive in 2001. In 2005, the EC issued the Good Clinical Practice Directive – 2005/28/EC. These two directives were instrumental in closing several gaps which existed in the regulation of clinical trial activities in the EU member states. These Directives specifically called for ICH E6(R2) to be taken into account in terms of clinical trial regulation. Many people therefore view ICH E6(R2) as essentially a legal requirement in the EU. While changes are underway in several aspects of the regulatory framework established under the two EU Directives they have served as the pillars of regulation for human clinical trials involving pharmaceutical drugs in the EU. Notwithstanding expected changes in other aspects of clinical trial regulation ICH E6(R2) will continue to be the key criteria for conduct of a clinical trial.

It is useful to point out that the regulation of human clinical trials involving medical device products in the European Union is addressed under separate Directives e.g. 93/42/EEC. The overall regulation of medical devices in the European Union is also in the process of change.

Policies developed or adopted by governments provide another source or format for requirements. Laws and regulations are often derived from important policy statements. For human clinical trials the fundamental principles and practices for the ethical treatment of subjects have been drawn from The Nuremburg Code, Declaration of Helsinki and Belmont Report which are generally recognized as being the "gold standards" for the protection of human subjects participating in clinical trials. Of the three the Declaration of Helsinki undergoes periodic updation. These documents will be mentioned a number of times in this text and you will study them in detail if you take courses in ethics and informed consent.

2.5 Guidelines and Guidance Materials

There are other types of documents which provide insight and understanding as to how regulatory authorities interpret compliance with laws and regulations. These include materials titled: good guidance practices, guidelines, reflection papers, best practices, standards, and notices. These documents do not generally have the legal standing of laws and regulations but they often represent the combined opinion of regulatory and scientific experts and therefore carry significant weight when assessing compliance with the law.

The exact definition for these materials does differ between regulatory authorities so it is important to review the definitions to be certain one understands whether they are essentially requirements or optional. For example in the European Union the EMEA offers the following on guidelines:

> The European Medicines Agency's Committee for Medicinal Products for Human Use prepares scientific guidelines in consultation with regulatory authorities in the European Union (EU) Member States, to help applicants prepare marketing authorisation applications for human medicines. Guidelines reflect a harmonised approach of the EU Member States and the Agency on how to interpret and apply the requirements for the demonstration of quality, safety, and efficacy set out in the Community directives.
>
> The Agency strongly encourages applicants and marketing authorisation holders to follow these guidelines. Applicants need to justify deviations from guidelines fully in their applications at the time of submission. Before that, they should seek scientific advice, to discuss any proposed deviations during medicine development.
>
> The guidelines are complementary to European Pharmacopoeia monographs and chapters: [1]

The FDA on the other hand states in their regulations defining Good Guidance Practices: *Good guidance practices (GGP's) are FDA's policies and procedures for developing, issuing, and using guidance documents. Guidance documents are documents prepared for FDA staff, applicants/sponsors, and the public that describe the agency's interpretation of or policy on a regulatory issue. Guidance documents include, but are not limited to, documents that relate to: The design, production, labeling, promotion, manufacturing, and testing of regulated products; the processing, content, and evaluation or approval of submissions; and inspection and enforcement policies [2].*

Best practices are usually published by industry or a professional organization. The importance of the content is linked to whether it receives any specific endorsement by a regulator or officials from regulatory agency. Very often best practices address topics that are not specifically found in laws or regulations. One example is handling regulatory inspections. Industry has developed their own set of best practices for interacting with regulatory inspectors during inspections with the goal of being forthright and compliant without being presumptuous. Another example of best practices might be recruiting and retaining subjects in clinical trials.

Notices are usually issued as one time alerts or reminders which are sent by regulatory authorities based on incidents which occur and which carry some importance in terms of protecting subjects or data integrity. Notices are also used by some regulatory authorities to advise sponsors, investigators, and others clinical trial players of regulatory interpretations they have made and which are enforceable. The country of India's Central Drug Standards Control Organization (CDSCO) uses Notices/Notifications in that manner.

Reflection papers are unique to the EU/EMA and they are a compellation of general issues on a topic which should be taken into consideration. An example is the EMA's *Reflection paper for laboratories that perform the analysis or evaluation of clinical trial samples*. Its purpose is to *provide laboratories that perform the analysis or evaluation of human samples collected as part of a clinical trial, with information that will help them develop and maintain quality systems which will comply with relevant European Union Directives, national regulations and associated guidance documents [3].*

Standards as such are not prevalent in the human clinical trial arena for pharmaceutical drugs. There are some clinical trial-related documents which have universal application and acceptance and are referred to as "standards." The ICH E6(R2) guideline being a primary example. Standard setting organizations such as the International Organization for Standardization (ISO) have played a role in setting globally accepted standards for medical devices for some time and the *Standard Clinical investigation of medical devices for human subjects – Good clinical practice, ISO 14155* [4] is an example that fits neatly with our discussion of human clinical trials.

The level of importance that is assigned to these various guidance materials is usually a function of who issues the document and what the issuing party says about its status and importance at the time of issuance.

2.6   Regulatory/Competent Authority Organizations

The second element in the regulatory environment matrix is the regulatory or competent authority. The regulatory authority is charged or assigned the task of implementing and enforcing the laws and regulations, i.e. regulatory requirements. ICH E6(R2) highlights the roles of application review and inspection for regulatory authorities. In fact their responsibilities include other tasks for example, inspecting clinical trial activities, enforcing the requirements, and educating regulated entities. Understanding the roles and responsibilities of the regulatory authority, how they are organized, and what their approaches are to implementation of the applicable laws and regulations adds value and is essential to conducting clinical trials in conformance with GCP.

There are internet resources which provide listings and links to many of the global regulatory authorities responsible for drug/device regulation in general and the oversight of clinical trials in particular. It is likely you have already accessed many of the webpages for global regulatory authorities.

While the US FDA does not serve as the single model for global regulatory authorities it represents one of the best known and seasoned regulators. If we look back at the introductory chapter you will note that many of the key events associated with the evolution of clinical trial and pharmaceutical product regulation took place in the United States and the growth of clinical trial regulation is directly linked to the growth of the US FDA as an organization.

Using the FDA's review process of applications for permission or authorization to conduct clinical trials does provide a somewhat generic blueprint for application review.

First a trial sponsor submits an application which is assigned to one of the three FDA headquarters' offices:

1) Center For Drug Evaluation and Research (CDER) – INDs
2) Center for Biologics Evaluation and Research (CBER) – INDs and IDEs
3) Center for Devices and Radiological Health (CDRH) – IDEs

Each of the FDA Centers has a scientific technical group assigned to receive, review, evaluate, and decide on acceptability of the applications submitted.

There are procedural aspects of the review process that must be followed including timeframes for decisions. It is the responsibility of the FDA and all regulatory agencies to determine whether there is adequate information from nonclinical as well as clinical information about an investigational product to support the plan for the proposed clinical trial. Information about the manufacturing aspects of the investigational product as well as details about the investigation plan and the ethics review process is also included in the application. Part of the authorization decision by the FDA is determining whether the ethics review process for the planned study is already completed or a commitment is made to do so before enrolling any subjects. If a proposed trial is approved the sponsor is advised and periodic reports will be required. The number of trial sites along with the proposed number of subjects is, or becomes part of the application file as the study progresses.

In the European Union, the application from the sponsor is evaluated by the individual member state's health authority. So if trials are to be conducted in five of the member states applications must be submitted to each. There is no common application forum as with the US FDA using the IND format. This lack of a central clinical trial authorization process is an issue that is being addressed by EU authorities and is expected to be resolved with the advent and full implementation of the European Clinical Trial regulation [5]. The European Medicines Agency (EMA) does play a role in facilitating coordination among the member states for clinical trial matters, e.g. inspections, but it does not serve as a central reviewer providing mutually accepted decisions. This text will not attempt to outline the regulatory review processes for all regulatory authorities/competent authorities but rather to point out that they exist and are the players in the regulatory environment.

2.7 Academic Medical Centers (AMCs)

What is an AMC and why do they fit in this matrix? The answer in part is found in the definition developed by the University of Pennsylvania – *At an academic medical center, education, research, and clinical care are combined to provide the best possible clinical care, that uses cutting-edge technologies, resources and therapies other community hospitals may not have available* [6]. AMCs are often affiliated with a college or university which pursues human clinical research through commercial sponsors via government agency grants or on their own as sponsors. Such institutions have established the infrastructure necessary to navigate the Federal, State and if needed foreign regulatory pathways to conduct human clinical trials in full compliance with national and local laws as well as meet all ethical expectations. A title for such a group at an AMC might be *Office of Research Conduct and Compliance.*

Since an AMC is a hospital environment patients receiving clinical care may also be recruited into clinical trials. Researchers, whether independent or affiliated directly with the AMC must abide by all applicable regulations, codes, and ethical review expectations in order to draw on the resources of the institution. In addition, the researcher must follow the internal procedures established by the institution many of which may be more rigorous above the baseline regulations imposed by the regulatory authority. AMCs also have a substantive measure of enforcement powers or sanctions which can be brought to bear swiftly if a researcher violates commitments made to the AMC and/or the regulator. For example revocation of medical privileges, economic sanctions, or being denied the ability to continue enrollment in a trial are the types of actions an AMC can take to address bad behavior by a clinical researcher.

AMCs also coordinate and support local IRB services in many cases so a researcher seeking to undertake a study can be directed to that resource. AMCs can be either nongovernmental or government affiliated. They wield important authority and impact in terms of ensuring that the Regulatory environment or matrix prevents uncontrolled human research study activity from occurring.

2.8   Professional Organizations

Not every medical practitioner belongs to a professional organization but most of those who are providing services in conformance with local licensing and professional credentialing requirements do belong to one or more professional organizations. Primary examples are medical associations who affiliate locally, nationally, and worldwide. Examples are the World Medical Association which developed and regularly updates the Declaration of Helsinki, and the, World Health Association which has its own set of Good Clinical Practices utilized throughout the globe. Those organizations promote and expect their members to comply with ethical and regulatory requirements. With their membership layered from global down through local states, regions and countries any transgressions in the conduct of human biomedical clinical trials or experimentation would be quickly identified and made visible to appropriate authorities. The reach of the international organizations is especially important in developing countries where the regulatory scheme is less mature.

2.9   Summary

There is no doubt that the primary force in the regulatory environment is the regulatory or competent authority. They are provided under law with the necessary authority to affect control over most clinical trial activities including evaluating compliance with GCP through laws, regulations, directives, and other legal instruments. There is a layering of this authority in many countries and regions. For example in the USA there are Federal and State authorities which may have a role depending upon the nature of the research. In the European Union, it would be the Central Government Directorates and the health ministries for the member states. Supporting the authorities are AMCs which work to ensure that clinical trials are conducted in conformance with requirements and ethical standards through their infrastructure. Professional organizations complete the regulatory matrix.

The regulatory matrix may be more complete in some parts of the globe than others but as a concept it continues to expand providing protection to subjects in human clinical trials and further ensuring the quality of data supporting application decisions.

Knowledge Check Questions

1) The regulatory matrix outlined in this chapter includes: Select all that apply
   _____ Regulatory authorities
   _____ Local Law enforcement organizations
   _____ Organizations that license/credential medical professionals
   _____ Standard setting organizations, e.g. ANSI
   _____ Academic Medical Institutions
2) Regulatory authorities create, publish, and enforce codes or requirements governing the conduct of clinical trials. True or False?
3) If a physician in the United States or an European Union member state was advertising for subjects to participate in a clinical research trial of an unapproved product without the approval of the regulatory authority what scenario do you think might occur once the regulatory authority (FDA or EMA) was alerted to the situation? (Brief narrative)
4) A physician practicing at an AMC decides to participate in a clinical trial. Do you think the trial protocol and/physician will need to obtain any internal approvals as well as external approvals for permission to participate? Who might be the first to act if it is found that the trial is being performed in nonconformance with GCP?
5) ICH E6(R2) E6 is considered a Guideline. True or False?

References

1 EMA Scientific Guidelines http://www.ema.europa.eu/ema/index.jsp?curl=pages/regulation/general/general_content_000043.jsp&mid=WC0b01ac05800240cb (accessed 27 January 2020)
2 FDA (2000). Good Guidance Practices/Guidance documents FDA Regs at 21 CFR 10.115. http://www.accessdata.fda.gov/scripts/cdrh/cfdocs/cfcfr/CFRSearch.cfm?fr=10.115 (accessed 27 January 2020)
3 EMA (2012). Reflection paper on laboratories that test clinical trial samples http://www.ema.europa.eu/docs/en_GB/document_library/Regulatory_and_procedural_guideline/2012/05/WC500127124.pdf (accessed 27 January 2020)

4 ISO (2011) ISO 14155:2011). *Clinical Investigation of Medical Devices for Human Subjects — Good Clinical Practice*. International Organization for Standardization https://www.iso.org/standard/45557.html (accessed 27 January 2020).

5 Regulation (EU) No 536/2014 of the European Parliament and of the Council of 16 April 2014 on Clinical Trials on Medicinal Products for Human Use, and Repealing Directive 2001/20/EC https://ec.europa.eu/health//sites/health/files/files/eudralex/vol-1/reg_2014_536/reg_2014_536_en.pdf (accessed 27 January 2020)

6 Penn Medicine (2020). What is an Academic Medical Center. https://www.pennmedicine.org/about/benefits-of-an-academic-medical-center (accessed 27 January 2020)

3

GCP in Context

P. Michael Dubinsky

GCP Key Point

Good Clinical Practice is only one of the "good" cultures in the drug development scheme. A culture of good practices is essential for compliance with USA and international regulatory authority expectations, and aids in ensuring quality data, and protection of trial participants.

3.1 Introduction

The drug development process depicted in Plate 1 is a lengthy and demanding endeavor. Good clinical practice is not an element in all of the steps, phases, and activities that makeup the full development process. However, keeping in perspective the fact that there are applicable regulatory requirements across the spectrum of the entire process and, at minimum best practices should be applied even when the step may not seem to involve regulatory oversight is a wise mindset to adopt. Applying the quality systems approach that is outlined in Chapter 30 as a guiding principle from the time a new drug concept is born to approval of a marketing application is a winning strategy.

3.2 Objectives

The objectives of this chapter are:

1) To put GCP into perspective with the other GXP. GXP is an acronym for Good Laboratory, manufacturing, and clinical practice requirements that are applicable during the drug development process.

The Fundamentals of Clinical Research: A Universal Guide for Implementing Good Clinical Practice, First Edition. P. Michael Dubinsky and Karen A. Henry.
© 2022 John Wiley & Sons, Inc. Published 2022 by John Wiley & Sons, Inc.
Companion website: www.wiley.com/go/dubinsky/clinicalresearch

2) To emphasize that clinical development must apply the "good" practices culture which evolved from drug and device manufacturing regulations.
3) To emphasize the importance of the cross connectivity of GXP requirements and the dependence of the overall drug development process on maintaining a compliance mindset while performing all steps, phases, and activities.. . .

3.2.1 Discovery

The first decision point in drug development is deciding to try and find a cure for or prevention of a disease. Medical researchers may pursue drug discovery based on learning about a disease process in a way that allows new approaches to slowing the disease down or possibly curing it. In the United States, there are government and nongovernmental organizations that pursue new cures and treatments for disease and injury for a variety of reasons. Profit-based decisions are often seen as the driving force behind seeking new and/or innovative treatments or procedures but that is probably not the primary driving force in place at early stages of discovery. One approach that has been successful is called repurposing [1]. Commercial industry and research-oriented academic institutions have been finding new applications for already approved or tested medicines. This approach to drug discovery has identified a number of innovative pathways. E.g. new uses for existing drugs, new uses for drugs whose development was cut short; and identifying side effects from tested drugs which may indicate useful new applications. Using scientific methods such as genetic testing also allows researchers to target a drug to a specific site in the human body thereby increasing drug efficacy. Repurposing existing drugs is also economically rewarding. One of the possible stumbling blocks encountered when pursuing this approach is when data and records from prior studies need to be resurrected for review and use in assessing the overall history of the drug's use in trials. If that data was not collected in conformance with GCP and other Good Practices (GXP) its use may be limited and may stand in the path of pursuing a new application. My experience in this regard was when a firm wanted to use data from studies which were performed 14 years prior. Not only were the records questionable in terms of completeness but the ability to demonstrate that the data was collected in conformance with good clinical practices and/or the applicable regulatory requirements was not clear.

3.2.2 1.4 Pre-Clinical Studies

The next step in the drug development continuum is for researchers to begin assembling data on whether the drug is toxic, i.e., is there laboratory data showing it might cause harm. The initial tests will be done via in vivo animal testing and/

or in vitro laboratory experiments. This nonclinical study activity places research-ers directly into the regulatory environment in that conducting such testing must be done following the Good Laboratory Practice (GLP) regulations at 21 CFR 58 if the drug is intended for the US market. *See Plate 1 Nonclinical Studies*-The ICH has developed safety guidelines addressing carcinogenicity, genotoxicity, and toxicity which form a basis for preclinical studies to be submitted to most global regulatory authorities including the FDA. These safety guidelines were one of the initial actions of the ICH when it was first founded and resulted in harmonizing many differing global approaches. The ICH safety guidelines are adopted by the US FDA as good guidance practices While there are provisions in the FDA's Investigational New Drug (IND) Applications regulations at 21 CFR 312, allowing use of data from animal studies not performed in compliance with GLP, once a firm has decided to pursue a drug development scheme they ought to be following the GLP regulatory requirements. Since many of the GLP animal studies, intended to be submitted to the FDA, are performed at a relatively small number of GLP testing facilities which are regularly inspected by the FDA it is likely that the laboratory's work will have been evaluated for conformance with the applicable regulations. If there are issues with the data gathered during the nonclinical phase of study it may stand in the way of moving to human administration of the investigational product.

3.2.3 Clinical Studies

Once sufficient data has been assembled to support administering the investiga-tional drug product to humans an IND is filed and barring FDA placing it (the IND) on hold, human studies begin. It is at this time, the GCP expectations come to the fore and are the subject matter of this text.

Once a firm has received approval of a new drug (or Biologic) they may decide to set aside most if not all clinical trials involving the product unless Phase IV tri-als have been ordered by the FDA. Of course in many cases, clinical trials are continued for a product and those trials whether ordered by FDA or not must be conducted in conformance with IND regulations and GCP expectations.

Post approval use of the product by the medical professionals is not governed by the FDA or GCP, at least not in any formal manner. States and local jurisdictions oversee activities associated with the prescribing of drugs by physicians and other health care professionals via their professional licensing programs. The Federal Food Drug and Cosmetic Act contains language which translates into FDA keep-ing its distance from the practice of medicine or regulating professional practices.

GCP is therefore only a part of the GXP regulatory scheme which is embedded in the drug development continuum. It represents a still evolving portion of the culture of quality that has been evolving in the clinical development arena for some time. It of course only applies to the authorized human biomedical clinical trials which are conducted to generate data of safety and efficacy but those are the trials where data integrity and subject protections are most important. Interestingly the FDA has not adopted the ICH E6(R2) as a formal regulatory requirement as have a number of foreign regulatory authorities. However, the FDA played a leading role in the development of the ICH E6 (R2) standard and references ICH GCP (R2) in several key spots of the governing investigational drug regulations. So the FDA certainly agrees with GCP and its use in guiding human trials. FDA refers to its regulations governing investigational drug studies as being GCP. Admittedly much of what is contained in ICH E6 (R2) was drawn from the FDA's existing regulations.

3.2.4 Manufacturing the Investigational Drug Product

Returning to Plate 1 we see the reference to current Good Manufacturing Practice (cGMP) regulations as it applies to the investigational drug product. The manufacturing of the investigational drug product must meet the cGMP regulations but on a graduating scale. FDA in 2008 published a guidance document describing its policy regarding the application of the cGMP requirements for Phase I investigational drugs. In summary, FDA provides some leeway for a manufacturer's compliance with the full range of 21 CFR 211 requirements in the earliest stages of clinical testing but that leeway starts to evaporate once Phase II begins and by Phase III of clinical testing of a new drug the manufacture of the investigational drug product is expected to be in full compliance with 21 CFR 211. Whether that is always the case may be up for debate since the FDA from a programmatic standpoint does not routinely or programmatically inspect the manufacture of new drugs being used in clinical trials. That said if the FDA were to find that an investigational drug product was not being manufactured in conformance with applicable cGMP or was adulterated or misbranded they can and will act to contain its use if the responsible firm does not do so.

3.2.5 Common Properties of GXPs

So what is it that ties the three GXP disciplines together? It is the culture of quality and building quality into all aspects and processes that are employed. If you turn to Chapter 30 and the diagram depicting the quality management system you can visualize that whether the investigational product is being manufactured, undergoing preliminary testing to assess its toxicity, or being administered to humans as part of a clinical trial the same set of quality characteristics are brought to bear.

Qualification of people, places, and things must be performed against a standard or set of criteria. Training must occur not only in the general aspects of the discipline but also in the details which apply, for example a clinical trial protocol. Written procedures must be in place, trained against and followed. Keeping written procedures current is one of the most demanding, but necessary aspects of this quality characteristic. Maintaining records and documentation which is accurate and complete cannot be overemphasized. Documenting data and events whether by hand or electronically is essential; however, it remains one of the quality activities that is the most difficult to convince people is critical. Keeping records is not viewed as fun by many people. Ensuring that all involved parties and systems are engaged when making changes is a management step that demands inclusiveness. Operating under a management system that has identified the risks associated with the trial and which represent a critical to quality categorization along with any planned mitigation is a characteristic which evolved from the medical device manufacturing arena but has become an accepted and necessary practice throughout GXP. Learning and making changes based on implementing a corrective and preventive action program is also a process which was born in the medical device regulatory scheme but adds value to the clinical trial endeavor because it forces systematic change not just one off corrections. From the Quality Assurance standpoint auditing programs either internally or by external parties highlights not just the issues but also the successes in a program. Lastly having the involvement of management that is empowered to make changes and is committed to doing so when needed is key to completing the GXP scheme in general and GCP is particular.

3.3 Summary

Once a firm has decided to pursue a drug development process it enters a regulated environment which includes GLP, GCP, and cGMP. The plans, actions, and decisions associated with the firm's drug development initiative must be in tune with and guided by these regulatory requirements. GCP is a part of the regulatory scheme not the entire regulatory scheme.

Knowledge Check Questions

1) GXP refers to what three regulatory concepts?
2) Repurposing of a drug is one approach to drug development. True or False
3) A drug being used in a Phase I study must meet all cGMP requirements according to FDA. True or False
4) Post approval prescribing of drug products is governed by state and local officials. True or False
5) ICH E6(R2) Is a regulatory requirement in the United States. True or False

Reference

1 Repurposing existing drugs for new indications. 1 January (2017). https://www.the-scientist.com/features/repurposing-existing-drugs-for-new-indications-32285?archived_content=9BmGYHLCH6vLGNdd9YzYFAqV8S3Xw3L5 (accessed 27 January 2020)

4

The Intersection of GCP and Regulation

P. Michael Dubinsky

GCP Key Point

GCP expectation intersects the entire functional scheme of clinical development for pharmaceutical medicinal products. Understanding the intersections is useful and enlightening.

The emergence of the ICH closely parallels with the emergence of current GCP because the ICH served as a catalyst for development of Standards such as the ICH E6(R2). The ICH-GCP (R1) was one of the first standards developed by the ICH. It was recognized that such a standard was needed. Regulatory Authorities had worked on building the GCP expectations into their regulatory schemes by detailing them in codes or regulations then interpreting the codes using mechanisms such as inspections and industry meeting presentations. The World Health Organization (WHO) had pursued developing principles of good clinical research practice as early as the late 1960s however the WHO was not a regulatory or standard setting organization so their guidance did not represent requirements nor was it mandated under any laws. The regulatory authorities were not working collaboratively to further their GCP thinking and as a result the requirements across countries and regions were evolving differently. It took an industry-regulatory authority initiative – The ICH – to open the door to establishing a pathway for harmonization of GCP as well as other drug development requirements. That initiative has flourished and expanded.

The Fundamentals of Clinical Research: A Universal Guide for Implementing Good Clinical Practice,
First Edition. P. Michael Dubinsky and Karen A. Henry.
© 2022 John Wiley & Sons, Inc. Published 2022 by John Wiley & Sons, Inc.
Companion website: www.wiley.com/go/dubinsky/clinicalresearch

4.1   Introduction

In Chapter 1 – History of GCP outlines key aspects of the birth of the ICH organization and its growth from 1990 to the present day. This chapter will not repeat that material but rather will outline how the ICH E6(R2) reflects the harmonized expectations of the industry-regulatory authority collaboration which began working to draft the GCP Efficacy Guideline almost immediately after the establishment of the ICH as an organization.

4.2   Objectives

The objectives of this chapter are to:

- Demonstrate how the ICH E6(R2) Guideline serves to underpin those practices which support subject safety and data integrity within the context of meeting regulatory authority requirements.
- Outline several ways the ICH guideline elements moved the conduct of clinical trials closer to meeting the expectation of regulatory compliance and best practices.

Since this text is devoted to explaining fundamental precepts for good clinical practice this chapter will not address each topic area but rather select several examples of how the ICH E6(R2) moves clinical research several steps higher than the regulatory expectations which are generally acknowledged to be the minimum requirements for compliance with a statute, directive, or code.

4.3   The Principles of ICH E6(R2)

The thirteen principles of ICH E6(R2) set a cultural tone which brings together ethical considerations, scientific requirements, and regulatory details in a succinct set of statements that are not always found in codes or regulations. In the United States, the FDA would have described such aspects in a preamble to a set of proposed regulations but would not have memorialized such principles in the regulations that are promulgated. However, having a set of principles to draw on gives the clinical trial players a set of cultural and ethical building blocks to use as they develop an investigational plan, prepare a protocol and train staff to conduct a clinical trial.

The high-level statements of principle that are found in this section of the ICH E6(R2) provide a reference point for just about every requirement that can be found in the lengthy and detailed requirements of the regulatory authorities. One could easily substitute the term *policy* for principles. The thirteen principles are the policies that will govern the entire scheme of a clinical trial activity from the time an application is submitted to a regulatory authority to the time the last subject is enrolled. See Chapter 6.

4.4   The Definition of GCP Embodies the Full Spectrum of Trial Activity – The Definition of GCP Reads

4.4.1   Good Clinical Practice (GCP)

A standard for the design, conduct, performance, monitoring, auditing, recording, analyses, and reporting of clinical trials that provides assurance that the data and reported results are credible and accurate, and that the rights, integrity, and confidentiality of trial subjects are protected.

Taking several of the functional steps included in this definition one can quickly understand how the contents of the Guideline/Standard are structured.

Design – The standard calls for the development of a scientifically sound protocol and investigator's brochure. The Standard then proceeds to list the content expectations for each document. The Sponsor of a trial need only follow the Standard.

Conduct – The Standard outlines expectations which inform the players how to conduct a trial. For example, obtaining approvals from the IRB as well as the appropriate regulatory authority prior to starting the trial; obtaining informed consent from subjects; maintaining data confidentiality and ensuring product accountability for the IMP. These are just a few examples.

Records and Record Keeping – Ensuring the integrity of data is a must. The ICH E6(R2) includes details about the types of records that are necessary and how to manage those records. Examples are the Case Report Forms, product accountability and the entire Section 8 which outlines the essential document needs for the three phases of the trial.

Reporting – There are a number of reporting requirements that are in place for a clinical trial to be in sync with the requirements of regulatory authorities. Reporting of adverse events, progress reports, final reports, reports of monitoring the trial sites and audit reports come to mind. The Standard references all these types of reporting expectations and others.

This is just a brief listing of the manner in which the Standard, through well-reasoned and thoughtful development, manages to encompass the full range of functional activities associated with clinical trial conduct.

4.5   Glossary

Suggesting that a list of definitions is important may seem trivial but having all the players on the same page calls for having everyone speak the same language, at least from the standpoint of meaning. Having a list of 65 terms that can be used by all and mean the same thing is a very important element. Clinical trials are complex undertakings requiring a broad range of specialists not all of whom are routinely involved in trials or who participate for certain parts and then leave to conduct their routine day-to-day business. Being certain that when terms are communicated, they mean the same to all parties in the conversation is important. The ICH E6(R2) Glossary accomplishes this objective.

4.6 Combining Key Elements

The ICH E6(R2) brings together the key functional areas of the drug development process that call for the application of the principles. If you wanted to study the requirements governing subject safety and data integrity from the FDA regulations you would need to organize the requirements from several different sections of the Code of Federal regulations. The ICH E6(R2) contains the information necessary to put in perspective the responsibilities of the sponsor, investigator, and IRB/EC all in one document. The applicable requirements of the respective regulatory authority are always referenced for details but the pathway for compliance with expectations that underpin subject safety and data integrity are available in one place.

4.7 Being Linked to an Organization That Is Respected and Authoritative

Standard setting organizations are generally seen as just that the "standard" setters. They have recognition as being thorough, authoritative, and quality oriented. The ICH is no exception and the ICH E6(R2) is hands down the final word when it comes to what constitutes good clinical practice. There are versions of the ICH E6(R2) good clinical practice guidelines published but for the most part they are renditions of the ICH E6(R2) which have been adapted to fit into the pharmaceutical regulatory scheme of a country, e.g. India. In addition organizations such as the World Health Organization (WHO) recognize the need for instructions such as that in ICH E6(R2) but are not standard setting entities themselves. The WHO has a handbook of GCP [1] but it is not advertised or promoted as a standard.

4.8 Standard Operating Procedures

The ICH E6(R2) lists the expectations for the development and use of Standard Operating Procedures (SOPs) in numerous sections. SOPs are generally viewed as a bedrock element in the requirements associated with the manufacturing and testing, labeling etc., for pharmaceutical medicinal products. However in the regulatory requirements promulgated by the US FDA defining the conduct of clinical trials at 21 CFR 312 – Investigational New Drug Applications the term procedures and/or standard operating procedures is not mentioned. Regulatory authorities such as the US FDA certainly expect sponsors and investigators to have written procedures for key processes and procedures in place but the requirements specifically stating that are just not there. The FDA's regulations for IRBs and informed consent do speak to written procedures. However is clear on the need and expectation for written procedures. It is apparent in numerous sections e.g. 5.18.15 Monitoring Procedures and Auditing Procedures. A quick survey of the guideline shows numerous instances where the term *procedures* is used and it refers to SOPs. Regulators can, if needed cite the ICG E6(R2) as the standard whereby written SOPs are necessary and required for virtually every functional aspect of a clinical trial.

4.9 Efficiency of Developing and Updating Materials

The ICH is not a regulatory agency or authority. It is however supported by regulatory authorities and regulatory authorities who were instrumental in establishing it as the organization which is looked to for investigative medicinal product standards. Industry trade organizations were partners in driving the establishment of the ICH. The members of those trade organizations committed scientific expertise and monetary support for the ICH so that the standards necessary to harmonize pharmaceutical drug development standards could be put in place. Those standards must then be translated into usable expectations which can be enforced as the must do or at a minimum held as the *should do* steps for pharmaceutical medicinal product development.

The ICH as a free standing nonaffiliated standard setting organization is in a position where it can develop a standard in an expedited manner compared to a regulatory authority. In particular the ICH, while its governance does include representatives from the regulatory authorities, does not need to go through lengthy and sometimes politically influenced reviews and challenges when developing a standard. The ICH follows a standard review process that reaches out to all parties, even the general public, but it is a process that is controlled and does not languish due to policy or political upheaval. The final work product must then be accepted and/or adopted by the regulatory authority but experience has already demonstrated that the regulatory authorities have found mechanisms to classify and categorize the ICH standards in a manner which lends relevance without having to translate them into law. The US FDA's approach of translating ICH guidelines into Good Guidance Practices is an example.

4.10 Value Added Practices and Principles are Adopted

The development of the and other standards by the ICH has moved the needle, so to speak, for furthering ethical and scientific best practices in the conduct of clinical trials throughout the world. A primary example is the country of Japan. When the ICH was founded circa 1990, Japan did not require that informed consent be given to trial subjects. This was a cultural matter however it did impact the usability/acceptability of clinical trial results by the regulatory authorities of other countries and regions because subjects had not been given informed consent. As an original founder of the ICH organization, Japan eventually fully adopted the ethical principle of informed consent. This adoption of the ethical principles inherent in the ICH E6(R2) is probably as important an outcome as any associated with the promulgation of the Standard.

4.11 Summary

In this chapter you have learned that the ICH E6(R2) Guideline/Standard contributes more than just a list of must or should do expectations as a sponsor, investigator, or IRB plays out their role in the clinical trial endeavor. The Standard serves a policy document where needed; it is more than just the combination of its parts in that it lays out the best practices for functional expectations in terms of how to: design a trial; conduct a trial; record the details of a trial and how to report trial activities in a way that data integrity is maintained. The Standard also serves as a benchmark for ethical expectations for a trial thereby building into the process a moral obligation that would be missing from most standards. The ICH E6(R2) standard is not in and of itself a law but it comes as close to being that as any standard applicable to the clinical trial process. It is really a unique and one of a kind Standard.

Knowledge Check Questions

1) The 13 principles found in the ICH E6(R2) were copied from the US FDA's regulations governing the conduct of investigation new drug studies found at 21 CFR 312. True ___ False ___

2) Would the maintenance of subject medical history and records confidentiality be categorized as a record keeping function or a trial conduct function? _____

3) Review the ICH E6(R2) Standard and prepare a list of 15 sections where the term procedures is listed. Can you find the same requirement/expectation in the regulations from a regulatory authority?

4) The author states that the ICH is a respected organization. Briefly describe several reasons why you believe the ICH is respected and its Standards seen as authoritative

5) The ICH E6(R2) Guideline calls for the clinical trial investigator to ensure that informed consent is given to each subject. Do you think that requirement was universal when the Standard was issued circa 1996? Do you know which benchmark ethical publication/policy document first called for informed consent of human subjects?

Reference

1 World Health Organization (2005). *Handbook for Good Clinical Research Practice (GCP): Guidance for Implementation.* World Health Organization https://apps.who.int/iris/handle/10665/43392 (accessed 13 February 2020).

5

Regulatory Affairs

P. Michael Dubinsky

GCP Key Point

GCP is grounded in the regulatory requirements of the participating members of the ICH. Understanding the regulatory lay of the land is therefore essential.

5.1 Introduction

The good clinical practice guidelines, which are the blueprint for this entire text, are a work product of the International Council for Harmonization of Technical Requirements for Pharmaceuticals for Human Use (ICH). The ICH, which was initiated circa 1990 by the US FDA, EC/EMA and Japan's MHLW along with corresponding pharmaceutical industry associations sought to pursue the harmonization of requirements leading to drug registration or approval. Their harmonization effort has led to the removal of unnecessary and often redundant requirements. The ICH has now evolved from a joint commitment of three government organizational units and three industry associations to a legal nonprofit international association under Swiss law. Understanding the ICH organization, its mission and roles is useful. However we suggest you visit the ICH Webpage [1] for insight into all of its history and accomplishments. The webpage is quite complete, easy to navigate, and transparent.

Since governmental requirements are the underlying foundation of ICH E6(R2) the there is merit in outlining some key points about the regulatory processes, leading to a successful drug registration or approval. The drug development process calls on a wide range of disciplines and while each may not appear to be a direct player in meeting GCP expectations they are all connected.

The Fundamentals of Clinical Research: A Universal Guide for Implementing Good Clinical Practice, First Edition. P. Michael Dubinsky and Karen A. Henry.
© 2022 John Wiley & Sons, Inc. Published 2022 by John Wiley & Sons, Inc.
Companion website: www.wiley.com/go/dubinsky/clinicalresearch

A key player or set of players in the drug development process will be from the sponsor's regulatory affairs group. Understanding their roles and responsibilities as they relate to clinical development is useful.

5.2 Objectives of the Chapter

1) To describe in general terms the roles and responsibilities of a regulatory affairs organizational unit and their role in meeting GCP expectations.
2) To reflect on the nature and purpose of interactions with competent authorities and the links that such interactions have to GCP.
3) To outline the important and sometimes challenging aspects of communicating with competent authorities during drug development.
4) To identify key times when meetings with competent authorities play an important role in the communications process about the development scheme.
5) To outline the general scheme of submissions associated with drug development activities and where they intersect with GCP.

5.3 Regulatory Affairs

The regulatory affairs organizational group in a drug/pharmaceutical firm is always assigned as the primary point of contact for interactions with competent authorities. Therefore, a representative from the group should be part of the clinical development core team from the beginning of any clinical development initiative. Regulatory affairs will not be the only group or person that communicates with a regulatory or competent authority but they must be aware of all communications and in most situations will review the substance of communications for consistency with company and regulatory policy.

The functional responsibilities that are assigned to Regulatory Affairs include all marketing and development related applications for a pharmaceutical drug including amendments and supplements to those applications. Regulatory affairs will also be responsible for coordinating the assembly of data and information used to support the various applications. In the case of drug development applications such as an FDA Investigational New Drug (IND) Application regulatory affairs will likely be the conduit for all communications with the regulatory authority whether electronic (e.g. video conference/phone), written, or face-to-face. Having a central point of contact and it being a regulatory affairs group is an approach which is favored by the regulatory authorities. They prefer to have one central point of contact for communications. It is also in the best interests of a firm to have communications processed through a central coordination point. That way there is institutional knowledge and awareness of what is being communicated, how it fits with what has been previously communicated and an understanding of the impact, if any, that the information being transmitted will have on the program, project, or application involved. There may be times when the information is communicated by an organizational group other than regulatory affairs an example being pharmacovigilance/ adverse experience reports. Even then the regulatory affairs group needs to be involved to ensure continuity and completeness.

So how does that intersect with meeting GCP expectations?

Basically, the regulatory affairs staff in a firm are charged with ensuring that the information and data reported on applications for pharmaceutical drug development is accurate, complete, original, and supported by facts. They are expected to sign off on all submissions to regulatory authorities and by doing so they guarantee the veracity and soundness of the information being submitted. In theory they could be held personally responsible for any inaccuracy, untruth, or omission found as part of a submission. Does that mean they double check all information? They might in some situations. The reality is that knowledgeable and seasoned regulatory affairs staff members have an in-depth working knowledge of all the elements of the drug development processes and they practice a policy of accept and verify. They receive and/or request information from members of the drug development team to populate a submission but then perform verification on a portion of the data to be sure of accuracy and completeness. It is part of their training and job to know, understand, and be fluent in GCP as well as other GXP requirements.

5.4 Interacting with Regulatory/Competent Authorities

There are a number of mechanisms utilized to communicate with regulatory authorities and while none are unique to drug development it is useful to reflect on them and on the manner, in which they are arranged, documented and records maintained. As mentioned earlier communications will occur through one of three means – electronic means such as videoconferencing or telephone; face-to-face in a meeting or in a written submission. E-mail would be considered as a written submission. The choice of which mechanism to use may take into consideration a number of factors. Factors such as the stage of development, the nature of the investigational product (IP), the circumstances prompting the need to communicate and the wishes of management can all be important forces when it comes to deciding which approach to choose. From the standpoint of GCP the sponsor is expected to establish and maintain the set of essential documents which represent the evidence that the trial was conducted in conformance with GCP and the applicable regulatory requirements. Records are kept by all the players in the clinical trial process, e.g. investigator, IRB, but the sponsor is responsible for the trial master file (TMF). The TMF is that central repository where the entire set of trial related documentation is maintained. Whether the records are hard copy or electronic the sponsor's regulatory affairs unit is generally in charge of those records being organized and up to date if and when needed. If you refer to Chapter 29 Essential Documents – the TMF is discussed in detail. It is worth mentioning, and we will several times in the text that the documents which populate the TMF represent the evidence that the trial was conducted in compliance with GCP.

Regulatory authorities have established ground rules for official communications and they live by those rules. For example the US FDA's Center for Drug Evaluation and Review has procedures defining types of meetings they will arrange with sponsors in terms of timing, topic, pre-meeting documentation, etc. [2] A trial sponsor should not expect to just send an E-mail or make a telephone call to arrange a meeting. Regulatory authorities have just so many people resources and those resources have a range of responsibilities, so requests for meetings are controlled closely.

Even with the complexities that accompany arranging a meeting they are an excellent framework for ensuring that the parties are on the same page about key aspects of the trial, such as the IP, the objectives, the entire nature, and scope of the endeavor. It is important for the sponsor to be certain their records of any meetings are as complete and clear as possible about any agreements, disagreements, and commitments made by the sponsor or the competent authority. Such factors play into the GCP arena in sometimes unexpected ways. For example if the sponsor makes commitments about the approach to monitoring, training or IP handling during meetings with the competent authority during a meeting prior to a Phase commencing and it is determined later that commitment was not kept it may prove very problematic. Such commitments actually become an element of GCP for the trial even if they are not specifically mentioned in the ICH E6(R2). It should be kept in perspective that GCP like the other GXP requirements are a baseline set of minimum requirements. Sponsors must meet the baseline requirements but the manner in which they implement them is usually left to the sponsor, IRB or site.

Applications for permission to initiate a clinical trial, e.g. IND or CTA, along with their amendments and supplements also bind the sponsor and other trial players to aspects of GCP. Competent authorities as part of their codified rules take the time to describe the expectations that are in place for sponsors, investigators, IRBs, and in some ways even subjects. Sponsors commit in writing to ensure compliance with all applicable requirements. If those commitments are not honored there are severe penalties which may be imposed. So compliance with GCP must become a cultural force in the entire scheme of conducting a clinical trial.

5.5 Communicating with Regulatory/Competent Authorities and Others

A good way to begin this portion of the discussion on communication is to recall ICH E6(R2) Principle 2.10 which reads: *All clinical trial information should be recorded, handled, and stored in a way that allows its accurate reporting, interpretation, and verification.*

Citing this principle makes sense here because recording, storing, and reporting on the large number of communications which will take place as part of the clinical trial scheme calls for training, a commitment to the record keeping fundamentals embodied in ALCOA [3] and a willingness on the part of staff to take the time to create a record. ICH E6(R2) does not use the terminology ALCOA but at section 4.9.0 states that source data should be attributable, legible, contemporaneous, original, accurate, and complete.

Earlier we noted the ways in which communication will occur with the regulatory authority. Meetings will generally involve a relatively small number of people and there will be a person appointed to act as the executive secretary or notetaker. During the course of a trial however there may be numerous times when a member(s) of the trial team will interact with a member(s) of the regulatory authority on a topic specific to their role on the trial team. It will be essential that those communications are recorded and made part of the TMF as well as being shared with all parties who need to know. It should not be assumed that every sponsor will have an SOP describing the process of documenting communications via phone (or otherwise) with representatives of a regulatory authority. Such procedures will usually be accompanied by a blank form to be used for documenting the specific of the call, meeting, etc. In times past, such records were made in pen and ink on three part carbonless forms which accommodated distributing the record, archiving it, and maintaining a personal copy. The blank form provided the user with places to record the basic elements of a communication such as names, titles, times, contact numbers, and substance of the communication. E-mail or a memo to the files would likely be used today but the parameters are the same. In order for the record, whether made in writing or electronically, to be in conformance with GCP, it must be legible, contemporaneous, original, complete, accurate, and clear as to who the author is. There is nothing more problematic than having an inspector from a regulatory authority, who is reviewing records of adverse experiences, find one with the word YIKES written across it in red ink! Try explaining that entry. The record must also be permanent so that any additions, changes or versions are clearly identified. In the case of meeting with or communicating with a regulatory authority it is sometimes appropriate to share the record of meeting with them. Doing so does not mean they consider it the only record or the "official" one but at least they will know you created a record and its content. This type of record keeping guidance and explanation will be mentioned in several places in the text and it is appropriate to do so because it is a fundamental requirement of applying GCP principles.

5.6 Meetings – When and How They fit-GCP

Meetings with regulatory authorities are encouraged for the Clinical Trial Sponsor at trial milestones. Those times are often just before submission of an application to conduct the trial and before embarking on each of the applicable phases. During such meetings topics such as complexities in the protocol, approach to compliance with elements of GCP can be on the agenda as well as the science of the IP and trial approach. After a trial a meeting may be scheduled to clarify outcomes prior to the submission of any marketing application. Regulatory authorities agree that meetings are useful. For example the US FDA includes specific references to meetings during the conduct of a clinical investigation in the controlling regulations.

In most situations the topics discussed are instrumental in the performance of clinical trial activities so documenting all outcomes, agreements, decisions, and follow-up steps via a meeting record is important. ICH E6(R2) section 8.3.11 serves as a catch all in the TMF for the written record of such meeting minutes.

Face-to-face meetings are usually the most effective forum for ensuring that there is clarity between parties on all aspects of an endeavor such as a clinical trial. Conformance with one or more aspects of GCP can and is on the agenda of many meetings between sponsor and regulatory authority as well as between the parties performing steps in the trial. Therefore, the records of meetings and all forms of communications are vital. An often overlooked benefit of well-documented communications is that they engender trust among the parties involved. Trust between parties goes a long way when issues arise and explanation must be made for decisions that impact a trial-related matter.

5.7 Applications

This text is not meant to serve as specific training for the regulatory affairs personnel in terms of application preparation and submission. Many other reference texts describe the ins and outs of that task. It is however useful to reflect on the importance of GCP when noncompliance with it can have a significant impact on the review and processing of applications.

All of the regulatory authorities who receive and process applications have established internal instructions regarding the evaluation of noncompliance with regulatory requirements. Serious deficiencies are evaluated for their impact on the continued review and evaluation of an application as well as whether the trial should continue to be conducted at a site(s) or be placed on hold. Any decision to place a trial on hold would be based on a risk-benefit evaluation to determine whether the risk factor may have changed due to the deficiencies. If, for example, adverse experience reports had not been made in a timely manner or at all, then the risk of the non-reporting will be weighed by the competent authority. Many such deficiencies are identified during inspections of sponsors and/or sites. Regulatory authorities also receive reports from sponsors of situations, e.g. in the UK a serious breach of the requirements impacting the safety of subjects must be reported.

5.8 Summary

The clinical development pathway which is navigated by a sponsor's regulatory affairs group is not a silo in terms of conformance with and adherence to GCP. The reach of GCP requirements runs throughout a sponsor's organization if they are involved and participating in some aspect of a clinical trial activity. Interactions with regulatory authorities via any communication mechanism must be appropriately documented, shared to the extent necessary and available for review as part of the evidence that the overall trial was conducted in conformance with GCP.

Knowledge Check Questions

1) Competent authorities prefer to have at least ten points of contact should there need to be communications between they and the sponsor about some aspect of a clinical trial. True or False?

2) The ICH E6(R2) Guideline calls for records of meeting and other relevant communications about a clinical trial to be maintained in section 5 6 8 9 (Circle the correct section)

3) Regulatory authorities support and encourage meetings to discuss issues which arise with clinical investigations. The US FDA reserves every Friday for such meetings. True or False?

4) Face-to-face meetings are a sound approach to discussing/communicating aspects of the conduct of a clinical trial with a regulatory authority. Such meetings also can build __?__ between the parties.

5) Nonconformance with GCP can be a rationale for placing a clinical trial or an investigational application on hold. True or False?

References

1 ICH. Website link for the international council for harmonization of technical requirements for pharmaceuticals for human use (ICH), https://www.ich.org/home.html (accessed 27 January 2020)

2 FDA (December 2017). Best practices for communication between IND sponsors and FDA during drug development. https://www.fda.gov/regulatory-information/search-fda-guidance-documents/best-practices-communication-between-ind-sponsors-and-fda-during-drug-development (accessed 27 January 2020)

3 Bargaje, C. (2011). Good documentation practice in clinical research. *Perspectives in Clinical Research* 2 (2): 59–63. https://www.ncbi.nlm.nih.gov/pmc/articles/PMC3121265/?report=printable (accessed 27 January 2020).

Part III

Good Clinical Practice

6

GCP Definition and Principles

Karen A. Henry

GCP Key Point

GCP and its principles are the foundational filters for performing any clinical trial activity or making any clinical trial-related decision.

6.1 Introduction

Experiments with and outright distribution and sale of products for the diagnosis, treatment, cure, or prevention of disease have resulted in a range of harmful effects to the safety and well-being of humans. Individual countries established regulatory requirements for clinical research in the development of a product to prevent such harmful effects. However, due to the cost of redundancies in resources, time, and additional exposure of an unapproved product to human subjects, a single guideline was developed with consideration of the current good clinical practices (GCPs) of the European Union, Japan, and the United States, as well as those of Australia, Canada, the Nordic countries and the World Health Organization (WHO). The objective of ICH E6 (R2) Guideline for GCP is to provide a unified standard for the European Union (EU), Japan, and the United States to facilitate the mutual acceptance of clinical data by the regulatory authorities in these jurisdictions. (ICH E6(R2) Introduction; Section on Good Clinical Practice History; Section on Drug Development in the Regulatory Environment).

The Guideline presents a set of international ethical and scientific quality standard for designing, conducting, recording and reporting trials that involve the participation of human subjects (ICH E6(R2) Introduction). The goal for anyone involved in the conception, planning, and execution of a trial is to conform with these standards that provide public assurance that the rights, safety, and well-being

The Fundamentals of Clinical Research: A Universal Guide for Implementing Good Clinical Practice, First Edition. P. Michael Dubinsky and Karen A. Henry.
© 2022 John Wiley & Sons, Inc. Published 2022 by John Wiley & Sons, Inc.
Companion website: www.wiley.com/go/dubinsky/clinicalresearch

of trial subjects are protected, consistent with the principles that have their origin in the Declaration of Helsinki, and that the clinical trial data are credible. The Guideline starts with definitions and principles as the foundation for the responsibilities and operational standards that are presented in the Guideline.

In this chapter, we will define GCP and present a practical interpretation of the GCP principles.

6.2 Objectives

The objectives of this chapter are:

1) Define GCP
2) Describe GCP principles and present a practical interpretation of the principles

6.3 The Definition of Good Clinical Practice

GCP is an international ethical and scientific quality standard for designing, conducting, recording, and reporting trials that involve the participation of human subjects. Compliance with this standard provides public assurance that the rights, safety and well-being of trial subjects are protected, consistent with the principles that have their origin in the Declaration of Helsinki, and that the clinical trial data are credible. (ICH E6(R2) Introduction).

6.4 Good Clinical Practice Principles

The Good Clinical Practice Guideline presents a set of principles which lay the foundation for the responsibilities and operational standards that are presented in the Guideline. We can think of the principles as those beliefs that will guide the behavior and chain of reasoning for all who are involved in the conception, planning, and execution of a clinical trial in order to protect human subjects and ensure the integrity of trial data.

There are 13 principles (ICH E6(R2) 2). Presented below are the principles and a practical interpretation of each principle to enhance understanding of the principle and facilitate its application in the conduct of clinical research.

2.1 *Clinical trials should be conducted in accordance with the ethical principles that have their origin in the Declaration of Helsinki, and that are consistent with GCP and the applicable regulatory requirement(s).*
- This principle is stating that clinical trials will follow those principles concerned with the safety, rights, well-being of research subjects and all other principles, guidelines, and regulations that are relevant to the conduct of clinical research.

2.2   *Before a trial is initiated, foreseeable risks and inconveniences should be weighed against the anticipated benefit for the individual trial subject and society. A trial should be initiated and continued only if the anticipated benefits justify the risks.*

- Considerations for benefit-risk to a trial subject and society occur before a trial is initiated as well as during the trial.

  Aside from the potential contribution to science and society, there is no guaranteed direct benefit to a volunteering clinical research subject in that,

  1) The researchers do not fully know if the investigational product will work
  2) While participating in a clinical trial, a subject will benefit from medical care for any adverse effects associated with their participation in the trial, but this benefit is their right
  3) While participating in the clinical trial, a subject may undergo procedures that diagnose or monitor their disease condition more regularly than standard care but this is because they are receiving an investigational product for which the safety profile is unknown.
  4) The subject may receive monetary compensation for participating in the trial, but this compensation should not be in amounts to influence or coerce the subject into taking part in the trial.

  However, *some* information about the efficacy/effectiveness of the investigational product may be already known from previous clinical or nonclinical experience and this information could be used in the assessment of benefit.

  The assessment of risk to the subject may largely be attributed to:

  1) Known and *unknown* adverse effects of the investigational product
  2) The burdens (e.g., adverse effects, physical, emotional, and mental) endured by the subject to undergo the study procedures
  3) The effects of the progressive course of the potentially untreated or under-treated disease depending on the effectiveness of available alternative care
  4) The chance for untreated or under-treated disease depending on the effectiveness of available alternative care in a placebo – or other approved comparator – controlled trial,

  The overall benefit-risk assessment will consider all the potential benefits and risks above (perhaps there are more). Given the limited known potential benefit, primarily, the known risk of the investigational product and the burden of study procedures will be weighed against the risk of the disease conditions and course to secondarily assess benefit-risk of the clinical trial. The safety and efficacy data from the ongoing study and all other ongoing and completed relevant nonclinical and clinical trials will be collected and evaluated with other risk factors for the on-going assessment of benefit-risk for study subjects. (Chapter 18 The Clinical Trial Protocol and Amendments; Chapter 19 Informed Consent and Other Human Subject Protection; Chapter 21 Safety Monitoring and Reporting; Chapter 22 Monitoring Overview)

2.3   *The rights, safety, and well-being of the trial subjects are the most important considerations and should prevail over interests of science and society.*

- This principle is essentially saying that the sponsor, investigator, IRB/EC and all of their representatives involved in the conduct of clinical research will first and foremost consider and prioritize the safety, rights, and well-being of clinical research subjects above all other considerations for a clinical trial. Any considerations for regulatory, scientific, business, or other objectives are secondary. If there is a potential for harm to any research subject as a result of a decision to comply with regulatory (e.g., complying with requirements of the protocol), other scientific, or business objectives (e.g., saving time or money), the decision should be modified in order to protect the research subject even if it means unfavorable consequences for regulatory compliance (e.g., a protocol deviation), or scientific or business objectives (e.g., losing time or money). (Chapter 19 Informed Consent and Other Human Subject Protection; Chapter 21 Safety Monitoring and Reporting; Chapter 22 Monitoring Overview)

2.4   *The available nonclinical and clinical information on an investigational product should be adequate to support the proposed clinical trial.*

- Any clinical study design and the choice of and dosing regimen for the investigational product and controls must be justified by results from nonclinical testing and previous clinical testing of the investigational product, and what is known about the drug class of the investigational product. As additional trial data are accumulated from other trials during overall development of the investigational product, these data may be used to contribute to the supporting information. If a clinical trial protocol is amended for study design or if additional indications will be studied with the investigational product, then nonclinical and clinical information should also be supportive of the changes. (Chapter 18 The Clinical Trial Protocol and Amendments; Chapter 16 The Investigator's Brochure)

2.5   *Clinical trials should be scientifically sound, and described in a clear, detailed protocol.*

- A clinical trial design should have its basis on relevant scientific principles and methods and be clearly described in a clinical trial protocol, what we may refer to as the "standard operating procedure" for the experiment on human subjects. The instructions should be clear, comprehensive, and accurate. Regulatory authority(ies), IRB/IECs, investigators, trial managers, monitors, and other stakeholders of the protocol may identify deficiencies during review and implementation of the protocol. If at any time it is discovered and determined that the instructions are ambiguous or incorrect, then the protocol should be amended to ensure clarity and accuracy. The protocol should also be amended if it is determined at any time that the trial design is inadequate to meet the protocol's, scientific, GCP, and and/or business objectives for the study. (Chapter 18 The Clinical Trial Protocol and Amendments)

2.6 *A trial should be conducted in compliance with the protocol that has received prior institutional review board (IRB)/independent ethics committee (IEC) approval/favorable opinion.*

- A clinical trial protocol may be implemented only if it has the prior review and approval/favorable opinion of an IRB/IEC. If the protocol is amended, the procedures as described in the amendment may only be implemented if it has the prior review and approval/favorable opinion of an IRB/IEC. The conduct of the trial must comply with the approved protocol.

In the real world, it is prudent for those involved in trial conduct to be attentive to approved versions of the protocol and to approved procedures before implementing those procedures. For example, a trial site may receive verbal notification from the IRB/IEC that a protocol/amendment has been approved, and with eagerness to enroll, may consent or administer a new procedure to a subject before receiving documentation of the approval. Upon receipt of the documentation of the IRB/IEC's approval, the date of approval was after the verbal notification and therefore the date of consent and new protocol procedure predated the approved protocol. The implementation of the protocol was therefore a violation of this principle and a violation of the effective protocol, if the scenario pertained to a protocol amendment.

Another example where keen attention is needed to prevent noncompliance is that protocol compliance means EXACT compliance with the protocol procedures as described. For example, if vital signs in the schedule of assessments are at 08:00 with a grace period ("window") of ± 5 minutes, and the vital signs were documented as obtained at 08:07, then this is a deviation from the protocol. For an auditor or inspector, rare instances of these deviations may be "acceptable"; however, multiple instances may be classified as chronic noncompliance and warrant a significant audit finding. The sponsor should monitor and note all deviations from the protocol, evaluate the root cause, implement corrective action, and/or amend the protocol as needed to ensure compliance. (Chapter 21 Safety Monitoring and Reporting; Chapter 22 Monitoring Overview)

2.7 *The medical care given to, and medical decisions made on behalf of, subjects should always be the responsibility of a qualified physician or, when appropriate, of a qualified dentist.*

- Only physicians who are qualified by education, training, and experience may provide medical care or make medical decisions on behalf of subjects. These physicians will be qualified not only by general training, but by specialty training if applicable. The local regulations will also determine what qualifications a physician may have to perform certain types of procedures. For example, consideration should be given to the qualifications of the investigator for a trial that evaluates a contrast agent that is administered via infusion for radiographical imaging of liver lesions; i.e., whether the investigator needs to be a radiologist or a hepatologist. Additionally, a busy clinical site should ensure that an individual who is recording adverse effects as reported by a study subject is not inadvertently diagnosing or making decisions about the clinical severity and treatment of the adverse effects. (Chapter 21 Safety Monitoring and Reporting; Chapter 22 Monitoring Overview; Chapter 9 Investigator and Sponsor Roles and Responsibilities)

2.8 *Each individual involved in conducting a trial should be qualified by education, training, and experience to perform his or her respective task(s).*

- Each individual, whether they are a sponsor, investigator, or IRB/IEC representative (employee or contractor) should have appropriate qualifications to perform their assigned tasks. The assignment of the tasks and the qualifications of each individual should be documented. There should also be documentation that the individual has been trained on the protocol-specific procedure or function. Documentation may be in the form of charts of the organizational structure for a team, lists of assigned tasks, current curriculum vitae with copies of certifications as required, and general and protocol-specific training records. If an individual changes roles during a trial or discontinues performing the trial task or function, the transfer and transition process of the responsibilities should also be documented. Consideration should also be given to conflicts of interest; e.g., someone with significant financial interest in the product or the trial site should not contribute to trial data. (Chapter 14 Trial Management; Start-up, On-Study, and Close-Out; Chapter 15 Trial Resourcing and Outsourcing; Chapter 21 Safety Monitoring and Reporting; Chapter 22 Monitoring Overview)

2.9 Freely given informed consent should be obtained from every subject prior to clinical trial participation.

- Careful consideration should be given to how trial subjects are consented. It is important to note that consenting is a process and does not only mean the subject's signing of the consent documents. Freely given; i.e., voluntary, consent means that there is no coercion either via verbal, body, or written language or via other medium; e.g., power, financial incentive. The inclusion of vulnerable populations in a protocol should be justified. Sponsor, investigator, IRB/EC institutions may have policies against recruiting staff as research subjects for a trial as their choice to participate may be unduly influenced by their superiors. (Chapter 19 Informed Consent and Other Human Subject Protection)

2.10   *All clinical trial information should be recorded, handled, and stored in a way that allows its accurate reporting, interpretation, and verification. This principle applies to all records referenced in this guideline, irrespective of the type of media used.*

- The clinical trial protocol provides the instructions for study procedures and additional procedures for study conduct are prescribed via standard operating procedures (SOPs), GCP, and applicable regulatory requirements. During the trial, all evidence of trial conduct will be maintained as Essential Documents. At the end of the trial, study conduct and results are reported in a clinical study report. All documentation of trial conduct from study start-up to study closeout will be documented as evident of trial conduct. The documentation should follow good documentation practices (be attributable, legible, contemporaneous, original, accurate, and complete), and be retrievable to retell the story of trial conduct as needed, during, immediately after, and several years after the ending of the trial. That trial data and information should be retrievable at any time is important to note: trial data and information should be maintained in a format, and storage formats should be updated as necessary, so that the data and information can be read or interpreted at any time in the future. (Chapter 29 Essential Documents; Chapter 21 Safety Monitoring and Reporting; Chapter 22 Monitoring Overview).

2.11   *The confidentiality of records that could identify subjects should be protected, respecting the privacy and confidentiality rules in accordance with the applicable regulatory requirement(s).*

- The IRB/IEC, investigator, and sponsor have responsibilities to ensure the protection of information that may identify research subjects (e.g., name, contact information, initials) in order to respect their privacy. IRBs/IECs and local regulatory requirements may dictate which, if any, personal identification for subjects may be used in trial data and documentation and with whom their personal information may be shared. Investigators and sponsors will implement procedures to ensure that unauthorized subject personal identification are not released and shared intentionally or inadvertently. (Chapter 19 Informed Consent and Other Human Subject Protection; Chapter 21 Safety Monitoring and Reporting; Chapter 22 Monitoring Overview).

2.12 *Investigational products should be manufactured, handled, and stored in accordance with applicable good manufacturing practice (GMP). They should be used in accordance with the approved protocol.*

- The sponsor will ensure that investigational products are manufactured, handled, and stored according to GMP. The sponsor will implement procedures for product handling, storage, and shipping from the distribution facility to investigators and for return, receipt, and destruction to the facility. The investigator will implement procedures for receipt, handling, storage, administration to subjects, and destruction or return of investigational product to the sponsor. The sponsor will also implement procedures to monitor the entire 'chain of custody' of the investigational products to ensure compliance with the protocol and applicable regulatory requirements. (Chapter 17 The Investigational Product (Clinical Supplies); Chapter 21 Safety Monitoring and Reporting; Chapter 22 Monitoring Overview).

2.13 *Systems with procedures that assure the quality of every aspect of the trial should be implemented.*

- All players, the IRB/IEC, investigator (and third parties), and sponsor (and CROs), will implement procedures that assure the quality of every aspect of the trial. Quality procedures include procedures for quality assurance and quality control, including establishing SOPs, training procedures, monitoring procedures, audit programs, ongoing quality control checks, and risk assessment and mitigation methods. (Source: ICH [1] Section on Quality in Clinical Trials).

6.5 Summary

The ICH E6(R2) presents a set of international ethical and scientific quality standard for designing, conducting, recording, and reporting trials that involve the participation of human subjects (ICH E6(R2) Introduction). The Guideline includes principles that lay the foundation for the responsibilities and operational standards of GCP. It is important to understand the application of principles to guide the behavior and chain of reasoning for all who are involved in the conception, planning, and execution of a clinical trial in order to protect human subjects and ensure the integrity of trial data.

Knowledge Check Questions
1) What is the definition of GCP? 2) What are the 13 principles of GCP? 3) How does each of the 13 principles of GCP apply to clinical research? 4) Overheard: "What is GCP?" Sponsor's associate responsible for filing documents in the trial master file. Comment and discuss: a) Why does the individual in this role need to know GCP? b) What aspect(s) of GCP would apply to his/her role?

Reference

1 International Council for Harmonisation of Technical Requirements for Pharmaceuticals for Human Use (ICH), Integrated Addendum to ICH E6(R1):Guideline for Good Clinical Practice, E6(R2) (2016). Current Step 4 version dated 9 November 2016. https://www.ich.org/page/efficacy-guidelines

7

Players Roles and Responsibilities Overview

Karen A. Henry

GCP Key Point
Clinical trials should be conducted in accordance with GCP and the applicable regulatory requirement(s).

7.1   Introduction

Who are the main players involved in the conduct of clinical research? To answer this question, let us first look at the reason clinical trials exist.

As we learned from the history of the evolution of clinical trials and drug development, there were incidents where many people were seriously or fatally harmed from using "medicinal" products that were sold on the market. The ensuing public outcry was heard by the government, and legislators created laws that evolved to ultimately require that a medicinal product must be proven to be safe and effective before it can be sold in the market place. (Chapter 1 Good Clinical Practice History)

Until a medicinal product is proven to be safe and effective, the product would be identified as "investigational." The laws also state that the entity to decide if a product is safe and effective would be a representative of the government and that the method for first proving that a product is safe and effective would be through the conduct of a series of well-controlled experiments, including trials on human subjects; hence, the requirement for clinical trials. The regulatory authorities established specific rules, regulations, and guidelines regarding clinical research for investigational products. The main players involved in clinical research conduct were identified as the Sponsor, Clinical Investigator, Institutional Review Board (IRB) or Independent Ethics Committee (IEC), the research participant,

The Fundamentals of Clinical Research: A Universal Guide for Implementing Good Clinical Practice, First Edition. P. Michael Dubinsky and Karen A. Henry.
Companion website: www.wiley.com/go/dubinsky/clinicalresearch

and the Regulatory Authority. The ICH E6(R2) guidance for Good Clinical Practice provides a unified standard for the generation of such clinical trial data that are intended to be submitted to regulatory authorities (ICH E6(R2) Introduction [1]).

ICH GCP Guidelines define roles and responsibilities for each player involved in the planning, executing, and reporting of a clinical trial: IRB/IEC, investigator, sponsor/CRO, regulatory agency, and research participant. This chapter will define the different types of players and describe their roles and interaction in clinical research. The details of each player's responsibilities are provided in the respective chapters for IRB/IEC (Chapter 8), investigator and sponsor (Chapter 9), the research volunteer (Chapter 10), and the regulatory authority (Chapter 11).

7.2 Objectives

In this chapter topic we will answer the following questions:

1. Who are the main players involved in the conduct of clinical research?
2. How do the main players interact with each other in the clinical research arena?

7.2.1 Main Players Involved in the Conduct of a Clinical Trial

The main players involved in the conduct of a clinical trial are: Sponsor, Investigator, IRB/IEC, Regulatory Authority, and Research Participant (Plate 3).

7.2.1.1 The Sponsor

The Sponsor is the "owner" of an investigational product. The sponsor is interested in studying the clinical use of investigational product to determine its pharmacological properties, safety, and/or effectiveness in humans. By definition, the sponsor is:

> An individual, company, institution, or organization that takes responsibility for the initiation, management, and/or financing of a clinical trial. (ICH E6(R2) 1.53)

A Sponsor can be, for example, a pharmaceutical or biotechnology company, a nongovernmental organization (NGO), a governmental agency, an academic institution, a single individual or any entity that wants to take responsibility for the initiation, management, and/or financing of a clinical trial.

The Sponsor often is the financial owner and/or the developer of the product being investigated; however, the Sponsor may simply have access to the investigational product through an agreement with the financial owner or developer. In all instances, the Sponsor does not actually conduct the investigation (i.e., administer the investigational product to research subjects and record data from the study assessments), but will be legally responsible for all handling and use of the investigational product in the trial, the integrity of the trial data collected, and the submission of the trial findings to the Regulatory Authority. A Sponsor will usually be ultimately interested in getting approval for marketing their product or for publishing new information about the product.

7.2.1.2 The Investigator

The Clinical Investigator is the qualified doctor (or dentist) who administers the investigational product to the research subjects. By definition, an Investigator is:

> A person responsible for the conduct of the clinical trial at a trial site. If a trial is conducted by a team of individuals at a trial site, the investigator is the responsible leader of the team and may be called the principal investigator (ICH E6(R2) 1.57).

A clinical Investigator is the physician who has access to and gives medical care to the research participant who is being administered the investigational product, or the control product, in the clinic. The clinic where the research participant is seen by the physician and undergoes trial procedures is known as the trial site. The Investigator can be practicing alone, be part of a clinical group practice or clinical research management organization, or a member in a hospital or other institution. Any of the different types of practices can be private or public.

In all situations, the Investigator will have responsibility for the medical care of the research participant and all activities of the trial at the trial site, regardless of who actually conducts those activities. If there are other individuals, such as a nurse, laboratory technician or other physicians, who conduct the trial procedures, the Investigator leading the team is typically called the Principal Investigator, and is legally responsible for the work of all those individuals and all trial conduct at the trial site.

7.2.1.3 The Subject/Trial Subject

The Subject/Trial Subject is a human who volunteers to participate in the clinical trial to receive the investigational product or control product. By definition, the Subject/Trial Subject is:

> An individual who participates in a clinical trial, either as a recipient of the investigational product(s) or as a control. (ICH E6(R2) 1.57)

The human research subject or Trial Subject, also known as clinical research subject, participant, or volunteer, is the individual who volunteers to participate in the clinical trial to receive the investigational product or to act as a control in the trial. The volunteer will be an individual from the population being studied in the trial; therefore, research participants can be healthy volunteers or someone who has the disease under study, and can be of any age, race, or gender. For all Trial Subjects, participation in a clinical trial is voluntary. The term Subject or Trial Subject is generally used to describe the person once they consent to being in a trial, although some prefer "patients" to refer to individuals who have the disease. Others also prefer the neutral term "volunteer" or participant' to refer to all types of trial participants.

7.2.1.4 The IRB/IEC

The ethics committee, which is formally known as Independent Ethics Committee (IEC) or IRB, is a body of individuals that ensures the protection of human research subjects (the term "IRB" is used in the United States regulations). By definition, an Independent Ethics Committee (IEC) is:

> An independent body (a review board or a committee, institutional, regional, national, or supranational), constituted of medical/scientific professionals and nonmedical/nonscientific members, whose responsibility it is to ensure the protection of the rights, safety, and well-being of human subjects involved in a trial and to provide public assurance of that protection, by, among other things, reviewing and approving/providing favorable opinion on the trial protocol, the suitability of the investigator(s), facilities, and the methods and material to be used in obtaining and documenting informed consent of the trial subject. (ICH E6(R2) 1.27)

An IRB is:

> An independent body constituted of medical, scientific, and nonscientific members, whose responsibility it is to ensure the protection of the rights, safety, and well-being of human subjects involved in a trial by, among other things, reviewing, approving, and providing continuing review of trials, of protocols and amendments, and of the methods and material to be used in obtaining and documenting informed consent of the trial subjects. (ICH E6(R2) 1.57)

An ethics committee that is responsible for the physical and psychological protection of human research subjects is known as an IRB or IEC, or ethical review board, depending on the geographical region or country, or institution. An institution where a trial is taking place, for example a hospital or academic center, may have a department dedicated to performing IRB activities for all clinical research studies that are executed at that institution. There are also IRBs that review a given trial for all the clinical sites participating in the given study and these IRBs are known as central IRBs. Additionally, a particular ethics committee may review research protocols for all studies conducted within its geographic region.

For all types of IRBs/IECs, the composition and functions remain the same per GCP (ICH E6(R2) 3). An IRB/IEC's review is independent of the influence of the investigator, sponsor or their representatives; however, for a given trial, some IRB/IECs may take into consideration the opinions of other IRB/IECs that are reviewing the same trial at other participating sites.

7.2.1.5   The Regulatory Authority

The regulatory authority is a public authority or government agency charged with overseeing clinical investigations that involve unapproved medicinal products. By definition, the Regulatory Authority is:

> A body having the power to regulate. In the ICH GCP guidance the expression "Regulatory Authorities" includes the authorities that review submitted clinical data and those that conduct inspections. These bodies are sometimes referred to as competent authorities. (ICH E6(R2) 1.49)

A regulatory authority is a public authority or government agency. There may be an agency named specifically to oversee the safety, effectiveness, quality, and security of medicinal products, such as the Food and Drug Administration (FDA) in the United States of America and the Medicines and Healthcare Products Regulatory Agency (MHRA) in the United Kingdom, or the function may fall under the general authority of, for example, a country's Ministry of Health.

The authority or authorities make rules to govern the activities for drug development, that is, manufacturing of the medicinal product, animal testing, and clinical testing. For clinical testing specifically, there are rules that govern the activities of the Sponsor, Clinical Investigator, and the IRB. Each of the clinical testing players has rules to follow and these rules are typically called "responsibilities." The Sponsor submits the data from clinical trials as part of an application for approval for marketing the test product. The Regulatory Authority reviews the application to assess a product's safety and efficacy, will conduct inspections to ensure that trials were conducted according to GCP and the applicable regulatory requirements, and will consider other factors prior to granting approval.

7.2.2   How the Main Players Interact

In the previous section, we defined the various main players involved in the clinical research conduct. The players are the Sponsor, Investigator, Trial Subject, IRB/IEC, and the Regulatory Authority. Figure 7.1 depicts the lines of communication between and among each of the main players.

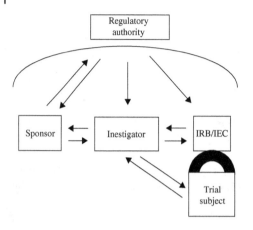

Figure 7.1 Players interaction.

We recall that the initiation of a clinical trial comes from the Sponsor, and the Regulatory Authority is a public authority or government agency that is essentially the gate-keeper between the Sponsor and the public who will eventually use the product.

Before a trial may be initiated, the Sponsor must communicate its intention to the governing regulatory authority or authorities who will provide feedback as to whether or not the trial may be conducted. The Sponsor reports the progress and the final outcome of the trial to the authority(ies) who review, ask questions, or request additional information as needed form the Sponsor. The Sponsor also engages the Investigator and provides them with the investigational product for the trial and all information they need to execute the trial at the trial site.

Prior to the Investigator initiating the clinical trial, the Investigator must obtain an approval from a duly constituted IRB/IEC to conduct the trial. The Investigator will communicate the progress and outcome of the trial to the IRB/IEC as well as the Sponsor. The Investigator, of course, will recruit the Trial Subject, who is asked to volunteer for the trial and to commit to following the trial procedures. The Trial Subject has the right to contact the IRB/IEC at any time if they have questions or concerns regarding the conduct of the clinical trial.

Lastly, the Regulatory Authority oversees all the players who have GCP responsibilities. We note that the Investigator and IRB/IEC do not typically communicate directly with the Regulatory Authority for routine trial conduct, but may certainly do so if the need arises.

7.3 Summary

In this overview, we answered the questions: Who are the main players involved in the conduct of clinical research? and, How do the main players interact with each other in the clinical research arena? The activities of the Sponsor, Investigator,

IRB/IEC, and Regulatory Authority are regulated; and the Regulatory Authority has complete oversight of the Sponsor, Investigator, and IRB. We note that they all are responsible in some way to ensure the protection of the rights, safety, and well-being of the research subject, for whom there are no regulatory "responsibilities" because their participation in a trial is completely voluntary, with the option to discontinue at any time. The GCP responsibilities of each of the players are be addressed in greater detail in separate chapters.

Knowledge Check Questions

1) Who are the main players involved in the conduct of clinical research?
2) What is the role of the IRB/IEC?
3) What is the role of the Sponsor?
4) What is the role of the Investigator?
5) What is the role of the Trial Subject?
6) What is the role of the Regulatory Authority?
7) How do the various players interact?

Reference

1 International Council for Harmonisation of Technical Requirements for Pharmaceuticals for Human Use (ICH), Integrated Addendum to ICH E6(R2):Guideline for Good Clinical Practice, E6(R2) (2016). Current Step 4 version dated 9 November 2016 https://www.ich.org/page/efficacy-guidelines

8

IRB/IEC Roles and Responsibilities

P. Michael Dubinsky

GCP Key Point

The absence or failure of researchers to follow or have in place ethical standards and safeguards resulted in several key policy documents, e.g. Declaration of Helsinki being developed. The IRB/IEC functionally implements ethical expectations contained in those documents.

8.1   Introduction

In other chapters the authors touch on some details about historical events which resulted in the development and issuance of policy documents which define the ethical expectations associated with the conduct of clinical trials. The Nuremburg Code, Declaration of Helsinki and Belmont Report were all developed and put in place in reaction to ethical abuses by researchers. Institutional Review Boards (IRBs) were the operating or functional demonstration of ethical oversight beginning in the US circa the 1960s. The US FDA put regulations in place circa 1971 and in 1974 the National Research Act formalized the requirements for having IRBs review planned clinical research. Regulations governing both the IRBs and requiring informed consent of trial subjects were in place circa 1981. The US IRB system was initially developed and implemented by academic medical institutions. In Europe the system of ethical oversight was largely developed by governments and became known as independent ethics committees (IECs). Since the ICH E6 (R2) was a work product of the both the US FDA and the EU EMA along with the Japanese health authority both titles were included in the ICH Glossary.

The Fundamentals of Clinical Research: A Universal Guide for Implementing Good Clinical Practice, First Edition. P. Michael Dubinsky and Karen A. Henry.
© 2022 John Wiley & Sons, Inc. Published 2022 by John Wiley & Sons, Inc.
Companion website: www.wiley.com/go/dubinsky/clinicalresearch

The roles and responsibilities of the IRB/IEC as spelled out in section 3 of the guideline involve a range of activities from making the decision as to whether a proposed trial is approved for implementation to what constitutes required record keeping for the IRB/IEC. The IRB/IEC roles and responsibilities section are fittingly at the very beginning of the guideline since without their approval the trial cannot begin.

8.2   Objectives

The objectives of this chapter are to review the requirements/expectations for IRB/IEC as found in the ICH E6 (R2) Guideline at section 3. The GCP expectations speak to:

1) Responsibilities of the IRB/IEC
2) Composition, functions, and operations of the IRB/IEC
3) Procedures for the IRB/IEC
4) Records that the IRB/IEC is expected to maintain

In addition, the chapter will highlight some of the areas where IRB/IECs have not adhered to these expectations. Such information should be useful as the risk assessment for a trial is prepared.

8.3   Responsibilities of the IRB/IEC

The IRB/IEC first and foremost is responsible for safeguarding the rights, safety, and well-being of the human subjects participating in the trial. If a trial involves a population that is considered vulnerable, e.g. children, then the IRB/IEC must apply an even more rigorous approach to their review and assessment of documents, people, processes, and places.

8.3.1   Documents

All the critical and essential documents which define the clinical trial are provided to the IRB/IEC for assessment and approval. That includes the Protocol, Informed Consent Form, Investigator's Brochure, subject recruitment materials such as advertisements, and the investigator's qualifications. Their conclusions about the acceptability of the investigational plan and the supporting materials are determinative when it comes to starting the trial. Absent their approval the trial cannot proceed. The IRB/IEC must provide their approval/favorable opinion. The IRB/IEC can require modifications to any of the essential documents as well as disapproving a study. In addition, their review must be ongoing which usually means annually but can differ if the IRB/IEC so decides. Vulnerable populations such as children call for the IRB/IEC to be even more attentive to details such as the circumstances under which the subject's consent is obtained and who may give consent on behalf of the subject. Compensation for participation in a trial is permitted in some form by most regulatory authorities. However, the method and monetary value of compensation associated with payment often calls for close review to ensure that subjects are not coerced or enticed in a manner which violates ethical standards. And it is not just the amount of a payment that could be problematic but also any claims related to the effect that the investigational product may have on the disease or injury being treated.

8.4 Composition, Functions, and Operations

Membership or makeup of the IRB/IEC as described in the guideline focuses on two aspects. A minimum number of members is set at five with one having a non-scientific background and one being independent of the institution or trial site. The investigator and sponsor must not have a voting representative on the IRB/IEC but can provide information about the trial as part of the IRB/IEC evaluation process. Outside experts can be invited to participate in the information gathering process if needed. The exact number of members and their credentials may be controlled by regulation or law for the country or region where the trial is to be conducted and those requirements must be followed.

The IRB/IEC should have written procedures (SOPs) in place to direct its operations. There should be written records of all meetings including decisions. Meeting minutes should list the members present and whether a quorum was achieved. The number of members constituting a quorum will be defined in an SOP.

8.5 Procedures

SOPs are a key part of meeting ICH E6(R2) across the board and the IRB expectations are no exception. The IRB/IEC's role in ensuring that ethical practices and policies are built into every trial is documented in part by having written procedures and records documenting that those procedures were followed. The procedures that are expected to be in writing include:

- Determining the composition such as qualifications for members and under what authority the IRB/IEC is established.
- How scheduling will be handled. This might include timing, notification procedures, and how members will be notified.
- How the Committee will conduct initial and ongoing reviews of trials.
- Criteria for ongoing review of trials.

- Special procedures such as expedited review
- Specifications that apply to every trial such as: not enrolling subjects until a written approval for the trial is given; deviations from an approved protocol cannot be made without IRB/IEC approval; items that must be reported to the IRB in a timely manner such as protocol changes, changes which might increase subject risk, adverse experiences that are unexpected or serious, and new information.
- The IRB/IECs timeline for reporting decisions on approvals as well as reasons for decisions and any criteria for appeals of decisions.

8.6   Records

The IRB/IEC should maintain all records for a retention period of 3 years. That is a minimum timeframe listed in some regulations. The retention period may vary. In the United States the retention period for IRB records is 3 years [1] after completion of the research however in the European Union the archiving requirement is for 25 years [2] after the end of the clinical trial.

8.7   Noncompliance by IRB/IECs – Areas of Risk

IRB/IECs are generally regarded and viewed as professional organizations established by government legislation or within the structure of academic medical institutions where clinical trial research may be centered. There are however commercial or independent IRB/IECs that operate globally which have found a niche in the business of clinical trial conduct. The independent IRBs have become a substantive presence in the review of clinical trials and the ethics of using a commercial or paid entity to conduct a review that is intended to determine if there are among other things any ethical concerns about a clinical trial plan may seem a dichotomy. However independent IRB/IECs have been around for some time and offer a sense of continuity to the review process especially when there are multiple trial sites involved as with large phase III trials.

Irrespective of whether the IRB/IEC is independent or affiliated with the institution where the trial is occurring inspections of IRB/IECs have shown noncompliance in a variety of areas. Many of the deficiencies might be described as administrative but the primary role of the IRB/IEC is in a way just that – Administrative. A list of the types of deficiencies follows and it should provide a basis for deciding whether to add any risk assessment regarding the IRB/IEC review process for a given trial.

- Inadequate meeting minutes
- Inadequate membership rosters

- Inadequate initial and continuing review of research
- Inadequate written procedures for prompt reporting of noncompliance, suspension, or termination
- Quorum issues
- Failure to promptly report noncompliance, suspension/termination of a site

It is useful to point out that from a practical standpoint IRB/IECs have established administrative control mechanisms due to the detailed requirements and record keeping that they must adhere to. This administrative staff is not the IRB/IEC per se but they (the staff) often know the details of the regulatory requirements better than the IRB members themselves. While not foolproof, having such organizational units overseeing and directing the IRB's functional activities can and does prevent noncompliance.

The US FDA publishes data from their inspections of the IRB/IECs that register with them. The items listed above are compiled from the inspections that the US FDA conducts and reported in FDA's Good Clinical Practices webpage [3].

8.8 Summary

The IRB/IEC represents the unbiased third-party reviewer for all the essential documents which comprise the clinical trial plan. The protection of the rights, well-being and safety of human subjects is the primary role of the IRB/IEC.

In order that this role is performed in a manner which is credible the ICH E6(R2) guideline calls for certain criteria to be in place so that as needed the procedures that were followed, the qualification of the people who followed the procedures and the records maintained of the work are complete, reliable, and accurate.

Avoiding ethical pitfalls should be inherent in the culture of the medical community that conducts human clinical trials, but history has shown that is not always the case. The IRB/IEC requirements are necessary and not likely to be set aside.

Knowledge Check Questions
1) Why do you think that the IRB/IEC requirements call for one member to be independent of the institutional/trial site? Please provide a brief narrative explaining your answer.
2) While not a common practice today, in the past prisoners were often called upon to participate in clinical trials. Would you consider prisoners to be a vulnerable population? If so, what might be some of the issues which would envision arising when an IRB/IEC is reviewing a protocol which allows them to be subjects in a clinical trial?

3) According to ICH E6(R2) the IRB/IEC must have written standard Operating procedures in place for all the functions they implement. True or False?
4) A quorum for an IRB is always three members being present, Correct? If not where is the number for a Quorum found?
5) According to regulatory authority reports one common deficiency for IRB/IECs is inadequate ongoing review of studies. Can you briefly explain how you might avoid such a deficiency if you were part of an IRB/IEC.

References

1 FDA (2002). Code of Federal Regulations Title 21 CFR 56.115 (b). https://www.accessdata.fda.gov/scripts/cdrh/cfdocs/cfcfr/CFRSearch.cfm?fr=56.115 (accessed 6 April 2020).

2 EU Regulation (2014). REGULATION (EU) No 536/2014 OF THE EUROPEAN PARLIAMENT AND OF THE COUNCIL of 16 April 2014 on clinical trials on medicinal products for human use, and repealing Directive 2001/20/ECEU Regulation 536, Article 58 - Archiving of the clinical trial master file. https://ec.europa.eu/health/sites/health/files/files/eudralex/vol-1/reg_2014_536/reg_2014_536_en.pdf (accessed 6 April 2020)

3 FDA Bioresearch Monitoring (BIMO)(2021). Inspection Metrics. https://www.fda.gov/science-research/clinical-trials-and-human-subject-protection/bimo-inspection-metrics (accessed 6 April 2020)

9

Investigator and Sponsor Roles and Responsibilities

Karen A. Henry

GCP Key Point
Clinical trials should be conducted in accordance with the ethical principles that have their origin in the Declaration of Helsinki, and that are consistent with GCP and the applicable regulatory requirement(s). Source: ICH [1]

9.1 Introduction

The ICH GCP guidance (E6(R2)), as it is today, reflects the attempt to prevent harmful consequences of experimentation on humans over centuries (Chapter 1 History). In societies, there have always been someone seeking to sell the next "wonder drug" and a "scientist" who is curious about how human bodies work and how they would respond to new or modified vaccines, treatments, or potential cures. Per ICH E6(R2), the sponsor is "an individual, company, institution, or organization which takes responsibility for the initiation, management, and/or financing of a clinical trial" (ICH E6(R2) 1.53) and the investigator is "a person responsible for the conduct of the clinical trial at a trial site" (ICH E6(R2) 1.34). ICH has provided guidance on the responsibilities of the sponsor (ICH E6(R2) 5) and of the investigator (ICH E6(R2) 4). Although the sponsor and investigator essentially collaborate to create and execute a clinical trial with an aim to discover new or improved vaccines, treatments, or potential cures new treatments, the sponsor and investigator have specific and independent responsibilities that are stipulated by ICH (E6(R2)) and perhaps regional or local regulatory requirements.

In this chapter, we will present the responsibilities of sponsors and investigators in the context of the general trial process and provide the reader with references to book chapters that describe the responsibilities in greater detail. Plate 4 Individual Clinical

The Fundamentals of Clinical Research: A Universal Guide for Implementing Good Clinical Practice, First Edition. P. Michael Dubinsky and Karen A. Henry.
© 2022 John Wiley & Sons, Inc. Published 2022 by John Wiley & Sons, Inc.
Companion website: www.wiley.com/go/dubinsky/clinicalresearch

Trial – Overview of Investigator and Sponsor Responsibilities displays the individual responsibilities in the context of the chapter content in the book and the reader may refer to the relevant sections of ICH E6(R2) for lists of the responsibilities by player.

9.2 Objectives

The objectives of this chapter are to:

1) Define sponsor and investigator and various forms
2) Describe sponsor and investigator responsibilities in the context of the clinical trial process

9.2.1 Definitions

Here are some important definitions for the sponsor and investigator players involved in conducting a clinical trial. A clinical trial will have,

a) The Sponsor:

   A sponsor who is "an individual, company, institution, or organization which takes responsibility for the initiation, management, and/or financing of a clinical trial" (ICH E6(R2) 1.53). The sponsor will be interested in collecting data from a series of clinical trials to prove the safety and efficacy of an investigational product so that they may apply to the governing regulatory authority(ies) for approval to market the product. The sponsor will seek out investigators who have access to the study population, i.e., healthy volunteers or the patients who have the indication being studied in the trial.

   The sponsor for a clinical trial may contract with a Contract Research Organization(s) (CRO), which is a person or an organization (commercial, academic, or other) contracted to perform one or more of a sponsor's trial-related duties and functions (ICH E6(R2) 1.20). The CRO will bear the GCP and regulatory responsibilities for the contracted tasks (Chapter 15 Trial Resourcing and Outsourcing).

b) The Investigator:

   The investigator is "a person responsible for the conduct of the clinical trial at a trial site. If a trial is conducted by a team of individuals at a trial site, the investigator is the responsible leader of the team and may be called the principal investigator" (ICH E6(R2) 1.34). The investigator, or a qualified designee, will administer the investigational product to the study subjects.

   The investigator may subcontract or delegate tasks to others; however, unlike the sponsor, the investigator maintains full GCP and regulatory responsibilities for the delegated tasks.

c) The Sponsor-Investigator:

An individual may decide to take responsibility for the supply of the investigational product and to test the investigational product on research volunteers as well. In this scenario, the individual or organization assumes the GCP and regulatory responsibilities as both sponsor and investigator. This sponsor-investigator is therefore an individual who both initiates and conducts, alone or with others, a clinical trial, and under whose immediate direction the investigational product is administered to, dispensed to, or used by a subject. The term does not include any person other than an individual (e.g., it does not include a corporation or an agency). The obligations of a sponsor–investigator include both those of a sponsor and those of an investigator (ICH E6(R2) 1.54). For example, an investigator at an academic medical research institution may be interested in testing an approved or investigational product for a new indication that the original sponsor may not pursue. The investigator will then procure the product, create the clinical trial protocol and conduct the trial as the sponsor as well as enroll the patients and administer the product to the patients.

An example of an Investigator–CRO combination is that of what is known as a phase 1 facility, where typically first-in-human testing is performed to obtain pharmacokinetic information of an investigational product. The sponsor may select such a facility because these facilities are equipped with on-site housing and hospital services and the phase 1 study is testing the investigational product on few individuals who must be constantly monitored for safety and pharmacokinetic results. This facility may not only perform investigator responsibilities, in that they will enroll and administer the product to the study subjects, but may also perform the pharmacokinetic testing and data analyses, and prepare the clinical study report for the sponsor. The facility has then also assumed sponsor responsibilities in that they are contracted as a central laboratory to perform the pharmacokinetic testing and as the writer of the clinical study report.

9.2.2 Sponsor and Investigator Responsibilities in the Context of the Clinical Trial Process

This chapter describes the responsibilities of sponsors and investigators in the context of the general clinical trial process (Plate 4 Individual Clinical Trial – Overview of Investigator and Sponsor Responsibilities). While some activities are necessarily sequential (e.g., IRB/IEC approval/favorable opinion of a protocol prior to consenting a human research subject), some activities may occur concurrently for efficiency (e.g., selecting investigators and selecting a CRO for data management).

9.2.2.1 Before the Clinical Phase of the Trial Commences
9.2.2.1.1 *The Sponsor*

- Implements a system to manage quality throughout all stages of the trial process (ICH E6(R2) 5.0 Quality Management). The sponsor will focus on those aspects of the trial to ensure human subject protection and the reliability of trial results when designing a protocol, preparing processes and procedures for data collection, processing, and reporting, and trial monitoring. The system will include:
  - Risk-based quality management methods to ensure that all aspects of the trial are operationally feasible and should avoid unnecessary complexity, procedures, and data collection. (Chapter 13 Risk Assessment and Quality Management)
  - Protocols, case report forms, and other operational and procedural documents that are clear, concise, and consistent.
  - The quality management system should be proportionate to the risks inherent in the trial and the importance of the information collected. (Chapter 31 Quality Responsibilities)

In practice, the quality management system will require, for example, policies that require all those involved in activities related to a clinical trial to be compliant with guidelines, practices, SOPs, regulatory requirements, and any other policies and procedures of the firm. Additional requirements may include the establishment of a core scientific team for the review and approval of proposed protocol designs and changes, an operations core team for review and approval of proposed SOPS and changes to systems, and a safety core team for the review and assessment of reported adverse events.

- Creates and implements procedures to assure and control the quality of the trial (ICH E6(R2) 5.1 Quality Assurance and Quality Control; Part V Quality in Clinical Trials). The sponsor will establish, ensure training on, and implement SOPs for activities related to planning, initiating, management and control, and audit and inspections of a trial.
- Prepares a clinical trial protocol (ICH E6(R2) 5.4 Trial Design; Chapter 18 The Clinical Trial Protocol and Amendments). The protocol is the Investigational plan and must be scientifically sound.
- Prepares the investigational product according to good manufacturing practices (ICH E6(R2) 5.13 Manufacturing, Packaging, Labeling, and Coding Investigational Product(S); Chapter 17 The Investigational Product (Clinical Supplies)).
- Prepares the investigator's brochure that contains all information known to date about the test article, including nonclinical testing (ICH E6(R2) 5.12 Information on Investigational Product(S); Chapter 16 The Investigator's Brochure).
- Identifies resources for all trial-related duties and functions, including designating appropriately qualified medical personnel who will be readily available to advise

on trial-related medical questions or problems, other qualified internal personnel and the selection and qualification of any CROs to assume any responsibilities of the sponsor. (ICH E6(R2) 5.3 Medical Expertise, ICH E6(R2) 5.7 Allocation of Responsibilities, ICH E6(R2) 5.2 Contract Research Organization (CRO); Chapter 15 Trial Resourcing and Outsourcing)

- Prepares and submits an application/notification to initiate a clinical trial to the regulatory authority(ies) for their review of the proposed investigational plan. (ICH E6(R2) 5.10 Notification/Submission to Regulatory Authority(Ies); Chapter 11 Regulatory Authority Roles and Responsibilities.)
- Prepares plans, systems, and procedures for managing trial operations, collecting and processing trial data, and maintaining trial records (Chapter 29 Essential Documents). (ICH E6(R2) 5.5 Trial Management, Data Handling, and Record Keeping). The plans and systems will include, but not limited to:
  - Case Report Forms (Chapter 20 Data Collection and Data Management)
  - Regulatory compliant data collection systems (Chapter 20 Data Collection and Data Management)
  - Informed Consent Template and other subject information and recruitment documents (Chapter 19 Informed Consent and Other Human Subject Protection)
  - Monitoring Plan (Chapter 22 Monitoring Overview)
  - Statistical Analysis Plan (Chapter 27 Study Design and Data Analysis)
  - Safety Management Plan (Chapter 21 Safety Monitoring and Reporting)
  - Audit Plan (Chapter 33 Quality Assurance Components)
  - Trial Management Plan (Chapter 14 Trial Management; Start-up, On-Study, and Close-Out)
  - Risk Management Plan (Chapter 13 Risk Assessment and Quality Management)
- Selects qualified investigator(s) (ICH E6(R2) 5.6 Investigator Selection, 5.23 Multicenter Trials; Chapter 23 Investigator/Institution Selection):
  - Assesses investigator and site qualifications for suitability to conduct the trial.
  - Provides investigators with information they need to conduct the trial, including the protocol, the investigator's brochure and other investigational product information, for their review and assessment prior to agreeing to conduct the trial.
  - Has signed written agreements with investigators to conduct the trial in compliance with GCP, the protocol, and applicable regulatory requirements. Ensures that the investigator knows of and agrees to regulatory and contractual obligations, including compliance requirements with GCP, the protocol, and the regulatory requirements, and permitting monitoring, auditing, and inspections, and retention of trial essential documents.
  - For multicenter trials, identifies a coordinating investigator, provides uniform sets of standards for data collection and laboratory assessments, and facilitates

communication between investigators (Chapter 20 Data Collection and Data Management).

- Has written agreements with investigator for access to source data and source documents trial records for monitoring, auditing, and inspections, (ICH E6(R2) 5.15 Record Access; Chapter 22 Monitoring Overview).
- Ensures possession of trial insurance and provisions for compensating subjects for trial participation (as applicable) and trial-related injury per applicable regulatory requirements. (ICH E6(R2) 5.8 Compensation to Subjects and Investigators; Chapter 19 Informed Consent and Other Human Subject Protection).
- Has agreements with the investigator/institution regarding financial arrangements for the trial (ICH E6(R2) 5.9 Financing; Chapter 23 Investigator/Institution Selection).

9.2.2.1.2 The Investigator

- Is qualified and agrees to specific stipulations prior to trial conduct (ICH E6(R2) 4.1 Investigator's Qualifications and Agreements; Chapter 24 Investigator/ Institution Initiation):
  - Is qualified by education, training, and experience to assume responsibility for the proper conduct of the trial.
  - Is thoroughly familiar with the appropriate use of the investigational product as described in the protocol and investigator's brochure.
  - Is aware of and complies with GCP and applicable regulatory requirements
  - Permits monitoring, auditing, and inspections
  - Trains site staff and maintains a list of appropriately qualified staff who are allowed to perform significant trial-related duties (i.e., record or change trial data).
- Has, supervises, and maintains adequate resources for trial conduct; i.e., subject recruitment, qualified and trained personnel and third parties, certified and adequate facilities, and time. Additionally, the investigator will implement procedures to ensure the integrity of trial activities and data that are generated (ICH E6(R2) 4.2 Adequate Resources; Chapter 22 Monitoring Overview; Chapter 25 Investigator/Institution Interim Monitoring)
- Obtains approval of trial protocol and subject information from a qualified IRB/ IEC. IRB/IEC approval must be obtained before implementing a new or amended or revised study protocol or subject information document. (ICH E6(R2) 4.4 Communication with IRB/IEC; Chapter 8 IRB/IEC Roles and Responsibilities).

9.2.2.1.3 The Sponsor

- Confirms qualification of investigator and site prior to initiation of the trial at the site (Chapter 24 Investigator/Institution Initiation).
- Confirms review and approval/favorable opinion of the trial by a qualified IRB/ IEC. Obtains IRB/IEC name, address, composition, registration, copy of approval,

and changes made to study documents by the IRB/IEC. (ICH E6(R2) 5.11 Confirmation of Review by IRB/IEC; Chapter 24 Investigator/Institution Initiation).

- Confirms approval/no objection from the regulatory authority(ies) to initiate the proposed investigational plan. (ICH E6(R2) 5.10 Notification/Submission to Regulatory Authority(Ies); Chapter 11 Regulatory Authority Roles and Responsibilities).
- Supplies investigational product and is responsible for the supply and handling of the product; i.e., the full chain of custody of the investigational product from shipment to the investigator to its return or destruction. (ICH E6(R2) 5.14 Supplying and Handling Investigational Product(S); Chapter 17 The Investigational Product (Clinical Supplies)).

9.2.2.2 During the Clinical Conduct of the Trial

9.2.2.2.1 The Investigator

- Ensures informed consent of trial subjects prior to the subject undergoing any study procedure at the start of and during the trial (ICH E6(R2) 4.8 Informed Consent of Trial Subjects) and provides adequate medical care to the subject for trial-related adverse events during and following a subject's participation in the trial, and ensures confidentiality of subject information (ICH E6(R2) 4.3 Medical Care of Trial Subjects; Chapter 19 Informed Consent and Other Human Subject Protection)
- Complies with protocol procedures and records, reports, and corrects any deviations (ICH E6(R2) 4.5 Compliance with Protocol; Chapter 25 Investigator/ Institution Interim Monitoring).
- Follows randomization procedures and procedures for any unblinding (ICH E6(R2) 4.7 Randomization Procedures and Unblinding; Chapter 25 Investigator/ Institution Interim Monitoring).
- Stores, handles, and administer the test article according to the protocol and IB, and accounts for receipt, use, return, and destruction of test article (ICH E6(R2) 4.6 Investigational Product(s); Chapter 25 Investigator/Institution Interim Monitoring).
- Reports adverse events to the sponsor (ICH E6(R2) 4.11 Safety Reporting, Chapter 21 Safety Monitoring and Reporting).
- Maintains source documentation and complete case histories for each subject in accordance with good documentation practices and the applicable regulatory requirements. Source documentation includes all activities from informed consenting to study completion. (ICH E6(R2) 4.9 Records and Reports, Chapter 25 Investigator/Institution Interim Monitoring; Chapter 29 Essential Documents).
- Permits monitoring and auditing by the sponsor (ICH E6(R2) 4.1 Investigator's Qualifications and Agreements; Chapter 22 Monitoring Overview).
- Communicates the study status and information per the IRB/IEC requirements and sponsor and regulatory requirements (ICH E6(R2) 4.10 Progress Reports; Chapter 29 Essential Documents; Chapter 25 Investigator/Institution Interim Monitoring; Chapter 8 IRB/IEC Roles and Responsibilities).

9.2.2.2.2 The Sponsor

Oversees and reviews the progress of the investigation to ensure protection of subject rights and safety, data integrity, and compliance with the protocol, SOPs, GCP, and regulatory requirements.

- Selects qualified monitors and implements procedures for on- and off-site and centralized monitoring of the progress of the investigation using a risk-based approach and methods as outlined in a Monitoring Plan for the trial (ICH E6(R2) 5.18 Monitoring; Chapter 22 Monitoring Overview)
- Collects, reviews, and assesses adverse events for ongoing risk-benefit evaluation of the investigational product and to notify all concerned investigator(s) and the regulatory authority(ies) of findings that could adversely affect the safety of subjects, impact the conduct of the trial, or alter the IRB/IEC's approval/favorable opinion to continue the trial (ICH E6(R2) 5.16 Safety Information). These notifications may be as single reports, protocol amendments, and/or updates to the investigator's brochure (Chapter 21 Safety Monitoring and Reporting; Chapter 25 Investigator/Institution Interim Monitoring; Chapter 16 The Investigator's Brochure; Chapter 18 The Clinical Trial Protocol and Amendments)
- Reports adverse drug reactions that are both serious and unexpected as per ICH E2A Guideline for Clinical Safety Data Management: Definitions and Standards for Expedited Reporting and applicable regulatory requirements [2] (ICH E6(R2) 5.17 Adverse Drug Reaction Reporting; Chapter 21 Safety Monitoring and Reporting)
- Assesses and manages risk for quality management (ICH E6(R2) 5.0; Chapter 13 Risk Assessment and Quality Management).
- Selects qualified independent auditors to conduct audits per the Audit Plan and/or for an unplanned cause (ICH E6(R2) 5.19 Audit, Chapter 33 Quality Assurance Components; Chapter 34 Regulatory Authority Inspections) and promptly secures compliance and implements corrective and preventive actions for deviations from the protocol, SOPs, GCP, and regulatory requirements that significantly impact or have the potential to significantly impact subject safety and data integrity. If monitoring or audit observations reflect serious or persistent noncompliance on the part of an investigator/institution then the sponsor should terminate the investigator's/institution's participation in the investigation and promptly notify the regulatory authority(ies). (ICH E6(R2) 5.20 Noncompliance, Chapter 25 Investigator/Institution Interim Monitoring, Chapter 33 Quality Assurance Components, Chapter 34 Regulatory Authority Inspections, Chapter 31 Quality Responsibilities).

9.2.2.3 After Completion or Termination of the Trial

9.2.2.3.1 The Investigator

- Submits reports of final trial status and outcome to IRB/IEC and regulatory authority(ies) as required (ICH E6(R2) 4.13 Final Report(s) by

Investigator; Chapter 29 Essential Documents; Chapter 26 Investigator/ Institution Close-out; Chapter 8 IRB/IEC Roles and Responsibilities).

- In the event of premature termination or suspension of a trial, promptly informs the trial subject, arranges for appropriate medical care follow-up for the subject, and informs the sponsor, IRB/IEC, and/or regulatory authority(ies) as applicable, (ICH E6(R2) 4.12 Premature Termination or Suspension of a Trial; Chapter 29 Essential Documents; Chapter 26 Investigator/Institution Close-out; Chapter 8 IRB/IEC Roles and Responsibilities).
- Permits audits/inspections by Sponsor, IRB, and Regulatory Authority(ies) at ANY time! (ICH E6(R2) 4.1 Investigator's Qualifications and Agreements; Chapter 24 Investigator/Institution Initiation)

9.2.2.3.2 *The Sponsor*

- In the event of premature termination or suspension of a trial, promptly informs the investigator(s), the regulatory authority(ies), and IRB/IEC as applicable, of the termination or suspension and the reason(s) for termination or suspension (ICH E6(R2) 5.21 Premature Termination or Suspension of a Trial; Chapter 18 Clinical Trial Protocol and Amendments; Chapter 26 Investigator/Institution Close-out; Chapter 8 IRB/IEC Roles and Responsibilities).
- Closes trial sites upon study completion (Chapter 26 Investigator/Institution Close-out).
- Prepares and submits clinical trial/study reports of trial results to the regulatory authority(ies) whether the trial is completed or prematurely terminated as required by the regulatory requirements. The clinical trial reports in marketing applications will meet the standards of the ICH E3 Guideline for Structure and Content of Clinical Study Reports [3,4]. (ICH E6(R2) 5.22 Clinical Trial/Study Reports; Chapter 28).
- Permits audits/inspections by Regulatory Authority(ies) at ANY time! (ICH E6(R2) 5.1 Quality Assurance and Quality Control; Chapter 31 Quality Responsibilities).

9.2.2.3.3 *The Sponsor and Investigator*

Maintain and archive records (evidence of trial conduct). Maintain records that demonstrate the conduct of the trial. Archive records so that they are retrievable and for the duration required by applicable regulations. The investigator will have access to trial data at all times. (ICH E6(R2) 4.9 Records and Reports, 5.5 Trial Management, Data Handling, and Record Keeping, Chapter 29 Essential Documents).

9.3 Summary

The sponsor and investigator are two key players in the clinical trial process. The sponsor is "an individual, company, institution, or organization which takes responsibility for the initiation, management, and/or financing of a clinical trial" (ICH

E6(R2) 1.53). The investigator is "a person responsible for the conduct of the clinical trial at a trial site. If a trial is conducted by a team of individuals at a trial site, the investigator is the responsible leader of the team and may be called the principal investigator" (ICH E6(R2) 1.34). The sponsor and investigator must comply with the GCP guidelines and regulatory requirements that clearly describe their respective trial-related duties and responsibilities. The sponsor may transfer any or all of their study-related duties to a CRO and the regulatory obligations that are associated with the transferred task; however, the sponsor retains regulatory responsibility for the oversight of the CRO and the overall safety of trial subjects and integrity of the trial data. The investigator may also delegate trial-related duties to staff or subcontractors; however, the investigator retains all regulatory obligations associated with delegated or subcontracted tasks.

Knowledge Check Questions

1) What is the role of the sponsor?
2) What other individuals or parties may assist the sponsor with trial-related duties, and under what conditions?
3) What is the role of the investigator?
4) What other individuals or parties may assist the investigator with trial-related duties, and under what conditions?
5) What are the sponsor's responsibilities before the trial commences, during the conduct of the trial, and after completion or termination of a trial?
6) What are the investigator's responsibilities before the trial commences, during the conduct of the trial, and after completion or termination of a trial?
7) Overheard:

"We should have ethics committee approval of the protocol tomorrow so we will enroll the patient the following day. We can then submit to the study to the regulatory authority."

Physician at a clinic who received donated study drug from a manufacturer to conduct their own clinical trial. This physician will otherwise wholly finance and resource the study.

Comment and discuss:
a) What are the GCP and regulatory responsibilities of this "investigator"?
b) Is the investigator violating any GCP requirement? If yes, which?

References

1 International Council for Harmonisation of Technical Requirements for Pharmaceuticals for Human Use (ICH), Integrated Addendum to ICH E6(R2):Guideline for Good Clinical Practice, E6(R2) (2016). Current Step 4 version dated 9 November 2016. https://www.ich.org/page/efficacy-guidelines

2 International Council for Harmonisation of Technical Requirements for Pharmaceuticals for Human Use (ICH), Guideline for Clinical Safety Data Management: Definitions and Standards for Expedited Reporting E2A (1994) Current Step 4 version dated 27 October 1994. https://www.ich.org/page/efficacy-guidelines

3 International Council for Harmonisation of Technical Requirements for Pharmaceuticals for Human Use (ICH), Guideline for Structure and Content of Clinical Study Reports E3 (1995). Current Step 4 version dated 30 November 1995. https://www.ich.org/page/efficacy-guidelines

4 International Council for Harmonisation of Technical Requirements for Pharmaceuticals for Human Use (ICH), Implementation Working Group ICH E3 Guideline: Structure and Content of Clinical Study Reports Questions & Answers (R1) Current version dated 6 July 2012. https://www.ich.org/page/efficacy-guidelines

10

The Research Volunteer

Karen A. Henry

GCP Key Point

The rights, safety, and well-being of the trial subjects are the most important considerations and should prevail over interests of science and society. (Source: ICH E6(R2) 2.3 [1])

10.1 Introduction

The goal of clinical research is to determine the safety and effectiveness of investigational products to diagnose, treat, cure, or prevent a disease or relieve the symptoms of a disease in humans. Given the risks of new products for which the safety and efficacy are unknown, it is unethical to expose more numbers of people than are necessary to obtain sufficient information to evaluate the benefits versus the risks of the investigational product. Fortunately, we are able to use the scientific method of testing the product on a representative subset of individuals from the entire population and infer the findings to the larger population.

An individual who participates in a clinical trial, either as a recipient of the investigational product(s) or as a control is known as the subject or trial/study subject (ICH E6(R2) 1.57). In practice, alternative terminology are used to refer to the trial/study subject, such as participant, subject, volunteer, patient (for trial subjects who have the disease that is being studied), healthy volunteers (for trial subjects who are generally healthy and without the disease being studied; e.g., typically phase 1 pharmacokinetic studies).

The trial subject will be recruited by the investigator and will be administered the investigational product by the investigator. Today, anyone participating as a

The Fundamentals of Clinical Research: A Universal Guide for Implementing Good Clinical Practice,
First Edition. P. Michael Dubinsky and Karen A. Henry.
© 2022 John Wiley & Sons, Inc. Published 2022 by John Wiley & Sons, Inc.
Companion website: www.wiley.com/go/dubinsky/clinicalresearch

research subject in a clinical trial has certain rights (Chapter 19 Informed Consent and Other Human Subject Protection):

a) Fully informed consent and voluntarily participate in a trial without coercion
b) Confidentiality of their identity and health information
c) Compensation for trial-related injury and for the time, effort, and expenses for their involvement in the study
d) Medical care for study-related injury or intercurrent illness(es)
e) The ability to withdraw from the study at any time

In addition to the sponsor and investigator, trial subjects also have a role to facilitate ensuring protection of their rights, safety, and well-being, the integrity of trial data, and trial compliance. Trial subjects do not have any formal GCP or regulatory obligations; however, they are *asked* to fulfill certain responsibilities during the consenting process for their participation in the trial. We must always keep in mind that that humans volunteering in a clinical trial are not *required* to and should not be coerced into doing anything. The investigator and sponsor do have the obligation to discontinue study treatment to a subject or withdraw the subject from the trial at any time if they determine that the subject's participation (or lack of participation and compliance with the protocol) puts the subject at risk for harm in the trial. It is also helpful if the trial protocol and trial operations are designed to facilitate the subject's compliance.

In this chapter, we will review the role and voluntary responsibilities of the trial subject, and quality by design concepts to facilitate the subject's compliance with trial requirements for their protection.

10.2 Objectives

The objectives of this chapter are:

1) Define and describe the role of trial subject
2) Describe the voluntary responsibilities of a trial subject regarding:
   a) Protection of rights, safety, and well-being
   b) Integrity of trial data
   c) Trial compliance
3) Describe Quality by Design Considerations to facilitate subject compliance with the trial requirements

10.2.1 The Definition and Role of Trial Subject

A trial subject is an individual who participates in a clinical trial, either as a recipient of the investigational product(s) or as a control (ICH E6(R2) 1.57).

Trial subjects are needed for a clinical trial to receive the investigational product to obtain data to evaluate the safety and efficacy of the investigational product for eventual approval of the product to diagnose, treat, cure, prevent diseases. The trial subject will be administered the investigational product at the clinical research facility by the investigator or a qualified designee.

10.2.2 Voluntary Responsibilities of a Trial Subject

While there are no formal regulatory or GCP obligations prescribed to a trial subject, as there are for the sponsor, investigator, IRB/IEC, the subject will be *asked* to comply with requirements of the protocol and other operational procedures. A subject who has a thorough understanding of what to expect from their trial participation, who provides complete and truthful health and other information to trial staff, who follows study procedures as instructed, and who knows of their rights for trial participation will help to assure protection of their of rights, safety, and well-being, integrity of trial data, and general trial compliance with SOPs, GCP, and applicable regulatory requirements.

NOTE: If the trial subject is a minor or has a legally authorized representative (LAR), then the parent/guardian/LAR will assume the voluntary responsibilities on behalf of the research subject.

We will describe examples of what subjects may do to facilitate their own protection and foster trial quality.

10.2.2.1 Voluntary Responsibilities for Protection of Rights, Safety, and Well-being

A subject may help to ensure the protection of their rights, safety, and well-being by following the study and operational requirements.

10.2.2.1.1 Prior to Volunteering for a Clinical Trial

Prior to volunteering for a clinical trial:

- A subject should understand what clinical research is and what to expect when they volunteer to take part in a clinical trial.
- The potential volunteer should know of their rights for participating in a clinical trial. The general GCP rights are:
  a) Fully informed consent and voluntarily participate in a trial without coercion
  b) Confidentiality of their identity and health information
  c) Compensation for trial-related injury and for the time, effort, and expenses for their involvement in the study
  d) Medical care for study-related injury or intercurrent illness(es)
  e) The ability to withdraw from the study at any time

Rights may be outlined in the consent form and/or in a separate document. In addition to GCP rights, sometimes rights are specifically stipulated by the institution or regional regulatory authority(ies).

- The potential volunteer should ensure that they receive a copy of the consent form that has been approved by an IRB/IEC to take with them to review before they sign the consent form. The consent form and any other subject information documents will be in a language that the potential volunteer can understand. They may review the consent documents with their family and friends and ask as many questions as they need to from the research staff at the clinic site, the IRB/IEC, or other sources to help them understand the information contained in the consent form. The subject should thoroughly understand the following, among other required elements of consent (Chapter 19 Informed Consent and Other Human Subject Protection):
  - That the trial is investigational and no claims of safety or efficacy can be made about the investigational product unless already proven and/or approved by the appropriate regulatory authority(ies)
  - Who is sponsoring the trial and who is the investigator and their contact information
  - The procedures involved in participating in the trial
  - What are the risks (side effects of all study procedures and study treatments, investigational or approved) and benefits for taking part in the trial
  - What alternatives they have to participating in the trial
  - Whom to contact in case of questions or concerns regarding study procedures, health, or rights issues
  - What happens if they experience adverse events or other harm from being in the trial
  - If, when, and how much they will be compensated for being in the trial
  - They cannot be coerced to volunteer for the trial and that their participation is completely VOLUNTARY and they may withdraw at any time

10.2.2.1.2 Volunteering to Participate in the Trial

The investigator or a qualified designee will administer consent to the subject in a language they can understand and, if necessary, with a witness (Chapter 19 Informed Consent and Other Human Subject Protection). The potential volunteer will have ample time for their questions to be answered before they sign consent for the trial.

10.2.2.1.3 Participating in the Trial

To ensure continued protection of their rights, safety, and well-being, subjects will ensure:

- They are not asked to sign any revised consent form that has not been approved by an IRB/IEC
- They are not asked to undergo any procedure for which they have not consented

- Their study records remain available only to those who are approved via the consent to see their records
- Their biological samples and diagnostic tests (e.g., imaging scans) are used only for the purposes of the study as they consented
- Their biological samples are properly labeled with their allowed identification information
- They are respectfully treated by research staff and not any differently from if they were clinic patients and not in a research study
- They truthfully provide medical and medication history as requested for the trial at screening
- Qualified personnel perform trial procedures as described in the consent form and record the findings in study records
- They are administered the investigational product by qualified personnel and as described in the consent form
- They are fully trained on how to self-administer study treatment(s) and the requirements for storage and handling of the study treatment(s)
- For self-administered study treatments, they use the study treatments only as directed and do not share or hoard study treatments
- They store, destroy, and ensure security (safeguard from pets or children or others not authorized to receive or handle the study treatments) according to the trial instructions
- They record (e.g., in a diary) and report adverse events as instructed, noting that for an event they will be asked for certain information about the event; e.g., medications or actions they took as a result of the event, when the event started and ended or the final outcome, and the severity of the event
- They follow requirements for forbidden concomitant foods, drinks, medications, procedures
- They receive a timely referral or timely and adequate medical care by a qualified healthcare professional for adverse events that occur as a result of their participation in the trial
- They receive trial compensation as described in the consent form
- Their questions are satisfactorily answered by qualified trial staff
- They are provided any new information about the study or alternatives for participating in the study
- Continue to undergo safety assessments as requested after discontinuation of study treatment(s)
- Continue to submit trial information as requested after discontinuation from the study
- They communicate as requested with trial staff and ask questions and express concerns about any trial issues as they arise
- They have the freedom to withdraw from the study at any time. It is helpful if a trial subject communicates their intention to the investigator or other staff member to withdraw from the study (if they are relocating, for health reasons,

other reasons) so that appropriate arrangements may be made to ensure continuity of their participation in the trial (e.g., relocate to another trial site) or continuation of safety follow-up.

10.2.2.2 Voluntary Responsibilities for Data Integrity

A subject may help to ensure integrity of trial data by following the study and operational requirements:

- They truthfully provide medical and medication history and information for adverse events as requested
- They complete study procedures per the protocol schedule
- They are fully trained on how to use and complete self-administered questionnaires and study diaries
- They truthfully complete study questionnaires and diaries as directed
- They respect the "blind" for blinded treatment and do not attempt to decode their blinded treatment
- They respect their randomization assignment and do not switch or share study treatment(s) with other study participants
- It is helpful if a trial subject communicates their intention to the investigator or other staff member to withdraw from the study to ensure safety follow-up and/ or continued collection of other study data

10.2.2.3 Voluntary Responsibilities for Trial Compliance

A subject may help overall trial compliance by following the study and operational requirements as outlined above. Additionally, as they follow study protocol and operational procedures, they can cross-check that the research staff is following study protocol and operational procedures as they interact with each other.

10.2.3 Quality by Design Considerations to Facilitate Subject Compliance with Trial Requirements

A number of principles and operational considerations that promote GCP, quality, and compliance may facilitate subject compliance with the trial requirements. Study protocol design and trial operations considerations to foster subject compliance include:

- Considerations for formulating and packaging study treatments for the simplest and easiest self-administration by the subject or care-giver
- Considerations for required storage and handling conditions for subject self-administered study treatment(s) and that the subject can comply
- Considerations for selecting and scheduling study procedures that are realistic for the research subjects to undergo
- Considerations for the design of informed consent forms and other subject information documents

- Considerations for the design and training of subjects on self-administered questionnaires and diaries so that they are easy to understand and fill out based on the subject's cognitive abilities and dexterities (Chapter 20 Data Collection and Data Management)
- Considerations for forbidden concomitant foods, drinks, medications, and/or procedures that are practical and easy for subjects to comply
- Considerations for study blinding procedures that are easy for subjects and research staff to comply

See chapters on protocol and data collection design considerations and study operational considerations for more strategies and details (Chapter 18 The Clinical Trial Protocol and Amendments; Chapter 14 Trial Management; Start-up, On-Study, and Close-Out)

10.3 Summary

A trial subject is volunteering to be administered an investigational product in a clinical trial. Those involved in the conduct of the trial must protect the rights, safety, well-being, and confidentiality of the trial subject. Although there are no formal GCP or regulatory stipulations for research subjects to follow, the trial subject can also help to facilitate these protections, as well as the integrity of trial data and the overall compliance for the conduct of a clinical trial if the subject complies with study protocol and operational procedures. Trial subjects are therefore asked to comply with protocol and operational procedures but cannot be penalized for not following or coerced into following those procedures.

There a several voluntary responsibilities for a subject to help facilitate the protection of their rights, safety, well-being, data integrity, and general trial compliance. Additionally the trial protocol, data collection methods, and study operations may be designed in a manner that also facilitates the protection of their rights, safety, well-being, data integrity, and trial compliance.

Knowledge Check Questions

1) Who is a trial subject?
2) Why are the responsibilities of a trial subject voluntary?
3) What are some of the voluntary responsibilities for a subject to help facilitate the protection of their rights, safety, well-being?
4) What are some of the voluntary responsibilities for a subject to help facilitate data integrity?
5) What are some of the voluntary responsibilities for a subject to help facilitate general trial compliance?

6) What are some quality-by-design principles that apply to protocol design that help to facilitate subject voluntary compliance?

7) What are some quality-by-design principles that apply to data collection methods that help facilitate subject voluntary compliance?

8) What are some quality-by-design principles that apply to study treatment(s) design that help to facilitate subject voluntary compliance?

9) Overheard:

They ask a lot of questions just for curiosity and I don't know all that is in the consent form anyway.

Investigator delegate who instructed a college student who volunteered as a healthy research subject to swallow the study medication (capsules) per the appointed clock time just as the subject was about to ask a question about the study. Beds for study subjects for the phase 1 first-in human study were lined up side by side in the research facility. A clock above each bed was used to record the time of the study procedure. A nurse took the subject's vital signs, followed by another who drew blood, and the subinvestigator physician followed with the cup of water and study dose to research subject. Comment and discuss:

a) Were any of the subject's rights violated in this scenario?

b) Are there any issues with investigator delegation of responsibility at this site?

Reference

1 International Council for Harmonisation of Technical Requirements for Pharmaceuticals for Human Use (ICH), Integrated Addendum to ICH E6(R1):Guideline for Good Clinical Practice, E6(R2) (2016). Current Step 4 version dated 9 November 2016. https://www.ich.org/page/efficacy-guidelines

11

Regulatory Authority – Roles and Responsibilities

P. Michael Dubinsky

GCP Key Point
Regulatory Authorities are part of the ICH team that draft ICH Guidance documents. They work to ensure that the guidance reflects the current regulatory expectations. Understanding their role is important.

11.1 Introduction

Among the players in the clinical trial endeavor, the regulatory authority has a unique and highly visible role. Understanding the roles of the regulatory authority whether it is as a gatekeeper approving a trial application or an inspector following up on a complaint, the regulatory authority is in a unique position of control and influence. Placing the roles and responsibilities of the regulatory authority in perspective is therefore meaningful.

11.2 Objectives

In this chapter, you will be introduced to the primary roles and responsibilities of the Regulatory Authority (or Competent Authority) in terms of those functions which are highlighted in the GCP framework. The primary roles, i.e. functions, of the regulator are:

- Reviewing and making decisions on clinical trial applications.
- Oversight and inspection of the other players involved in the clinical trial endeavor to ensure conformance with GCP, investigational plans, and applicable regulations.

The Fundamentals of Clinical Research: A Universal Guide for Implementing Good Clinical Practice, First Edition. P. Michael Dubinsky and Karen A. Henry.
© 2022 John Wiley & Sons, Inc. Published 2022 by John Wiley & Sons, Inc.
Companion website: www.wiley.com/go/dubinsky/clinicalresearch

As noted in the Players and Interactions topic, the regulator performs these functions through interactions with sponsors, investigator sites, and IRBs/IECs.

In addition, you will gain insight into why the regulator has responsibility for these functions and is therefore accountable for implementing them.

11.3   Definition and Overview

When one reviews the ICH E6(R2), the number of references to the regulatory authorities (regulators) is limited and there is no specific section devoted to delineating roles or responsibilities for this important player in the clinical trial process. Regulatory authorities are of course mentioned several times in the body of the ICH E6(R2) guideline. Examples include Section 5.10 Notification/Submission to Regulatory Authority (ies) and Section 5.20.2 – Noncompliance – which speaks to the need for regulatory authorities to be notified if an investigator is terminated from participation in a trial. Therefore, one needs to look elsewhere to fully frame out and define the roles and responsibilities of the regulatory authority from a GCP standpoint.

The ICH E6(R2) guideline does, however, include a definition of a regulatory authority and it is useful to reflect on it because it sets the stage for how these entities fit, from a GCP standpoint into the clinical trial arena. The definition reads in part: *Regulatory Authorities: Bodies having the power to regulate.* In the ICH E6(R2) guidance, the expression "Regulatory Authorities" includes the authorities that review submitted clinical data and those that conduct inspections (see Section 1.29). These bodies are sometimes referred to as competent authorities. Note: The terms Regulatory Authority, regulator, and competent authority all are used in this topic write up interchangeably.

The roles of regulatory authorities in the oversight of clinical trials have been an evolutionary process often driven by tragic events. As noted in Chapter 1 History, the topic the birth defects caused by the product Thalidomide in many newborns was instrumental in moving legislative bodies worldwide to require substantial evidence of safety and effectiveness before allowing a new drug product on the market. Such events and the failure of industry or professional groups to self-regulate in an effective manner have all too often been the match that lit the fire of regulatory change.

The regulator's clinical trial responsibilities are assigned and founded in the laws, statutes, regulations, and directives that are put in place by a country or region's legislative bodies. Well-known examples of such laws are the USA's Federal Food Drug and Cosmetic Act and the EU's Clinical Trial Directive 2001/20/EC and the EU's Clinical Trial Regulation 536/2014 which supersede the Directive.

This chapter's discussion of the regulatory authority will focus on how they intersect with the other key players in performing their roles in the conduct and implementation of the clinical trial process as well as the underlying responsibilities for which they are held accountable.

Figure 11.1 depicts the Regulatory Authority's interaction with the other players in the clinical trial arena.

11.4 Trial Approval – Submission of Applications

The scheme for undertaking a clinical trial process begins with a sponsor who has developed and prepared, in the form of a clinical trial plan including a scientifically sound protocol, an approach to conducting human research to gather data demonstrating that an investigational product is safe and effective for a specified indication. In all countries and regions with established regulatory authorities, the sponsor must obtain the agreement of the regulatory authority before activating that clinical trial plan and protocol for pharmaceutical drug product clinical trials.

The agreement of the regulatory authority is usually given in the form of an approval or permission to proceed. In the United States, the U.S. Food and Drug Administration implements this permission pursuant to the regulations governing Investigational New Drug Applications (IND) – 21 CFR 312. In the EU, the competent authority for each of the 27 member State implements the permission as part of their Clinical Trial Authorization (CTA) process. Under the EU CTR 536, the trial authorization process has been harmonized to increase efficiency. In these and in most similar situations, the regulatory authority is the decision maker. Therefore, it is up to the applicant or sponsor to submit a complete and convincing submission requesting permission to undertake the clinical trial investigation and providing the information and data specified by the regulations governing the application process. The sponsor or applicant is the primary point of

Figure 11.1 Regulatory Authority's interaction with other players.

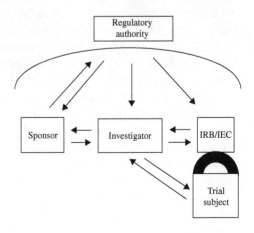

contact for the regulator in the application submission process since that entity, be it a firm, institution, or person, is held responsible for the study being conducted in conformance with regulatory requirements including GCP.

11.5 Communication, Reporting, and Oversight

Communication is a key role for the regulator as well as the sponsor in terms of a successful CTA application and the regulators generally accommodate, in a reasonable manner, a variety of lines of communication including telephone conversations, letters, facsimile, online message, or meetings. Obviously, such communication will be consistent with the available technology as long as appropriate confidentiality is maintained. It is useful to remember that there is one regulatory authority serving a large number of sponsors/applicants so at times a queue may form. The responsibility for effective lines of communication is a shared one with the sponsor. The regulator must maintain a full and complete administrative record of their interactions with a sponsor if they are to be accountable for making decisions about such matters as starting a clinical trial in humans with a new investigational drug product or other investigational article. The content of the administrative records documenting communication may well be reviewed and evaluated by others and by panels of experts who might be called upon to assist the regulator at some point in making a decision impacting the application.

The regulator will usually identify one central point of contact (POC) for the applicant/sponsor. That POC will be organizationally located in a group which is responsible for such applications or in a group whose responsibilities are grounded in the area of therapeutic treatment being researched. That POC person or office serves as the gateway, either electronically or physically, for communications with the regulator. Regulators almost always enforce the use of a central POC or the potential for miscommunications and misunderstandings is magnified. The POC is not, however, the only person with whom the applicant's staff will communicate. The regulator's professional experts in topics such as chemistry, statistical analysis, safety evaluations, etc., will interact as needed with the sponsor's counterparts but always working through or with the central POC. This approach ensures that the lines of communication remain centralized, complete, and up to date.

By ensuring the centralization of submissions and communications, the regulatory authority has in one place the body of information needed to conduct overall reviews and evaluations should it be necessary. Such evaluations might be needed if a safety issue arose or if a report, e.g. complaint of noncompliance with the protocol were received. ICH E6(R2) speaks to the regulatory authorities' role in receiving and evaluating such reports especially as it relates to safety information. Most regulators have rules specifying the timing of serious and unexpected safety and adverse drug reaction reports. Such reports may generate additional communications between the regulator and the sponsor/applicant. It is essential that the regulator obtain and review the full body of information concerning adverse reactions which are serious and unexpected so they can weigh, along with the sponsor/applicant, whether the risks associated with the trial have changed and if that change warrants enrollment being halted.

There is a continuous and viable line of communication about the conduct of a clinical trial for which the regulator shares responsibility. This is not to imply that communication is daily or weekly, although that might occur from time to time, but the communication must be timely for the topic or issue at hand.

The regulatory authorities have through regulation and policy a responsibility to ensure that appropriate periodic reports are received from sponsors/applicants about the status of the clinical trial endeavor. These reports are usually termed progress reports and the review and evaluation of them is a role that the regulator is expected to perform. Depending upon the content, or lack thereof the regulator may need to consider some follow-up action regarding the application. Progress reports must be adequate and complete since they represent a key component of the regulator's oversight role in clinical trials. Such reports are usually required on an annual basis unless they are specified at different times. If required reports are not received or are found to be inaccurate or incomplete, the regulator may take steps to terminate the study or penalize the sponsor. In most such situations, the regulator, through its POC, will attempt to resolve such matters through communications both informal and formal and documented in the regulator's file on the study.

Taking and documenting actions on an application throughout its lifecycle is expected of the regulator.

11.6 Inspections and Oversight

Most regulatory authorities will be performing inspections as part of their clinical trial oversight role. Some regulators have a defined responsibility for conducting inspections of clinical trial related, i.e. GCP activities during the time period that the study is underway and some do not.

Clinical trial activities can be inspected at any time; however, such inspections are usually not conducted on a routine or programmatic basis but generally are driven by events. One such event is the successful completion of the overall clinical study which results in the submission of a marketing application. Another is to follow-up on reports of noncompliance or complaints which are received either from the sponsor or some other source knowledgeable about the study. The nature and scope of such inspections are covered in Chapter 34 Regulatory Authority Inspections in some detail but suffice it to say that if inspections are scheduled and conducted, they will be rigorous and demanding.

Regulators, having the decision-making responsibility for applications, want to ensure they make valid, supportable, and accountable decisions. Inspections are a mechanism of oversight that regulators use to aid in ensuring that clinical trial activities being conducted in their jurisdiction are performed in compliance with the investigational plan, the regulations, and GCP. Inspections can have a number of outcomes but it is important to keep in perspective that unlike audits conducted by a sponsor's quality assurance staff, an inspection which documents significant noncompliance can result in legal/administrative penalties or sanctions being applied. The regulatory authorities have a responsibility to act on significant noncompliance in part to punish and in part to demonstrate that such behavior will not be tolerated.

Regulatory authority inspections of clinical trial activities are not mandated in all global regions or countries. For example, GCP inspections became a responsibility for EU member states when the EU Clinical Trial Directive 2001/20/EC became effective in 2004. In the United States, GCP inspections are authorized but not mandated by law or regulation. Whether mandated or not, inspections are a key role performed by regulators as part of their oversight activities. Inspections which are GCP in nature include inspections of trial sponsors, investigational sites, and institutional review boards. Inspections of the manufacturing of investigational articles may also be conducted but they would be categorized as GMP inspections. Inspections of animal and in-vitro studies supporting CTAs are inspected but are categorized as Good Laboratory Practice (GLP) and are not addressed in this text.

With regard to investigator sites, regulators depend in large measure upon sponsors to serve as the primary go-between with sites during the course of a study unless it becomes apparent that the sponsor is not exercising control over the site(s). If the application involves an investigator-sponsor, then the situation is different; however, most of the discussion points above would apply since that person is also the sponsor. The one area of difference would be the matter of inspections. Regulators recognize that the investigator sites are where all of the key steps associated with the trial occur. Drug is administered, adverse reactions are recorded and reported, records are made and maintained, and subjects are given informed consent. Therefore, it is the inspections of sites where regulators spend the bulk of their available inspectional time when it comes to GCP compliance. Regulators will want to interact directly with the principal investigator at a site if they are aware of, or document noncompliances at the site. Clinical investigators are viewed as having a direct responsibility to ensure conformance with the protocol, the applicable regulations, and GCP at their site. Admittedly, they work through the sponsor on critical items such as reporting serious unexpected adverse reactions; however, the regulators usually have some administrative or legal mechanism available to bring to bear against noncompliant investigators. Administrative provisions granting regulators the ability to put clinical holds in place, disqualify clinical investigators, terminate sites, or limit enrollment are tools that regulators have available if serious noncompliance is documented during inspections.

11.7 Summary

In this topic area, we have outlined the roles and responsibilities of the regulatory authority within the context of the GCP Guidelines. It is meaningful to keep in perspective that while the regulatory authority is a player in the clinical trial process, as defined in GCP and has roles and responsibilities, it (the regulator) is not in large measure the focus of the GCP requirements.

The responsibilities of the regulatory authority are founded in law, regulations, and directives and are carried out by governmental agencies or their designees. It is the role of the regulatory authority to act as a gatekeeper, overseer, and evaluator using the legally mandated requirements including GCP.

The regulatory authority has a responsibility to be accountable for its actions through documentation, transparency, and clear communications with sponsors, investigators when appropriate, and IRBs/IECs.

Knowledge Check Questions

1) A primary role/responsibility of the regulatory authority is to review clinical trial applications and then advise the independent ethics Committee whether the trial can begin. True _____ or False____?

2) Regulatory Authorities are called upon to inspect the ICH as well as sponsors and clinical trial sites. True_____ or False_____?

3) Unlike the quality assurance audits conducted by clinical trial sponsors, the inspections conducted by regulators can result in enforcement action if: 1) the inspection uncovers significant noncompliance_____; 2) The sponsor or site refuses to allow inspection_____; or 3) The sponsor or site has made significant changes to the study plan without notifying the regulator___; 4) all three situations apply.

4) Communication between the sponsor and the regulator is essential. The regulator will therefore provide the sponsor with several – up to five – points of contact (POCs) within their organization who can be contacted about important changes to the clinical trial plan. Correct? If not how many are considered acceptable?

5) You have recently been hired by a large pharmaceutical drug manufacturer to oversee several of their clinical trial projects. Upon reviewing your assigned projects, you determine that the annual reports to regulators are overdue for every one of the trials. What steps should you be taking on an immediate basis? Prepare a brief plan to serve as an agenda for your meeting with your supervisor and/or the regulatory authority.

Part IV

Individual Clinical Trial

12

Individual Clinical Trial Overview

Karen A. Henry

GCP Key Point

Knowledge and clear understanding of the regulatory requirements for the conduct of a trial and management of risks and resources assure compliance with the protocol, GCP, and applicable regulatory requirements.

12.1 Introduction

The individual clinical study is only one of many studies that will be conducted as part of the clinical development plan (Chapter 3 GCP in Context; Plate 1 Drug Development Methodology). The results of the individual clinical trial, therefore, will be expected to provide further information about the product's safety and efficacy for its target indication in its target population (Chapter 2 Regulatory Environment).

The components and activities are similar from one study to the next, regardless of its phase in the development plan, because all trials must be conducted according to GCP and applicable regulatory requirements, which are generally similar across regulatory agencies (Chapter 2 Regulatory Environment; Plate 2 Significant Dates in GCP History). These components and activities consist of:

1) Players' roles and responsibilities:
   GCP guidelines address principles for trial design, the protection of subject rights, safety, and well-being, maintaining data integrity, trial oversight and compliance, and reporting of trial conduct. Each trial will, therefore, consist of a specific set of players (Plate 3 Players Roles and Responsibilities: IRB/EC, Investigator, Sponsor/ CRO Regulatory Agency) who have prescribed responsibilities (Chapter 7 Players

The Fundamentals of Clinical Research: A Universal Guide for Implementing Good Clinical Practice, First Edition. P. Michael Dubinsky and Karen A. Henry.
© 2022 John Wiley & Sons, Inc. Published 2022 by John Wiley & Sons, Inc.
Companion website: www.wiley.com/go/dubinsky/clinicalresearch

Roles and Responsibilities Overview; Plate 4 Individual Clinical Trial – Overview of Investigator and Sponsor Responsibilities).

2) Key trial documents

Each trial will generally consist of a standard set of key trial documents that are interdependent (Plate 8 Data Framework/Information Flow Among Key Trial Documents):

- Investigator's brochure (IB): a description of what is known to date of the safety and efficacy of the investigational product (IP) (Plate 9 Investigator's Brochure).
- Clinical trial protocol: a document that describes the "recipe" for conducting the trial (Plate 10 Clinical Trial Protocol).
- Informed consent form: a form which provides the potential research subject with a description of the procedures that they will undergo, the benefits and risks of being the study, and a description of their rights as research subjects (Plate 11 Informed Consent Form).
- Statistical analysis plan (SAP): a description of the methods to analyze the study data (Plate 12 Statistical Analysis Plan).
- Case report form: a form used by the investigator to report the collected study data to the sponsor (Plate 13 Case Report Form).
- Clinical study report: the final report describing the actual trial conduct and the trial results (Plate 14 Clinical Study Report).
- Standard operating procedures or other procedural guidelines: written procedures describing how trial activities, including quality control and quality assurance procedures, and risk management will be performed.

These documents are interdependent and therefore have a domino effect for consequences on each other if any document is deficient or is changed; for example:

1) The clinical, nonclinical, and properties information about the IP in the IB will inform:

   a) The sponsor on, e.g. the risks associated with the use of the IP, the expectedness of adverse events associated with the use of the IP to guide safety management and reporting requirements, and how to determine the objectives and design of the protocol; i.e. the available clinical and nonclinical safety information in the IB must support the proposed trial design, including the IP dosing and dosing regimen to be used in the trial.

   b) The investigators of, e.g. the risks associated with the use of the IP, how to handle and administer the IP, expectedness of adverse events associated with the use of the IP to guide safety management and reporting requirements, and the risks that must be included in the subject informed consent form.

   c) The IRBs/ECs and regulatory authorities of the known safety and efficacy profile of the IP to assess the benefits versus risks for the implementation of the proposed protocol objectives and design.

2) The objectives described in the protocol will determine the endpoints, which, in turn, determine the assessments that will be performed to obtain the data for analysis. This information will be used to develop:
   a) The case report form
   b) The informed consent form
   c) The SAP
3) The SAP will describe the format and definitions for the variables that will be analyzed, the methods for analyzing the data, and provide a list of statistical reports that will present the data for the clinical study report.
4) The design of the case report form will be based on the format and definitions for the variables as described in the SAP.
5) The clinical database will be designed based on the case report form.
6) The clinical study report will use the statistical reports to present the final results of the study.
7) Any deviations from the planned design or analysis of the study or from the planned study procedures will be documented and described in the clinical study report.
   Consideration should be given to the domino effect on criteria for informing study safety and efficacy decisions, on planned study procedures, and on planned study analyses when there is a deviation or change from the contents of any of the key study documents.

Although the documents that form the foundation for the various trials may be created by different parties (individuals or contract research organizations [CROs]) during the course of the development cycle of the IP, individuals responsible for designing and executing an individual trial within the development plan should consider that the results of the "registration" studies (Chapter 2 Regulatory Environment) will eventually be integrated for analysis and reporting in the application for marketing authorization (Chapter 3 GCP in Context). It is therefore prudent that, as much as possible, basic elements of study design and conduct (such as, clinical supplies formulations and dosing schemas, endpoints that are common to multiple studies, and, as applicable, criteria for subject eligibility, analysis populations, and protocol deviations) remain consistent across all studies to facilitate the merging of the data for integrated analysis.

3) Key trial activities
   Each trial will require a standard set of activities, such as the selection of qualified investigators/institution; resourcing and trial staff training; trial and investigator initiation; consenting and enrollment of research subjects; shipment, use, and accountability of the IP; trial monitoring; safety monitoring and reporting; and final trial closeout and reporting.
   The responsibilities for sponsors and investigators as prescribed by GCP are carried out via these similar components and activities, which are discussed in

other chapters of this book (Plate 4 Individual Clinical Trial – Overview of Investigator and Sponsor Responsibilities). The sponsor and investigator have responsibility for oversight of their respective activities.

12.2   Objectives

The objectives of this chapter are to describe the key trial responsibilities and describe:

1) Trial Management
   a) Defining trial initiation
   b) Describing trial activities for
      i) Pre-study
      ii) On-study
      iii) End-study
2) Risk and Quality Management
3) Resourcing and Outsourcing
4) Investigational Product
   a) Investigator's Brochure
   b) Clinical Supplies
5) Clinical Trial Protocol and Amendments
6) IC and ICF, Other Subject Information, and Recruitment Documents
7) IRB/EC and Regulatory Authority Communication
8) Data Collection and Data Management
9) Safety, Pharmacokinetics, and Pharmacodynamics Laboratory Testing
10) Safety Monitoring and Reporting
11) Trial Monitoring
    a) Investigator and Site Selection
    b) Trial Initiation
    c) Interim Monitoring
    d) Investigator/Institution Study Close-out
12) Statistics and Data Analysis
13) Clinical Study Report
14) Essential Documents
15) Study Closeout
16) Consequences of Inadequate Trial Conduct

12.2.1   Trial Management

Clinical trial management staff in the respective sponsor and investigator domains will be responsible for coordinating and managing trial activities and for the documentation of all components of a clinical trial to ensure subject safety, data integrity, and compliance with the protocol, GCP, SOPs, and applicable regulatory requirements (Plate 4 Individual Clinical Trial; Plate 15 Monitoring Overview Checklist). These components include:

- Thorough oversight of trial personnel and activities with prospective identified risks and procedures to manage and mitigate risks associated with critical trial outcomes in tangent with quality assurance and quality control systems (Chapter 14 Trial Management; Start-up, On-Study, and Close-Out).
- An IB that is generated by the sponsor and provided to the investigator and that is current with all available information about the IP for the indication being studied in the protocol (Chapter 16 The Investigator's Brochure).
- A clear, detailed, and well-designed study protocol or amendments that are generated by the sponsor and provided to the investigator (Chapter 18 The Clinical Trial Protocol and Amendments).
- Protection of the rights, safety, and well-being of clinical research subjects, including duly administered and comprehensive informed consent for research participants at the clinical trial site and maintenance of confidentiality of subject's identity by all parties involved in trial conduct (Chapter 19 Informed Consent and Other Human Subject Protection).
- Qualified facilities and trained and qualified personnel with clear delegation of responsibilities to qualified personnel, and written agreements that describe compliance requirements and include protection of sponsor propriety information (Chapter 15 Trial Resourcing and Outsourcing).
- Procedures to record source study data and maintain case histories according to good documentation practices, CRFs to collect the data needed for analysis of protocol endpoints, and data collection and management systems that ensure validity and reliability of data (Chapter 20 Data Collection and Data Management).
- IP manufactured per Good Manufacturing Practices, and stored, handled, and accounted for from manufacturing by the sponsor to administration to trial subjects at the clinical investigator site to destruction by the clinical investigator site or the sponsor (Chapter 17 The Investigational Product (Clinical Supplies)).
- Laboratory testing of specimens collected from subjects per established health standards and management by the investigator and sponsor to ensure confidentiality of subject identification, and accountability, and tracking of all specimens (Chapter 22 Monitoring Overview).
- Collection, timely assessment, reporting, tracking, and reconciliation of safety events by the investigator and the sponsor (Chapter 21 Safety Monitoring and Reporting).
- Complete and continuous reporting to a qualified IRB/EC and to the regulatory authority(ies) by the investigator and sponsor, respectively (Chapter 9 Investigator and Sponsor Roles and Responsibilities).

- Sponsor interactive selection (Chapter 23 Investigator/Institution Selection), training and initiation (Chapter 24 Investigator/Institution Initiation), monitoring (Chapter 25 Investigator/Institution Interim Monitoring), and close-out (Chapter 26 Investigator/Institution Close-out) of investigator staff and activities to ensure adequacy of resources and implement timely corrective and preventive actions to address any protocol deviations or noncompliance.
- Final review, reconciliation, and organization, and archiving of final study records (essential documents) at clinical investigator sites and for the study so that the records are retrievable and readable for the minimum required retention period (Chapter 29 Essential documents).
- Appropriate statistical and data analyses per *a priori* specifications by the sponsor (Chapter 27 Study Design and Data Analysis).
- Final study status reports to IRB/ECs by the investigator (Chapter 9 Investigator and Sponsor Roles and Responsibilities) and a clinical study report generated by the sponsor that accurately and completely reflects the conduct and results of the trial (Chapter 28 The Clinical Study Report).
- Maintenance in the investigator and sponsor domains of accurate and complete study records (essential documents) that individually and collectively permit evaluation of the conduct of the study and quality of the data produced (Chapter 29 Essential Documents).
- Final study closeout of all trial activities to ensure documentation and retention of all evidence of trial conduct (Chapter 14 Trial Management; Start-up, On-Study, and Close-Out).

Trial management will coordinate and monitor all of the above in accordance with desired timelines and budget constraints. Trial management will also prepare for and manage all study activities from the decision to execute a trial through archiving the records that reflect study conduct (Plate 4 Individual clinical trial). Figure 12.1 displays the milestones for a clinical trial.

12.2.1.1 Defining Trial Initiation and Subject Enrollment
Generally, trial start-up is the process between the decision to execute a trial and the milestone of "trial initiation." ICH E6(R2) makes several references to activities and

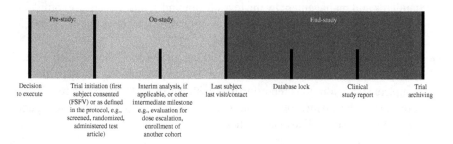

Figure 12.1 Milestones for a clinical trial.

essential documents that are prerequisites to "trial initiation," and also refers to "enrollment" of research subjects, but these concepts are not specifically defined in the Glossary and have mixed interpretations, thereby resulting in inconsistent applications in practice, which can impact GCP compliance and trial results.

Several trial initiation and enrollment milestones are involved in the trial start-up phase of a clinical trial. Let us look closely at how each of these milestones may impact GCP and trial results.

- *Submission of the final protocol to the regulatory authority(ies) and ethics committees*: the trial is essentially a proposal at this time and has not been approved for implementation, so there is no trial.
- *No objections or approval from the regulatory authority(ies):* While no objections or approval from the regulatory authority(ies) is required prior to the implementation of a trial, the trial may not be implemented until an ethics committee (EC) has approved it or given its favorable opinion.
- *Ethics committee approval:* EC approval of the trial protocol and the subject-informed consent information is required before any trial procedures may be executed. Once ethics approval is obtained, subject recruitment may commence. However, it does occur that a trial site can have ethics approval and no trial subjects are recruited because of any of the many reasons discussed in the Chapter 19 (Chapter 19 Informed Consent and Other Human Subject Protection). Therefore, in this situation there is no impact on humans or trial data.
- *The first recruitment activity for the first potential participant:* Protection of the rights, integrity, and confidentiality of a human subject are triggered upon the first contact with the potential trial participant; however, there is no impact on trial data.
- *Informed consent of the first trial participant:* Once a volunteer has agreed to participate in the trial and has signed the consent documents, this signals that the subject may undergo trial procedures. However, it does happen that a subject may "withdraw consent" or choose not to continue in the trial and so no trial protocol procedures have been carried out. While there is impact on humans at this stage, there is no impact on trial data.
- *Screening of the first trial participant:* A volunteer must sign consent before undergoing any trial protocol procedure, including "screening procedures." Most trials have screening procedures, the results of which determine if the subject is eligible to continue in the trial and receive the test article. If a subject undergoes screening procedures, then we are impacting their rights, safety, and well-being, and we have also collected data that tell us that something about the eligibility criteria in the protocol. However, not every participant meets the protocol eligibility criteria and it does happen that a consented participant may never receive the test article. At the same time, we need to consider that a subject would not be undergoing the screening procedures if they were not in the trial, so strictly speaking, the trial, per protocol, has commenced.

- *Randomization of the first trial participant:* If the trial design is such that subjects will be "randomized" to one of the different arms/groups/cohorts of a trial, then the randomization assignment usually occurs after it is determined that the subject is eligible to participate in the trial. However, it does happen that the randomization assignment takes place operationally but the subject withdraws consent prior to receiving the test article or for some other reason does not receive the test article. Technically, the trial has commenced because protocol procedures have been carried out, but the test article has not been administered, which is the primary purpose of the trial.

- *Administration of the test article to the first trial participant:* The last milestone in the trial start-up process to consider is the administration of the test article to the research participant. It is clear that upon administration of the test article, we are impacting all of the GCP and trial objectives. However, depending on the type of test article, its administration may involve multiple steps, such as anesthesia and incision for surgical implantation of a test device or drug in the body or the subject may receive a standard-of-care treatment prior to receiving the test article. In such cases, we note that it is controversial if the preparatory procedures or pretreatments are considered one and the same as administration of the test article. If the preparatory procedures or pretreatments are completed but the test article itself it not administered for any reason, it is clear that in such cases the protection of the human subject participant is impacted and we have started to collect trial data; however, it is not clear if we have actually impacted the trial objectives.

Based on the descriptions provided above, let us now look more closely at which milestones are most appropriate to meet trial objectives. Let us first interpret the meaning of "trial initiation." ICH E6(R2) requires that certain documentation and systems are in place before the "clinical phase" of the trial commences (ICH E6(R2) 8.2). What does the "clinical phase" of the trial mean? In practice, this means any clinical procedure that is effected by the human subject. Since it is very common that the first clinical procedure will be performed on the same day as when signed informed consent is obtained from the research subject to participate in the trial, in this book we therefore assign the milestone of "trial initiation" to when:
The first research subject has provided signed consent to participate in the trial.

Summarily, all documentation and systems that are prerequisites to trial initiation must be in place prior to the administration of the first consent for the trial.

The next interpretation to discuss is that of "enrollment." It is important that all involved in the planning, tracking, review, approval, analysis, and reporting of a clinical trial are synchronized regarding the definition of "enrollment" for a clinical trial subject because subject enrollment numbers are integral to the integrity of the study analyses and results. In practice, "enrollment" of a subject is variably employed, for example, a subject is considered "enrolled" in the trial at the time of:

- Signed informed consent of the trial subject.
- The start of the first screening procedure for the trial subject.
- The completion of all screening procedures for the trial subject.
- Completed randomization, if applicable, of the trial subject.
- Administration of the test article to the trial subject.

However, the prevailing acceptable definition for subject "enrollment" is:
The subject completed all screening procedures and meets all study eligibility criteria so that they can be enrolled in the trial; i.e. randomized and/or receive first study treatment, depending on the study design and planned analyses.

As we can see, the various interpretations of "trial initiation" or "enrollment" may impact GCP compliance and trial results, so it is crucial that these milestones for the trial are clearly defined in the study operations procedures and all persons involved in the conduct of trial are trained on and understands exactly what they mean.

12.2.1.2 Trial Activities

The three major phases of the life cycle of a clinical trial are as follows:

1) Pre-study
2) On-study
3) End-study

We break down the GCP responsibilities of the sponsor and investigator and group the resulting activities into these three phases.

12.2.1.2.1 Pre-Study

In practice, pre-study (also referred to as clinical trial start-up) refers to the period from the decision to execute the trial to initiation of the first investigator/institution for the trial. During this period, the sponsor will

1) Prepare the trial protocol, bearing in mind risk and quality issues while designing the trial.
2) Identify qualified sponsor personnel to be responsible for trial conduct.
3) Set up the infrastructure for the trial, based on decisions regarding resources and outsourcing, and assess risks and plan for risk mitigation.
4) Evaluate and qualify CROs, if any are to be used for the trial.
5) Select central laboratories and set up laboratory procedures.
6) Train sponsor trial conduct personnel.
7) Determine standard operating procedures that will be used for the trial.
8) Create other written procedures to be used for the trial.
9) Prepare other key study documents needed for the trial (e.g. IB, ICF).

10) Submit the application for the trial to regulatory authority(ies) and obtain approval/no objection.
11) Procure the IP.
12) Design the CRF and set up data collection and management processes and databases.
13) Select investigators/institutions.
14) Provide investigators/institutions with all trial information and supplies.
15) Execute regulatory and business agreements with investigator/institutions and CROs.
16) Initiate investigator/institutions.

During this period, the investigator will:

1) Identify qualified institution personnel to be responsible for trial conduct.
2) Set up the infrastructure for the trial, based on decisions regarding resources and outsourcing.
3) Evaluate and qualify subcontractors, if any are to be used for the trial.
4) Select laboratories and set up laboratory procedures.
5) Submit the trial application to the IRB/EC and obtain approval/favorable opinion.
6) Train investigator trial conduct personnel.
7) Determine standard operating procedures that will be used for the trial.
8) Create other written procedures to be used for the trial.
9) Execute regulatory and business agreements.
10) Other activities that are relevant to the specific trial and that are needed for trial implementation.

12.2.1.2.2 On-Study

In practice, on-study refers to the period from the consent of the first study subject across all sites until the investigator's collection of data for the last subject's last visit or contact across all sites in the study. During this period, the sponsor will

1) Monitor the progress of the trial, and mitigate risks.
2) Oversee CROs, if any are used for the trial.
3) Train new or retrain trial personnel.
4) Amend the protocol and update other key study documents as needed.
5) Ensure that investigators/institutions have updated trial information.
6) Release and ship clinical and other trial supplies to the investigators/institutions.
7) Communicate clinical trial status updates to the regulatory authority(ies).
8) Communicate safety information to investigators and regulatory authority(ies).
9) Collect and review trial data via CRFs.
10) Submit CRF queries to the investigator and review and collect query resolutions.
11) Conduct interim study analyses, if applicable.
12) Update written procedures for the trial as needed.
13) Update regulatory and business agreements as needed.

During this period, the investigator will:

1) Oversee all personnel who are delegated trial-related duties.
2) Oversee subcontractors, if any are used for the trial.
3) Train new or retrain trial personnel.
4) Recruit, consent, screen, and enroll eligible subjects into the trial.
5) Administer an IP to eligible subjects and account for the IP.
6) Collect and track subjects' biological samples.
7) Provide medical care to research subjects as needed.
8) Complete CRFs and address CRF queries and submit them to the sponsor.
9) Report safety information to the sponsor.
10) Communicate clinical trial status updates to the IRB/EC and the sponsor.
11) Update written procedures for the trial as needed.
12) Update regulatory and business agreements as needed.
13) Other activities that are relevant to the specific trial and that are needed during the trial.

12.2.1.2.3   End-Study

In practice, end-study refers to the period from the sponsor's collection of data for the last subject's last visit or contact in the study until all study documentation are archived. During this period, the sponsor will

1) Complete processing CRF queries and collection of query resolutions from the investigator.
2) Reconcile safety reporting databases.
3) Lock the database after all data queries are resolved.
4) Unblind a blinded study, if applicable, analyze the study data, and prepare the clinical study report.
5) Track stored subjects' biological samples.
6) Retrieve or approve for destruction any remaining clinical and other trial supplies from trial sites.
7) Close out clinical sites.
8) Close out CROs, if any are used for the trial.
9) Communicate final clinical trial status to the regulatory authority(ies).
10) Make final payments to investigators/institutions and CROs.
11) Host regulatory inspections.
12) Archive trial files of essential documents.

During this period, the investigator will:

1) Complete the processing of CRF data queries.
2) Close out subcontractors, if any are used for the trial.
3) Track and ship subjects' biological samples to be retained by the sponsor.
4) Return to the sponsor or destroy any remaining clinical and other trial supplies.

5) Communicate final clinical trial status to the IRB/EC.
6) Host final investigator/institution close-out monitoring by the sponsor, sponsor audits, and regulatory inspections.
7) Archive trial files of essential documents.
8) Other activities that are relevant to the specific trial and that are needed to close out the trial.

12.2.2 Risk and Quality Management

Obtaining reliable trial data while ensuring the protection of human subjects volunteering to be administered an IP is the first concern for all persons involved in the conduct of a clinical trial. Implementation of systems with this focus and to manage quality throughout all stages of the trial process is therefore the responsibility of all players. The quality management system should use a risk-based approach where applicable.

The relationship among the various players and the quality control and quality assurance activities are presented in Plate 5 Quality Assurance and Quality Control and greater details regarding risk and quality control processes are discussed in Chapter 13 Risk Assessment and Quality Management. Both the sponsor and the investigator have responsibilities for oversight of trial conduct. Quality assurance and quality control processes will be described in written standard operating procedures that all personnel involved in trial conduct will follow. These procedures will include requirements for sponsor trial staff qualifications and training as a quality assurance activity and for investigator monitoring as a quality control activity. Furthermore, quality assurance will include audits of both the sponsor and investigator, and trial oversight of risk and quality management as a quality control measure.

Quality management by the sponsor includes the design of efficient clinical trial protocols and tools and procedures for data collection and processing, as well as the collection of information that is essential to decision-making. The methods used to assure and control the quality of the trial should be proportionate to the risks inherent in the trial and the importance of the information collected. The sponsor should ensure that all aspects of the trial are operationally feasible and should avoid unnecessary complexity, procedures, and data collection. Protocols, case report forms, and other operational documents should be clear, concise, and consistent. The sponsor is also responsible for implementing and maintaining quality assurance and quality control systems with written SOPs to ensure that trials are conducted and data are generated, documented (recorded), and reported in compliance with the protocol, GCP, and the applicable regulatory requirement(s) (ICH E6(R2) 5.0 and 5.1).

Quality management by the investigator is reflected in the investigator's responsibility to implement procedures to ensure the integrity of the trial-related duties and functions performed and any data generated by any individuals or party to whom the investigator delegates trial-related duties and functions (ICH E6(R2) 4.2.5 and 4.2.6).

12.2.3 Resourcing and Outsourcing

All parties involved in trial start-up and execution must ensure that they have qualified and sufficient resources. Resources (personnel, facilities, equipment, and time) may be drawn from within the organization or outsourced.

All resources must be reviewed for adequacy before and during the trial to ensure their pre- and continued qualification for the duration of the trial. Study personnel will be qualified by experience and formal training (including certifications and licensing as applicable) on the therapeutic area, GCP, regulatory requirements, SOPs, and the clinical trial protocol, IB, and other protocol and institutional procedures that support the conduct of the trial. All facilities and equipment used for the trial will have to be reviewed for adequacy and compliance with study requirements.

When a sponsor outsources trial-related activities that are regulated, the contractor who will be taking over those regulated activities is referred to as a Contract Research Organization (CRO). The CRO is a person or an organization (commercial, academic, or other) contracted by the sponsor to perform one or more of a sponsor's trial-related duties and functions (ICH E6(R2) 1.20). The sponsor will have written agreements describing the specific trial-related duties and functions with each CRO, and the sponsor is responsible for any trial-related duties and functions that are not contained in a written agreement with a CRO. While CROs assume the regulatory responsibility of the contracted trial-related activities and functions and are expected to comply with the relevant protocol, GCP, and regulatory requirements, the sponsor continues to have responsibility for oversight of the CRO to ensure safety of the research subject, integrity of trial data, and compliance with all applicable requirements.

In contrast to the sponsor, although the investigator may delegate trial-related activities and functions, the investigator maintains all regulatory responsibility for all trial-related functions and activities that are stipulated as responsibilities of the investigator by the protocol, GCP, and regulations. The investigator, therefore, must ensure that all individuals and facilities are trained and qualified to perform delegated activities that are stipulated as investigator responsibilities and must oversee all those personnel and activities of the trial at their clinical site and that are subcontracted by the clinical site. And similarly to the CRO, the sponsor continues to have responsibility for oversight of the investigator's activities and functions to ensure safety of the research subject, integrity of trial data, and compliance with all applicable requirements.

See Chapter 15 Trial Resourcing and Outsourcing for details.

12.2.4 Investigational Product

There are two primary entities that pertain to the IP in a clinical trial: the product itself and any other clinical supplies that are used in conjunction with the product, and the IB.

12.2.4.1 Investigator's Brochure

The IB is a document that contains a description of what is known to date of the product characteristics, and the safety and efficacy of the IP (Plate 9 Investigator's Brochure). This document is the precursor to the approved label for a medicinal product so it contains similar information while the product is used as an investigational article.

12.2.4.2 Clinical Supplies

The sponsor will provide the investigator with the IP and other clinical trial supplies. A product that is being used in a way that has not been approved by regulatory authorities is, by definition, investigational. Investigational means that the safety profile has not been evaluated and approved by a regulatory authority, and more likely, that we do not yet know its full safety (and efficacy) profiles for its intended use. The IP, therefore, must be carefully controlled and monitored with respect to its exposure to humans, other animals, and the environment.

The sponsor will ensure manufacturing, packaging, labeling, and management of the IP in accordance with Good Manufacturing Practices and track the shipment of all investigational supplies to and from clinical investigator sites in accordance with regulatory requirements. The investigator is responsible for the administration of the IP to research participants in accordance with the protocol. They must also ensure appropriate handling and storage and maintain accountability of all supplies received from the sponsor, administered to research subjects, used and unused, and disposed of or returned to the sponsor (Chapter 17 The Investigational Product (Clinical Supplies)). At the end of the trial, the sponsor will account for all manufactured, shipped, returned, and destroyed IP.

In addition to the instructions for IP dosing, administration, handling, and storage, the investigator will receive the IB, which contains all known clinical and nonclinical information about the IP. The IB is a key trial document (Plate 8 Data Framework/Information Flow Among Key Trial Documents) that includes information to help the investigator to make decisions about subject eligibility and medical care and reporting of adverse events (Chapter 16 The Investigator's Brochure; Plate 9 Investigator's Brochure Contents).

The IP may be used only for the sole purpose of the trial.

12.2.5 Clinical Trial Protocol and Amendments

The Clinical Trial Protocol is an essential trial document (Plate 10 Data Framework/ Information Flow Among Key Trial Documents) that clearly describes the objectives, design, methodology, statistical considerations, and organization of a trial and is the basis for all trial procedures and activities (Chapter 18 The Clinical Trial Protocol and Amendments; Plate 10 Protocol Contents). The protocol design will be scientifically sound and supported by currently available nonclinical and clinical information on the IP and it will be initiated only if the foreseeable risks and inconveniences do not outweigh the anticipated benefit for the individual trial subject and society (ICH E6(R2) 2.0).

The sponsor of the clinical trial is responsible for selecting qualified investigators who will have access to the appropriate clinical research participants who make up the protocol's study population. The investigator must also have adequate qualified staff, facilities, equipment, and time to conduct the trial. The sponsor will provide a copy of the protocol to the investigator and the investigator, in turn, will confirm agreement to comply with the protocol for trial conduct (ICH E6(R2) 5.6). The protocol must have the favorable opinion or approval of an IRB/EC and submitted to a regulatory authority as required before execution of any of its procedures. The trial should be conducted in compliance with the approved protocol and will be continued only if the anticipated benefits continue to justify the risks (ICH E6(R2) 2.0).

12.2.6 Human Subject Protection

Human subject protection refers to the protection of the rights, safety, and well-being of a research subject (Chapter 19 Informed Consent and Other Human Subject Protection). The investigator will have access to the study population needed for the trial. These research subjects will be recruited as volunteers based on their potential for meeting eligibility requirements for the protocol. All study information (including advertising materials, informed consent materials, and other study information) must have favorable opinion or approval of an IRB/IEC before it is given to a research subject. The informed consent form is a key study document (Plate 8 Data Framework/Information Flow Among Key Trial Documents; Plate 11 Informed Consent Contents).

After being given all known study information in a language that they understand, and after having had opportunity to consider the trial and have all their questions answered, potential subjects will voluntarily sign consent to participate prior to undergoing any trial procedures, including so-called screening procedures to determine their eligibility to be administered the IP. During the trial, research subjects will continue to be provided with any information known about the IP (including alternative treatments or therapies that become available) that may influence their willingness to continue participating in the trial (ICH E6(2) 4.8). Additionally, although not a GCP or regulatory requirement, study subjects may be supplied information about the IP that may have long-term potential harm or benefit after they discontinue trial.

During the trial, the investigator will be responsible for the medical care of the subject. The investigator will make trial-related medical decisions and ensure that the participant receives adequate medical care for intercurrent illness(s) or for the treatment of trial-related adverse events (ICH E6(2) 4.3). Sponsor and investigators will have written agreements regarding payments for the treatment of trial-related injury (Chapter 15 Resourcing and Outsourcing), and the method and manner of any compensation to trial subjects should comply with applicable regulatory requirement(s) (ICH E6(2) 5.8.3).

The identity of research subjects must be protected throughout the trial and after the trial. Individual trial countries or regions may have specific requirements for protection of research subjects' identification and information and research subjects will consent as to which aspects of their identity may be used for trial documentation and who may have access to their trial information. The investigator will maintain a code list that links the full identity of the subject and the identification code used for the subject in the trial. The code list will be have secure access and be used to verify a subject's existence and may be used for as necessary for the management of a subject's safety. Published study results may present information in only aggregate for subjects and may not reveal the identity of any individual subject.

12.2.7 IRB/EC and Regulatory Authority Communication

Before any clinical may be initiated, that is, before any research participant may be consented to participate in a trial, the trial's protocol must be granted the favorable opinion or approval from a qualified Institutional Review Board (IRB) or EC whose responsibility is to ensure the protection of the rights, safety, and well-being of human subjects involved in a trial. Additionally, the regulatory authority (sometimes referred to as competent authority) that governs the region where investigational sites are located will require their receipt or approval of the protocol. Throughout the duration of the trial, the sponsor will continue to update the regulatory authority(ies) and the investigator will update the IRB/EC with study status and new study information as required for their continuing review. Regulatory authority(ies) and IRBs/ECs are expected to respond to evidence of potential or actual harm to research volunteers, or of sponsor or investigator noncompliance with the protocol, Good Clinical Practice (GCP), or regulations via investigations and warranted actions. At the end of the study, whether the study completed or prematurely terminated, and regardless of the outcome of the study's objectives, the investigator will inform the IRB/EC and the sponsor will inform the regulatory authorities of the final status of the study. IRB/ECs and regulatory authorities may have different requirements for the contents and timelines of those reports (Chapter 9 Investigator and Sponsor Roles and Responsibilities).

12.2.8 Data Collection and Data Management

Inherent in the definition of a clinical trial is the collection and analysis of data with the object of ascertaining its safety and/or efficacy. The sponsor will design a

CRF, a key trial document (Plate 8 Data Framework/Information Flow Among Key Trial Documents; Plate 13 Case Report Form), that will collect only data necessary to evaluate the study endpoints and other data to support compliance and that is conducive to accurate data entry for each type of user. The investigator will set up procedures to record and maintain source data of protocol procedures and case histories for study participants. The medium(ia) and structure used to collect data will be set up prior to trial start and may vary within a trial. A host of different systems may be used to collect data (e.g. directly from the clinical site, the subject, clinical laboratory(ies), IP depot) but all systems must individually and collectively be designed and managed (when merged) to ensure the integrity of the data (Chapter 20 Data Collection and Data Management).

12.2.9 Safety, Pharmacokinetics, and Pharmacodynamics Laboratory Testing

The collection and laboratory testing of biological specimens from research subjects is important to analyze the pharmacokinetics, pharmacodynamics, and genetic effects of the administration of the IP to research subjects. A clinical trial protocol will require the collection of specimens only when they are needed to measure the endpoints outlined in the protocol. These specimens should be collected and used only as directed by the protocol. Research subjects may be asked to provide new or additional samples that are not required by the protocol but for future research testing.

Research subjects will consent for the collection of all samples. Subjects may be required per applicable local regulations to provide a separate and distinct consent for the collection of specific types of biological specimen (e.g. invasive biopsy samples) or for the type of use of the specimen (e.g. for genetic testing).

All biological samples will be collected, processed, stored, and shipped per scientific and health authority standards and all specimens will be tracked and accounted for at all times during and after the trial, as required by the IRB/EC.

12.2.10 Safety Monitoring and Reporting

In addition to understanding how well an IP alleviates, cures, or prevents a disease, the primary goal of conducting clinical trials is to determine the safety profile of the use of the IP in humans. All trials have to be monitored for safety: the investigator is identifying and reporting safety events, and the sponsor is analyzing those events across all investigator sites and across all trials using the same IP. The investigator is also responsible for reporting safety information to the governing IRB/EC and the sponsor is responsible for reporting to the regulatory authority(ies) and all investigators.

An adverse event is defined as "any untoward medical occurrence in a patient or clinical investigation subject administered a pharmaceutical product and which does not necessarily have a causal relationship with this treatment. An adverse event (AE) can therefore be any unfavorable and unintended sign (including an abnormal laboratory finding), symptom, or disease temporally associated with the use of a medicinal (investigational) product, whether or not related to the medicinal (investigational) product" (ICH E6(R2) 1.2). When adverse events are serious (e.g. life threatening or meet other criteria as defined in ICH E6(R2) 1.50), these events may be required to be expeditiously reported to the sponsor, IRB/EC, and regulatory authority(ies) (see additional GCP requirements for safety reporting are outlined in ICH E2A Guideline for Clinical Safety Data Management: Definitions and Standards for Expedited Reporting).

The sponsor will provide the IB to all investigators. The IB will include what is currently known of the safety profile of the IP and will be updated as new information (from clinical, nonclinical, or CMC sources) is obtained. During the trial, the sponsor will analyze all reported safety events as individual events, by subject, by investigator, by trial, and in aggregate for the IP. New, worsening, or recurring events should also be analyzed by the sponsor to identify possible safety signals associated with the use of the IP.

See the Chapter 21 Safety Monitoring and Reporting for details.

12.2.11 Trial Monitoring

The sponsor has responsibility for monitoring the investigation to ensure that all trial activities and procedures are conducted in compliance with the protocol, GCP, and applicable regulatory requirements, and trial conduct is by qualified and trained personnel. Monitoring is a quality-control activity. The sponsor will select qualified monitors to conduct monitoring activities before, during, and after the study and will establish a Monitoring Plan to guide those monitoring activities. The Plan will be built on determination of critical aspects of the trial that need to be reviewed and will describe what, when, and how those aspects will be reviewed. Monitoring may be conducted on- or off-site, depending on access to the documentation of trial information and procedures, and facilities. The method(s) used must not compromise the ultimate goal of compliance with the protocol, GCP, and applicable regulatory requirements. The sponsor will ensure that corrective and preventive actions are taken for identified deviations to secure compliance with the protocol, GCP, and applicable regulatory requirements. All review and results of monitoring will be documented and reported to a qualified sponsor representative who has responsibility for oversight and management of the trial (Plate 7 Trial Monitoring; Plate 15 Monitoring Overview Checklist; Chapter 22 Monitoring Overview).

12.2.11.1 Investigator/Institution Selection

Investigator/Institution selection involves the sponsor ensuring that the investigator/institution is qualified to conduct the trial prior to trial initiation. The trial sponsor has responsibility for selecting the investigator and trial site. The Sponsor will identify qualified physicians or dentists who will perform the role of clinical investigators. The clinics or institutions where the qualified physicians or dentists will administer the test article to trial subjects will also be selected as trial sites. The clinical investigators will be able to recruit and provide appropriate medical care to the study subjects and have adequate time and resources (personnel, facilities, and equipment) to conduct the trial per the protocol, GCP, and applicable regulatory requirements. A written agreement regarding trial obligations and conduct must be in place between the sponsor and investigator prior to start of the trial (Chapter 23 Investigator/Institution Selection).

12.2.11.2 Investigator/Institution Initiation

Investigator/Institution initiation involves the sponsor ensuring that the investigator/institution is prepared to conduct the trial prior to enrolling subjects in the trial. The sponsor is responsible for ensuring that the investigator is provided with all trial information, supplies, and resources that are needed and that the investigator and trial site are qualified for trial conduct. In turn, the investigator is responsible for ensuring that trial staff are trained and qualified to perform delegated trial duties. In practice, because the sponsor is responsible for overseeing all investigator activities, the sponsor will typically train the investigator and trial staff on all trial procedures and requirements. At the same time, the sponsor will also confirm that the investigator/institution, including staff and facilities, are ready and prepared to start enrollment (i.e. consenting) of trial subjects (Chapter 24 Investigator/Institution Initiation).

12.2.11.3 Interim Monitoring

Interim monitoring is a quality-control activity that involves the sponsor ensuring that the investigator/institution is conducting the ongoing trial in compliance with the protocol, GCP, and applicable regulatory requirements. The sponsor will continuously review documentation of qualifications of investigator and staff, delegation of trial duties, consent and enrollment of trial subjects, storage, handling, administration and use of IP(s), completion of trial procedures, and reporting of safety and trial information, and will ensure that corrective and preventive actions are taken for identified deviations to secure compliance with the protocol, GCP, and applicable regulatory requirements (Chapter 25 Investigator/Institution Interim Monitoring).

12.2.11.4 Investigator/Institution Close-out

Investigator/Institution close-out involves the sponsor ensuring that documentation of all study conduct by the investigator/institution is complete, reconciled with the sponsor's records, and appropriately archived; used and unused IP have been accounted for; unused product and remnants of used product have been appropriately returned to the sponsor or destroyed by the investigator/institution; finances are reconciled; final study status has been reported to the sponsor and the IRB/EC; and the investigator knows of their obligations for any outstanding follow-up (e.g. safety, pregnancy outcomes, availability of records for regulatory inspections) (Chapter 26 Investigator/Institution Close-out; Plate 16 Investigator/Institution Closeout).

12.2.12 Statistics and Data Analysis

Statistical requirements for a trial will be outlined in the protocol and additional details may be described in a SAP (ICH E6(R2) 6.9). The clinical trial protocol will specify the endpoint variables that will be used to assess the objectives of the trial, and the CRF will be designed to collect the data from the measurements for the variables that will be analyzed. The SAP is a written procedure that will provide the minimum information that is required for the CSR (Chapter 28 The Clinical Study Report), including the following and other details about how the data collected will be analyzed:

- Definitions of all variables that will be used to measure the primary, secondary, and other endpoints.
- Definitions of the sets of subjects to be analyzed (e.g. all randomized subjects, all dosed subjects, all eligible subjects, evaluable subjects).
- The timing for interim analyses.
- The methods for randomization, if applicable.
- The methods for blinding, if applicable.
- A detailed description of the statistical methods to be used for data analysis.

The SAP, an essential trial document (Plate 8 Data Framework/Information Flow Among Key Trial Documents; Plate 12 Statistical Analysis Plan), should be finalized prior to unblinding the data for blinded trials or prior to locking the database for open label trials. Any changes to the finalized plan must be explained and dated and it should be noted that any changes to the planned analyses after the unblinding of blinded trials may introduce bias in the data analysis.

Once the CRF data are cleaned and the database is locked, reports based on the planned analyses will display the data results as summary tables, figures, or in listings of the values for variables of interest. As much as possible, the use of manually calculated or compiled reports should be avoided and these reports should instead be outputs of computer programmed and validated algorithms to ensure accuracy of the data results in the reports. The collection of statistical reports, along with other documentation from the trial, will form the basis for presenting the study results in the clinical study report.

12.2.13 Clinical Study Report

The Clinical Trial/Study Report (CSR) is a key trial document (Plate 8 Data Framework/Information Flow Among Key Trial Documents; Plate 14 Clinical Study

Report) that contains a written description of a trial/study of any therapeutic, prophylactic, or diagnostic agent conducted in human subjects, in which the clinical and statistical description, presentations, and analyses are fully integrated into a single report (ICH E6(R2) 1.13). The CSR may contain full study analyses, or may be abbreviated per applicable regulatory requirements (Chapter 28 The Clinical Study Report).

The CSR, with all of its attachments and appendices, must completely and accurately reflect study conduct. An individual reading the study report should be able to glean from its contents exactly how the trial was planned to be conducted, how it was actually conducted, and the results and conclusions of the data analyses. The report will not only include presentation of study data as analyzed per the SAP, but also a compilation of the administrative structure of the trial, the names and locations of investigators, trial sites, and IRBs/ECs used for the trial, accountability for all subjects who consented for the trial at each trial site (subjects who signed consent, screened, enrolled, discontinued, completed), the amount of exposure each subject had to the IP(s), the reason for each subject who did not receive all study treatment or did not complete the study, a complete report and analysis of safety events, descriptions of deviations from the protocol, GCP, or regulatory requirements, and results of any audits of sponsor, CROs, or investigators.

The CSR will be signed by the investigator or coordinating investigator, and a sponsor representative, as applicable, and will be submitted to the regulatory authority(ies) as required.

12.2.14 Essential Documents

Essential documents are the evidence of trial conduct. These documents reflect the processes and decisions of trial conduct, and data collected during the trial. They also individually and collectively permit evaluation of the conduct of a study and the quality of the data produced. The ICH defines all documents that must be retained, by whom, and for how long (ICH E6(R2) 8). Plate 6 Individual Clinical Trial – Essential Documents displays ICH-required essential documents based on their respective activities by the phase of trial conduct.

12.2.15 Study Closeout

Study closeout occurs after all trial data from subjects are entered and accounted for, all individual investigator/institution sites are closed, and the database of all trial data is locked. Study closeout ensures that all trial processes and procedures are completed and all the documentation that reflect trial conduct are organized and in place and ready for archiving. Study closeout involves accounting for all clinical supplies, and reconciliation of finances and essential documents. All trial players will archive and retain essential documents per GCP and applicable regulatory requirements (Plate 17 Study Closeout).

12.2.16   Consequences of Inadequate Trial Conduct

In clinical research, our aim is to prevent the sponsor's or investigator's failure to comply with the protocol, GCP, and regulatory requirements. There is potential risk to a subject's rights, safety, and well-being, the quality and integrity of the data, or compliance with regulatory requirements if there is noncompliance. Additionally, we want to avoid opposing effects on the business objectives. The goal of the design and implementation of a scientifically sound and detailed protocol is to ensure that all sponsor and investigators and their representatives are qualified, trained, managed, have sufficient resources, have knowledge of the trial protocol, IP, and trial procedures, GCP, and applicable regulatory requirements, and that all staff involved in trial conduct are complying with those requirements. A clinical trial is at high risk for noncompliance with the protocol, GCP, and applicable regulatory requirements, or business objectives if,

- The sponsor does not adequately:
  - Manage resources and oversee the trial to ensure compliance while meeting the business timelines and budget.
  - Execute written agreements with investigators and CROs as required by GCP and the applicable regulatory requirements.
  - Make payments to investigators and CROs per written agreements.
  - Obtain trial insurance, indemnify investigators of non-negligent trial-related liability, and compensate trial subjects for trial-related injury according to applicable regulatory requirement(s).
  - Perform risk assessment and quality management prior to and during the course of the trial.
  - Employ qualified staff and CROs to perform trial duties in accordance with the protocol, GCP, and applicable regulatory requirements.
  - Train all staff involved in trial conduct on the trial information that is related to their trial duties.
  - Manufacture, release, ship, and handle the IP per Good Manufacturing Practices and regulatory requirements, and account for all use, return, and destruction of the IP.
  - Design and describe the study in a detailed and complete protocol that includes all elements required by GCP and applicable regulations.
  - Describe all aspects of the properties and known clinical and nonclinical safety and efficacy information of the IP in a current IB that includes all elements required by GCP and applicable regulations.
  - Provide the investigator with all trial information and supplies needed to adequately conduct the trial.
  - Ensure that the trial protocol and other study documents as required are reviewed and approved by or receive no objections from the governing

regulatory authority(ies) for the location(s) where the IP will be tested prior to initiation (i.e. implementation) of the study.

- Ensure that the trial protocol and other study documents are reviewed and approved by or given the favorable opinion of a duly constituted and qualified IRB/EC prior to its initiation (i.e. implementation) at the clinical site.
- Design a CRF and data collection, correction, and management methods that allow for collection of accurate study data as required to meet the objectives of the protocol from the investigator.
- Ensure the appropriate collection and tracking of biological specimens as directed by the protocol.
- Collect, analyze, and report safety events per the protocol, GCP, and applicable regulatory requirements.
- Employ risk-based processes and qualified monitors to monitor of the investigation before, during, and after completion of the trial, and implement corrective and preventive actions for identified deviations.
- Analyze the study data as described in the SAP.
- Completely and accurately describe the planned conduct of the study, the actual conduct of the study, deviations from the planned conduct or planned analysis of the study, the study results in a final clinical study report that is submitted.
- Collect and retain all required essential documents per the protocol, GCP, and applicable regulatory requirements.
- Comply with standard operating procedures, the protocol, GCP, and applicable regulations.
- And/Or if the investigator/institution does not adequately:
  - Manage resources and oversee the trial to ensure compliance with GCP, the protocol, and the applicable regulatory requirements, and budget and contractual obligations.
  - Execute written agreements with sponsors and regulatory authority(ies) as required by GCP and the applicable regulatory requirements.
  - Make payments to subcontractors per written agreements.
  - Employ qualified staff and subcontractors to perform trial duties in accordance with the protocol, GCP, and applicable regulatory requirements.
  - Train all staff involved in trial conduct on the trial information that is related to their trial duties.
  - Handle and administer the IP per the protocol, IB, and applicable regulatory requirements, and account for all use, return, and destruction of the IP.
  - Understand the requirements of the protocol and the information about the IP as described in the IB.
  - Submit to and obtain the approval/favorable opinion of a duly constituted and qualified IRB/EC of the trial protocol, informed consent materials, and other study documents prior to initiation (i.e. implementation) of the trial.

- Administer and obtain informed consent using an IRB/EC-approved informed consent form from each potential trial subject prior to the subject undergoing any trial-related procedure.
- Compensate trial subjects for trial participation as approved by the IRB/EC.
- Maintain confidentiality of subject information throughout the trial and thereafter, except as necessary for the management of subject safety.
- Provide medical care to subjects for study-related adverse events and ensure medical care is provided to subjects for intercurrent illnesses.
- Enroll only subjects who meet the eligibility criteria for the trial.
- Maintain source documentation of case histories and study data, and submit CRFs of complete and accurate study data to the sponsor in a timely manner.
- Collect, process, store, ship, and track biological specimens as directed by the protocol and scientific and health authority standards.
- Identify, review, and report safety events per the protocol, GCP, and applicable regulatory requirements.
- Allow monitoring, auditing, inspections of trial conduct and implement corrective and preventive actions for identified deviations.
- Collect and retain all required essential documents per the protocol, GCP, and applicable regulatory requirements.
- Comply with standard operating procedures, the protocol, GCP, and applicable regulations.

Some common consequences of inadequate compliance with the protocol, GCP, and/or regulatory requirements are:

Subject:
- Violation of rights; e.g.
  - Failure to administer or inadequately administer consent to a subject.
  - Breach of subject confidentiality.
  - Misrepresentation of the IP as safe and/or effective.
- Violation of safety; e.g.
  - Improper administration of the IP.
  - Failure to identify and treat adverse events.
  - Administration of damaged or contaminated IP.

Regulatory:
- Violation of protocol procedures; e.g.
  - Failure to perform protocol procedures as described and at the time they are required.
  - Failure to maintain blinding or following randomization procedures.
  - Failure to address protocol deviations.

- Violation of IRB procedures; e.g.
  - Failure to submit to the IRB/IEC for initial and/or continuing review.
  - Inadequate communication of study status with the IRB.
- Violation of regulatory requirements; e.g.
  - Implementing the protocol and/or consent forms that are not approved by the IRB/IEC.
  - Failure to maintain adequate case histories and other source documents.
  - Documenting what did not happen.
  - Investigator's failure to oversee the investigation.
  - Unqualified personnel performing study duties.
  - Failure to report safety events as required.
- Misuse/handling of IP; e.g.
  - Inadequate accountability for the IP.
  - Improper storage of the IP.

Business:
- No or slow enrollment at the clinical investigational site.
- Increased costs of operations by the sponsor.
- Increased costs of operations at the site.
- Costs related to addressing issues due to negligence.

Everything perfect?!
- If the investigator site produces perfect data, and there are no protocol deviations, and no adverse events reported, this may be a sign of a "too good to be true" situation. While this situation is certainly possible, it is highly improbable, given the nature of clinical trials; i.e. they involve human beings as research participants and as conductors of the trials. It is prudent for the Monitor(s) to carefully review such circumstances, and if there are no findings, Bravo!

12.3 Summary

All parties involved in the design and conduct of a clinical trial (i.e. the sponsor and investigators and their representatives) are required to follow GCP and applicable requirements. These requirements call for the creation of key study documents, the conduct of specific activities, and the implementation of procedures and processes to guide the creation of the documents and the conduct of trial activities. Sponsors and investigators have GCP and regulatory responsibilities to which they must abide. When there is noncompliance with these responsibilities, the subject's rights, safety, and well-being, the quality and integrity of the data, or the business objectives may be compromised. It is prudent, therefore, that individual clinical trials are designed, planned, and managed with the eventual goal of obtaining credible data to critically assess the benefit versus risk of the IP.

Knowledge Check Questions

1) What are three activities that are performed during the pre-study phase of the study, by the sponsor? By the investigator?
2) What are three activities that are performed during the on-study phase of the study, by the sponsor? By the investigator?
3) What are three activities that are performed during the end-study phase of the study, by the sponsor? By the investigator?
4) What is the definition of trial initiation?
5) Who has responsibility for trial oversight?
6) What are some of the considerations by a sponsor to assure the best quality for a trial?

Reference

1 International Council for Harmonisation of Technical Requirements for Pharmaceuticals for Human Use (ICH), Integrated Addendum to ICH E6(R1):Guideline for Good Clinical Practice, E6(R2), Current Step 4 version dated 9 November 2016. https://www.ich.org/page/efficacy-guidelines.

13

Risk Assessment and Quality Management
P. Michael Dubinsky

GCP Key Point

Assessing possible risks that may be encountered is a business and industry practice that has been applied across all disciplines and endeavors. The clinical trial process can benefit from such an assessment and undertaking a risk determination is a demonstration of quality management.

13.1 Introduction

The revisions to the ICH/GCP Guideline from November 2016 specifically call for the sponsor to integrate quality management into their planning and conduct of clinical trials by conducting a set of coordinated and documented activities around the topic of risks that might be encountered during the conduct of the trial. The process of risk assessment and management is inherently part of quality management, however we saw placing the discussion in this Chapter as appropriate because it should be undertaken at the earliest stage of trial planning and development.

13.2 Objectives

This chapter is not meant to be formal training in risk assessment and management. The objective is to ensure that this new and sometimes confusing assessment process is embraced and applied.

Training of staff in risk assessment and management or employing trained mentors to guide staff in the process should be undertaken to the extent necessary

The Fundamentals of Clinical Research: A Universal Guide for Implementing Good Clinical Practice, First Edition. P. Michael Dubinsky and Karen A. Henry.

for the trial that is being planned. Do not forget the application of ICH E6 (R2) principles and meeting ICH E6 (R2) expectations are not restricted to Phase III clinical trials.

13.3 Risk Assessment

There has been considerable discussion in the clinical trial community about building quality into the overall process and terminology such as Quality by Design has emerged as a lead strategy for ensuring that risks are understood and their impact minimized. That is not to say that risks are eliminated but by adopting the risk assessment and management approach that is outlined in the 2016 ICH/GCP Revision 2 Part 5, a sponsor follows a pathway that strives to avoid the occurrence of events which might adversely impact those aspects of the trial conduct that are critical to the quality of the outcome. Risks that might adversely impact a trial have always been considered by sponsors however in our view we see the expectation that sponsors will now be establishing a written plan which describes those risks and how best to assess and manage them. In addition, this will be a documented activity becoming part of the archive of materials for the trial. A check of ICH E6 (R2) Section 8, Essential Documents does not list a risk-related review and report as being expected but if a sponsor is implementing such a process they should have a written procedure for it, training for staff and records documenting that the task was performed.

13.3.1 Risk Identification and Evaluation

Risk is possible harms or adverse consequences which could occur placed in perspective with the likelihood of the harm occurring. Identifying risks associated with a trial calls for the sponsor to gather together key participants in the trial development to consider what risks may be present. Risks can be at the system or trial level. For example failure to provide adequate validation to a trial management computer application would be a system level risk. Failure to train properly for administering informed consent to subjects would be a trial level risk. Placing the risks in perspective must begin before the implementation of the trial; so conducting the risk identification step is part of pre-study activities. Having the research, medical, biostatistical, vendor management, quality, and other staff involved in trial development brainstorming possible risks as they structure essential documents such as the protocol is one approach which works. Risks are described then categorized or qualified as to: severity; internal vs. external; likelihood of occurring; impact of it occurring; and whether it represents a critical to quality (CTQ) factor. CTQ factors are aspects of the trial that are critical to generating reliable data and providing appropriate protections for research participants [1].

13.3.2 Risk Documentation

Table 13.1 gives an example of how information gathered during risk identification might be documented.

13.3.3 Risk Management

Risk management involves controlling the risks, communicating the risks encountered to all parties that need to know and reviewing the risks on a planned and regular basis.

Depending upon the nature and scope of the trial the number and type of CTQ risks that are identified for assessment and management will differ. The risk management process will also identify or classify some risks as not CTQ. Those risks determined to be not CTQ will not receive the management or other attention that CTQ risks will receive.

In Table 13.1 the mitigation steps briefly stated in the far right column represent the types of actions and activities that will be put in place depending upon the classification of the risk, its likelihood to occur and the severity of impact if it does occur. Controlling the emergence of risk is dependent upon a number of factors such as complexity of the trial, experience of the site and investigator, available resources training and qualifications of the clinical operation staff and the level of management support in giving quality management and quality systems a place at the table as the trial is designed and implemented.

It is useful to keep in perspective that while risk assessment and management calls for some risks to be accepted and resources not directed toward those risks, if the frequency, duration, and scope of an accepted risk changes dramatically, its classification may also change.

Communication of risk can likely be integrated into the overall trial communication plans that already exist. For example events such as the investigator's meeting, periodic clinical team conference calls, periodic updates with a CRO(s), all can and should include discussion of the items included on the risk management plan. Risks may be removed or added to the plan as appropriate.

Several mechanisms that can be instrumental in avoiding risk are conducting several quality assurance audits early on in a trial at key sites to ensure that the site staff members are well trained on the protocol and that the protocol is clear to users. Secondly, if CROs are involved in the trial that a quality agreement be in place and that single points of contact be identified at the sponsor and CRO to ensure that lines of communication are kept open and flowing throughout the trial.

Table 13.1 Documentation of information gathered during risk identification.

Risk/harm	Severity/CTQ	Likelihood to occur/impact	Mitigation steps
Failure to record key patient vital sign value at time of enrollment (external)	High/yes	Unlikely/loss of eligible subject	Retrain staff
Failure to report unexpected AER by a site (external)	High/yes	Unlikely/failure to communicate important information in timely manner. Possible harm to other subjects.	Build importance of reporting all AERs into site contract and training
Complaint filed by whistleblower (external)	Medium/no	Unlikely/possible follow up by regulator or IRB	Establish and publish reporting hot line to all involved in the trial
Site fails to make screen failure reports in timely manner per contract.(external)	Medium/no	Likely to occur from time to time/ records will be untimely and possibly deficient.	Make the topic a required agenda item for each clinical development conference call.
Financial support is withdrawn from trial (internal)	High/no	Unlikely/trial comes to end	Keep management up to date on trial progress
Certain site activation milestones not met (Internal)	Low/no	Likely/time for gathering data is extended. Cost goes up.	Place more emphasis on identifying sites that specialize in the patient population needed.
Key subject vital sign data is not being reported correctly or data appears skewed from one or more sites (external)	High/yes	Likely/may result in inaccurate or incomplete trial data base	Establish tolerance levels for remote monitoring of data being gathered via computer data entry.
Failure to specify whose SOPs will be used to guide informed consent and adverse experience reporting	High/yes	Unlikely/may result in significant noncompliance and place subject safety at risk	Ensure that the Site Initiation plan includes reminders about specifying whose SOPs will be controlling across all major processes

Risk assessment and management is a discipline that pursuant to ICH E6 (R2) should be integrated into the trial activities. It may involve drawing on a subject matter expert or outside expert however it is important that the players in the day to day trial activities be partners in this aspect of the quality management scheme. There may or may not be a specific risk manager assignment in a trial however an owner should be identified with each risk for which mitigation steps are taken. It is more likely that at least one member of the clinical development team will have been trained in risk management and be assigned to serve as the point person for ensuring that the risk process is performed according to procedure and records maintained. It may be a collateral duty. No matter how it is identified it needs to occur in place as part of GCP.

13.4 Summary

The nature and scope of a clinical trial will be the key factor in the magnitude of the risk assessment and management process that is pursued. This section focused on what the sponsor of a trial needs to implement in terms of compliance with ICH-GCP's new expectations for identifying, assessing and as needed managing trial-related risks. Risk assessment and management is now an important and expected element of overall quality management for the sponsor. From the author's standpoint this represents another example of how innovations in the pharmaceutical/biotech/medical device manufacturing industry have been transferred to the development side of the timeline.

> **Knowledge Check Questions**
>
> 1) Conducting a risk analysis is the responsibility of the site investigator. True or False
> 2) Risk identification and management as a process needs a written standard procedure. True or False.
> 3) Failure to conduct remote monitoring according written procedures would be a system level or trial level risk?
> 4) CTQ factors must be addressed as part of the risk identification and management process. True or False
> 5) Name one approach to communicating high severity, likely to occur risks.

Reference

1 Clinical Trials Transformation Initiative Recommendations (2015). Quality by Design. https://www.ctti-clinicaltrials.org/sites/www.ctti-clinicaltrials.org/files/CTTI%2520Quality%2520by%2520Design%2520Recommendations_FINAL_1JUN15.pdf (accessed 25 May 2021).

14

Trial Management; Start-up, On-Study, and Close-Out

Karen A. Henry

GCP Key Point
The sponsor is responsible for the initiation, management, and/or financing of a clinical trial and the investigator must have adequate resources for conducting a clinical trial.

14.1 Introduction

A sponsor is defined as an individual, company, institution, or organization which takes responsibility for the initiation, management, and/or financing of a clinical trial (ICH E6(R2) 1.53). The sponsor should utilize appropriately qualified individuals to supervise the overall conduct of the trial, to handle the data, to verify the data, to conduct the statistical analyses, and to prepare the trial reports (ICH E6(R2) 5.5.1). The sponsor will also have appropriate management and staff responsible for trial and site oversight (ICH E6(R2) 5.18.6(e)). In summary, the sponsor will utilize qualified individuals to plan, organize, and control resources for the initiation, management, and financing of a trial to meet the research and business objectives of the trial. Similarly, the investigator must have adequate resources for conducting a clinical trial; i.e., the investigator should have sufficient time, adequate number of qualified and trained staff, and facilities to properly conduct and complete the trial within the agreed trial period (ICH E6(R2) 4.2).

Effective initiation, management, and financing of a trial are key factors to the success of a trial. Effective initiation, management, and financing of a clinical trial means that the business and scientific objectives are achieved while adhering to the protocol, Good Clinical Practice (GCP), and applicable regulatory

The Fundamentals of Clinical Research: A Universal Guide for Implementing Good Clinical Practice, First Edition. P. Michael Dubinsky and Karen A. Henry.
© 2022 John Wiley & Sons, Inc. Published 2022 by John Wiley & Sons, Inc.
Companion website: www.wiley.com/go/dubinsky/clinicalresearch

requirements during the course of the trial. There are finite resources, timelines, and multiple activities across various disciplines that must be planned, organized and controlled for the sponsor and investigator to execute a clinical trial.

To put a familiar perspective on trial management, let us think of a family party as a possible metaphor for a clinical trial. For a family party, there is a host, and children and their parents are the guests. The host funds the party, determines the venue, guests (parents and children), and activities, and provides the supplies. The parents and children participate in the activities while the parents ensure their children's wellbeing and safety. Now let us compare with a clinical trial: the Sponsor is the host, and the guests are the Investigators and trial subjects as parents and children, respectively. In a clinical trial, the Sponsor funds, provides the investigational article and other trial supplies, and determines the trial locations. The Investigator controls the administration of the investigational article and is responsible for the wellbeing and safety of the trial subjects.

As for a party, ethics, norms or "best practices" and rules that are enforceable by law, also apply. Given that clinical research is the conduct of an experiment on human subjects, for a clinical trial, these rules are codified by the regulatory authorities (Chapter 2 Regulatory Environment; Chapter 11 Regulatory Authority Roles and Responsibilities), ethics have been outlined as principles (Chapter 6 GCP Definition and Principles), and additional conventions of conduct have evolved as norms or best practices throughout the industry. Those involved in the activities for management of a trial must have knowledge and clear understanding of the relationships and responsibilities of the various players and of the various levels of governance (see Chapter 7 Players Roles and Responsibilities Overview).

In this chapter, we will review principles/assumptions for the initiation and management of a clinical trial; i.e., determining resources, timelines, and the multiple activities across various disciplines that must be planned, organized, prioritized, and controlled to execute a clinical trial. (Details on resourcing are addressed in the Chapter 15 Trial Resourcing and Outsourcing.) Additionally, in order to provide the complete picture of functions and activities involved in managing a trial, we will look at the functions and activities of both the Sponsor and the Investigator who are the players responsible for the execution of the trial.

14.2 Objectives

The objectives of this chapter are to:

1) Define trial management and the objectives of trial management
2) Describe the infrastructure for trial management
    a) Provide an overview of trial functional areas
        i) Functions of the Sponsor
        ii) Functions of the Investigator
    b) Describe the qualifications and role of the Study lead
    c) To discuss tools for trial management

3) Provide an overview of trial management activities
  a) Trial initiation
     i) Describe trial initiation activities
     ii) Describe the process for trial initiation
  b) On-study
     i) Describe on-study activities
     ii) Describe the process for on-study management
  c) End-study and study closeout
     i) Describe end-study and study closeout activities
     ii) Describe the process for end-study management and study closeout
  d) Purpose of study closeout
  e) Timing for study closeout
  f) The study closeout checklist
  g) Archiving Essential Documents
4) Discuss the typical issues in Trial Management

14.2.1 Definition and Objectives of Trial Management

The definition of a sponsor is an individual, company, institution, or organization which takes responsibility for the initiation, management, and/or financing of a clinical trial (ICH E6(R2) 1.53). The sponsor should utilize appropriately qualified individuals to supervise the overall conduct of the trial, to handle the data, to verify the data, to conduct the statistical analyses, and to prepare the trial reports (ICH E6(R2) 5.5.1). The sponsor will also have appropriate management and staff responsible for trial and site oversight (ICH E6(R2) 5.18.6(e)). That is, the sponsor will utilize qualified individuals to plan, organize, and control resources for the initiation, management, and financing of a trial to meet the research and business objectives of the trial. Similarly, the Investigator must have adequate resources for conducting a clinical trial; i.e., the investigator should have sufficient time and adequate qualified and trained staff, and facilities to properly conduct and complete the trial within the agreed trial period (ICH E6(R2) 4.2).

In practice, clinical trial management refers to planning, organizing, and controlling resources to meet the research and business objectives of the trial. Although not a role or title specified by ICH E6(R2), a sponsor will typically employ a leading individual to manage the initiation and conduct of the trial. This "study lead" manages the functional team members, activities, timelines, and budget for a trial.

The objectives of trial management are to implement trial operation procedures that ensure:

- Achievement of the scientific and business objectives of the trial, while prioritizing subject safety, welfare, and integrity
- Collection of accurate and complete data
- Trial activities comply with requirements of the protocol, regulatory, GCP, and standard operating procedures (SOPs)

- Achievement of desired quality outcomes
- Trial conduct by trained and qualified personnel
- Tracking, management, and control of resources
- Clear and timely communication of trial information
- Complete and accurate documentation of trial conduct

14.2.2   The Infrastructure for Trial Management

The infrastructure of trial management here refers to understanding the roles and functions involved and how they are organized. The sponsor and investigator have different roles in the conduct of clinical trials and therefore have different regulatory responsibilities for carrying out their roles. Each player will set up functional areas of individuals who have the required expertise for the responsibilities of its function. Each function has specific contributions for trial initiation, on-study, and end of the study activities so it is important that an infrastructure is in place to facilitate communication between and among functions for collaboration, transmittal and receipt of information.

14.2.2.1   Overview of Functional Areas Involved in a Trial
A variety of specialized expertise is required to perform trial-related duties and functions. As described in this topic's introduction, both the Sponsor and Investigator have responsibilities for activities involved in trial execution.

14.2.2.2   Functions of the Sponsor
The following describes the functional individuals or teams that are relevant to the Sponsor's conduct of the trial and their general responsibilities (Table 14.1).

14.2.2.3   Functions of the Investigator
The following describes the functional individuals or teams that are relevant to the Investigator's conduct of the trial and their general responsibilities (Table 14.2).

14.2.2.4   Qualifications and Role of the Study Lead
Trial management is a responsibility of the Sponsor (see Chapter 9 Investigator and Sponsor Roles and Responsibilities) who should utilize appropriately qualified individuals to supervise the overall conduct of the trial (ICH E6(R2) 5.5). A sponsor will typically assign one qualified individual, the study lead, to have responsibility for oversight of the entire trial. The study lead coordinates all activities of the trial, and many of the activities are carried out by other functional individuals or teams.

A study lead needs to have knowledge of GCP, applicable regulatory requirements, and, preferably, of the therapeutic area that is being studied. The study

Table 14.1 Functions of the sponsor.

Sponsor function	General responsibility
Medical monitor	Medical personnel who will be readily available to advise on trial-related medical questions or problems. Outside consultant(s) may be appointed for this purpose (ICH E6(R2) 5.3). In practice, the medical monitor customarily leads the creation of the trial design, and is the lead decision-maker and contributor of clinical information to the trial protocol, clinical investigator's brochure, the clinical study report, and submissions to the regulatory authorities.
Trial manager	Individual who supervises the overall conduct of the trial (ICH E6(R2) 5.5). The trial manager will also lead and contribute to the creation of processes and documents that support trial conduct.
Biostatistician	Individual who conducts the statistical analysis. The biostatistician is also a key contributor to trial design.
Data management	Individual or team that handles the trial data. The data management staff creates the medium for data collection and provides training and instructions for data collection, and processes the trial data.
Regulatory affairs	Individual or team that communicates with and submits reports to the regulatory authorities on behalf of the sponsor. Regulatory affairs staff provides guidance on the regulatory requirements regarding general format and timelines for the submission of information to the regulatory authorities.
Clinical trial site monitor(s)	Individual(s) who act(s) as main line of communication between the sponsor and the investigator, verifies trial data at the trial site, and ensures that the trial is conducted and documented per the protocol, GCP, applicable regulatory requirements, and standard operating procedures (ICH E6(R2) 18.4).
Quality assurance	Individual or team responsible for planned and systematic actions that are established to ensure that the trial is performed and the data are generated, documented, recorded, and reported in compliance with GCP and applicable regulatory requirements (ICH E6(R2) 1.46).
Contracts and budgets	Individual or team that prepares, negotiates, and maintains contracts and budgets. Contracts are executed between the sponsor and clinical trial sites and between the sponsor and contract research organizations or other vendors.
Safety data processing	Individual or team that receives, reviews, and prepares reports of safety events to be submitted to participating investigators and regulatory authorities, and as applicable to IRBs/IECs.
Legal	Individual or team that reviews contracts and other trial documents, as appropriate, for consistency with applicable law and regulatory requirements.

(Continued)

Table 14.1 (Continued)

Sponsor function	General responsibility
Nonclinical testing	Individual or team that conducts or oversees the conduct and reporting of nonclinical trials.
Drug assessment (pharmacokinetics and pharmacodynamics)	Individual or team that conducts or oversees the conduct and reporting of pharmacokinetics and/or pharmacodynamic studies.
Project management	Individual or team that provides project management services for all trials in the development program for a product or indication, or for a single trial.
Outsourcing/vendor management	Individual or team that identifies and manages the selection and contracting of contract research organizations or vendors.
CMC/clinical supplies	Individual or team that oversees the manufacturing, packaging, and distribution of the investigational article.

Table 14.2 Functions of the investigator.

Investigator function	General responsibility
Principal investigator	A person responsible for the conduct of the clinical trial at a trial site (ICH E6(R2) 1.34).
Subinvestigator(s)	An individual member of the clinical trial team designated and supervised by the investigator at a trial site to perform critical trial-related procedures and/or to make important trial-related decisions (e.g., associates, residents, research fellows) (ICH E6(R2)) 1.56. Subinvestigators typically perform physical exams, assess adverse events, or perform specialized clinical assessments.
Clinical research coordinator (CRC)	The member of the investigator team at the clinical trial site who coordinates and manages the trial activities and related functions, such as ethics committee submissions, contracting, pharmacy and laboratory subject recruitment, enrollment, subject visits, documentation of trial data. The CRC may also prepare submissions for the ethics committee and communicate with the Sponsor's representative. (Chapter 9 Investigator and Sponsor Roles and Responsibilities)
Pharmacist	The individual or team responsible for handling, storage, and preparation of the investigational article for its dispensation or administration.
Contract and budget reviewers and approvers	Individual or team responsible for contract and budget review, negotiation, and execution.

lead must plan, organize, and control the resources and operations, being mindful that the trial conduct must always be in compliance with GCP and applicable regulatory requirements. Having knowledge of the requirements is critical to making decisions that produce compliant outcomes during initiation, on-study and at the end of the study. Multiple disciplines contribute to the execution of a clinical trial and the study lead is responsible for coordinating input of the various functions. The study lead, therefore, needs to have clear understanding of the roles of different functions involved in trial conduct, how these functions interact, and the regulatory impact of each function.

Preexisting knowledge of the therapeutic area and population under investigation allows a study lead to anticipate the clinical needs and logistics required to address the clinical needs and issues for a trial. For example, a trial that is being conducted with patients who have advanced debilitating disease will need to provide logistical support not only for the patient, but also for their caregiver; the consent process differs for different populations (see Chapter 19 Informed Consent and Other Human Subject Protection); and a trial protocol to perform surgery on children with brain cancer is more complex than a headache remedy protocol that is designed to measure pharmacokinetics on healthy adult volunteers.

The successful study lead is skilled at coordinating people and organizing, juggling, and tracking multiple tasks. There are several activities being carried out by many individuals and teams from multiple disciplines during the course of executing a trial. The study lead, therefore, needs to be able to track different types of activities that occur parallely and sequentially relative to each other. Equally, the study lead will be skilled at budget and time management to ensure that the conduct of the trial meets the business objectives of the firm.

14.2.2.4.1 *Tools for Trial Management*

We note from the preceding overviews that there are numerous activities, documents, and specialized functions that contribute to trial conduct. There are many tools that can assist a study lead and other trial personnel to manage the various activities, documents creation and collection, and functional personnel involved in trial conduct. SOPs and the various trial-specific plans and instructions intrinsically guide trial personnel on who does what, when, and how. At the same time, we want to track the trial activities, deliverables, timelines, and costs to ensure that the trial is conducted in accordance with the research and business objectives.

The typical items that we want to track for a trial are the deliverables, status in time, and cost. Tools for trial management may extend from all-encompassing clinical trial management systems to simple spreadsheets, or other prepackaged or customized tools. Trial management tools vary considerably in design and cost and new tools are constantly being developed. As a detailed discussion is beyond the scope of this book, here are a few examples of general designs that are used.

Comprehensive clinical trial management systems (e.g., Figure 14.1) can be used to track several levels of clinical development activities in an organization or can be customized to collect only those items that may be of interest to an organization depending on its size or economic resources. These types of systems not only assist the trial management team to plan and track activities, but also let other stakeholders such as senior management access the status of a trial or of all of clinical development at a given point of time.

Gantt charts (a type of bar chart developed by Henry Gantt in the 1910s) or similar tools can be used to map the start, stop dates, and "owner" for each trial activity while depicting the dependency relationships between activities. These scheduling

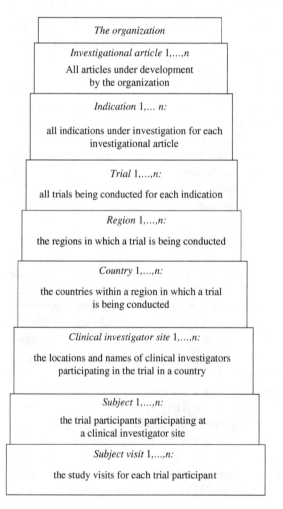

Figure 14.1 Example of items tracked in a clinical trial management system for all clinical development activities in an organization.

tools are helpful to anticipate resources, bottlenecks or critical paths, and ultimate completion times.

Simple tools, such as spreadsheets, can be used to track trial details such as those depicted in Figure 14.2.

All tools used for trial management should be interpretable not only to the trial management team, but also to other stakeholders such as senior management who at any time may want to know the status of a trial or all clinical development. Tools that can generate metrics and summary reports can be most helpful for the team.

A report generated from the clinical trial management system may service to communicate the organization, personnel, deliverables, and timelines for a trial. This communication can also be made via a document that is typically known as a Trial Management Plan, Project Management Plan, Project Operations Plan, or Trial Operations Plan. The typical table of contents for such a plan is shown in Figure 14.3.

The trial level
• Team contact information
• Essential documents and their versions
• Budget and expenses
• Study decisions
• Safety events
• Study advertising

Per subject information	Per site information
• Projected and actual dates of subject study visits, consenting, screening, randomization, administration of investigational article, and disposition	• Projected an actual dates of site selection, site initiation, interim monitoring, and close-out visits dates
• Reasons for subjects failing screening	• Ethics committee submissions, approvals, and communications
• Reasons for discontinuation of the study or administration of the investigational article	• Investigational article shipping and accountability
• Amounts of administration of investigational article to subject	• Investigator delegation of responsibilities and investigator staff qualification
• Case report forms completion, collection, and data queries	• Qualification of facilities
• Payments to subjects	• Payments to investigators
• Subject biological samples	• Protocol deviations and their correction and preventive actions
• Outcomes for study endpoints	

Figure 14.2 Examples of other operational items tracked for a specific trial.

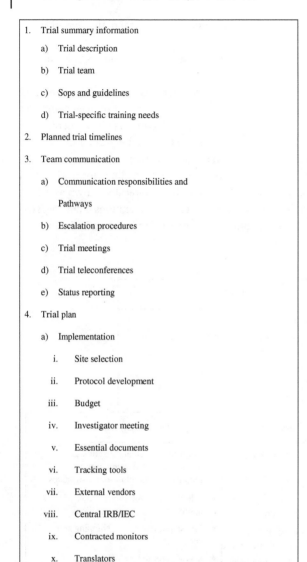

1. Trial summary information
   a) Trial description
   b) Trial team
   c) Sops and guidelines
   d) Trial-specific training needs
2. Planned trial timelines
3. Team communication
   a) Communication responsibilities and
      Pathways
   b) Escalation procedures
   c) Trial meetings
   d) Trial teleconferences
   e) Status reporting
4. Trial plan
   a) Implementation
      i.   Site selection
      ii.   Protocol development
      iii. Budget
      iv.   Investigator meeting
      v.   Essential documents
      vi.   Tracking tools
      vii. External vendors
      viii. Central IRB/IEC
      ix.   Contracted monitors
      x.   Translators

Figure 14.3 Example of table of contents for trial operations plan.

```
        xi.     Other External Vendors

        xii.    Study Supplies

        xiii.   Screen Failure Subjects

        xiv.    CRFs/Diary Cards

     b)  Monitoring

         i.     Routine monitoring

         ii.    Responsibilities for ancillary departments and

                equipment

         iii.   Monitoring - protocol deviations

         iv.    Safety monitoring

         v.     Crf and query flow / process

     c)  Data management / statistics

         i.     Data management responsibilities

         ii.    Data transfer specifications

         iii.   Data coding

         iv.    Biostatistics programming and analysis

         v.     Medical writing

     d)  Quality assurance requirements

     e)  Close-out phase

         i.     Final activities

 5.  Appendices
```

Figure 14.3   (Continued)

14.2.2.5   Overview of Trial Management Activities

Figure 14.4 depicts the general timeline and milestones for trial activities. Trial activities are considered in three phases: Pre-study or trial initiation (also known as "start-up") is the period from deciding to execute a trial up to the consent of the first trial participant, On-study continues until the last visit of the last trial participant, and End-study refers to those activities that occur until the trial records are archived. In this topic, we will provide greater details of the activities involved in each of the three phases.

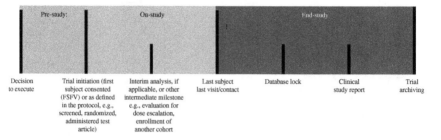

Figure 14.4 Milestones for a clinical trial.

It is important for realistic timelines to be set for study completion. In practice, the duration of a clinical trial from initiation to study closeout depends on several factors:

1) Duration of initiation
   a) Early phase studies will typically have a single investigational site and less complex protocol designs and may therefore take one to three months for initiation once the clinical trial protocol is final.
   b) Later phase trials with randomization, blinding, and several investigational sites may take three to six months for initiation once the clinical trial protocol is final.
   c) Large randomized controlled trials with investigational sites that span the globe may take 6–12 months for initiation once the clinical trial protocol is final
2) Duration of the on-study portion of the trial
   a) Participation for each subject
      i) The on-study portion of a trial will be at least the total duration of study participation for a single subject. The duration of subject participation starts with informed consent prior to screening procedures and concludes at the time of the last study procedure or contact with the research subject.
      ii) All subjects will be followed (e.g., for safety) until the last subject completes the study
   b) Rate of subject enrollment
      i) If all subjects are enrolled at the same time, then the on-study portion of the trial is the duration of participation for a single subject.
      ii) If the subject enrollment is spaced (most often the case), then the on-study portion of the trial will be determined by the timing and rate of subject enrollment.
   c) End-study as defined in the protocol, depending on the scientific objective of the protocol; for example
      i) The last protocol procedure or contact for the last subject enrolled in the study
      ii) Event-based endpoint, in which case, the sponsor may not have to wait for all subjects to complete the trial

iii) Survival-based endpoint, in which case, the trial ends after survival data are obtained for all subjects

3) Duration of the end-study portion of the trial
   a) Database lock occurs once the study has been closed and all data have been collected and cleaned (Chapter 20 Data Collection and Data Management). The duration of database lock depends on how up-to-date are trial monitoring and data cleaning once the data for the last subject's last visit are collected.
   b) Data analysis will occur after database lock. The duration of data analysis and the production of statistical reports (tables, figures, and listings (TFLs)) depends on how well the study results align with the anticipated data analysis plan (Chapter 27 Study Design and Data Analysis) or if unanticipated outcomes are identified and additional unplanned analyses will have to be performed.
   c) Preparation of the clinical study report (CSR) occurs after the statistical reports are available. While portions of the (CSR) may be written in advance of database lock (Chapter 28 The Clinical Study Report), presentation of study results must wait for the completion of statistical analyses and production of the TFLs.
   d) Final study closeout of study activities and archiving of the essential documents (see Section 14.2.2.6.3).

4) Availability of resources
   a) The duration of the trial also completely depends on the availability of resources; i.e., personnel, money. A trial that has extensive available resources can take advantage of employing several sites to expedite the overall enrollment rate and can also assign abundant resources for monitoring and data management to always be current with the flow of CRF data from the trial sites. Similarly, the files of essential documents may always be up-to-date (which should be always "inspection ready") and advance preparation of the CSR and statistical programs for statistical analyses can help expedite the time to final CSR and study closeout.
   b) Availability of trial materials and clinical supplies.

5) The acceptable quality level based on a risk assessment
   a) A risk-based approach may be used for trial monitoring (Chapter 22 Monitoring Overview). This approach allows for the focus of resources to specific trial characteristics based on identified critical elements that will ensure adequate compliance with the protocol, GCP, and applicable regulatory requirements.

When timelines for a trial are unrealistic, the quality of the trial may be compromised and limited resources could be wasted if trial activities and materials have to be repeated. A trial that is not conducted according to GCP or regulatory requirements is at risk of disregard for its study efficacy and/or safety results by a regulatory authority during its review of an application for marketing authorization.

14.2.2.5.1 *Trial Initiation Activities*

Pre-study or trial initiation is an important phase in the conduct and management of a clinical trial. This phase includes planning, identifying resources, and organizing. We may want to compare trial initiation to planning any event: There are fixed (e.g., budget, timing, venue, and attendees) and variable or optional activities (e.g., food, music, and attractions), and while there are unforeseen circumstances, the homework done to plan and organize an event is directly related to the efficiency and quality of the event. Similarly, the homework done to plan, resource, and organize a clinical trial is directly related to the quality of the trial data and compliance with GCP, the protocol, and regulatory requirements. This phase also includes fixed, variable, and optional activities, some of which are regulated procedures so it is crucial that these are managed and executed well to ensure compliance.

Prior to initiating a trial, the sponsor should define, establish, and allocate all trial-related duties and functions (ICH E6(R2) 5.7). The practical goal of the initiation activities is to, let us say, build the airplane, before we fly it; otherwise, many inefficiencies and errors may occur during the conduct of a trial if we try to build the airplane while we are flying it. The following is a list of some typical activities that are part of the process.

- *Trial Management:* Although trial management is the responsibility of the Sponsor per GCP, its formality and design depend completely on the business practices and resources of a firm and/or the trial team. The infrastructure for managing coordination and control of the trial, including identifying tasks, resources and timelines, will be outlined prior to trial start and will be modified as needed during the course of the trial. A trial management plan, including plans for trial communication, should be provided and applicable staff trained on the procedures.
- *Resourcing:* Resourcing, that is, identifying human, financial, and technological resources for the trial, includes regulated and nonregulated factors. For example, all staff members and facilities that perform regulated Sponsor responsibilities must be qualified by training and experience and comply with applicable regulatory requirements. On the other hand, the processes for nonregulated activities may be more flexible, although it is essential that all trial personnel are qualified to perform their assigned duties. Regulatory oversight of financial resourcing is largely limited to ensuring that there is no financial incentive that could potentially influence the results of the trial documents (Chapter 15 Trial Resourcing and Outsourcing)
- *Training:* Training of all trial personnel is a quality function (see Chapter 30 Quality Systems in Clinical Research) that responds to the GCP principle that each individual involved in conducting a trial must be qualified by education, training, and experience to perform his or her respective task(s). Training is done prior to trial start and during the trial as needed. Study manual(s) with

instructions for study conduct should be provided and applicable staff trained on the procedures.

- *Clinical Supplies* (investigational and comparator product(s)): The investigational product(s) will be procured during the initiation phase of the study. The study drug or investigational product will have been manufactured, packaged, and labeled per regulatory requirements. If the sponsor will supply marketed comparators for the trial, those must be procured or systems set up for their delivery to the investigator. Any systems to pay for clinical supplies (e.g., if the investigator will obtain for the subject or if the subject will self-supply (note applicable regulatory requirements for such situations) must also be established. Import, export, and shipping permits should be secured during this period to avoid delays in shipping clinical supplies to the investigator. Investigational product will be released and shipped in time for the investigator's receipt for trial initiation. Pharmacy manual(s) with instructions for storage, handling, preparation, administration, destruction, and return of used and unused supplies of investigational product(s) should be provided and applicable staff trained on the procedures. (Chapter 17 The Investigational Product (Clinical Supplies); Chapter 24 Investigator/Institution Initiation).
- *Laboratory Testing and Supplies:* Laboratories that will perform centralized testing or analysis of biological specimen or other laboratory testing media must be evaluated for qualification of the scientists, technologists, and facilities. Necessary collection and shipping supplies must be procured and provided to the investigator. Systems for tracking and reviewing laboratory samples and test results should be established. Laboratory manual(s) with instructions for the collection, preparation, storage, and shipping of specimen and media should be provided and applicable staff trained on the procedures. (Chapter 19 Informed Consent and Other Human Subject Protection).
- *Key Trial Documents:* GCP and clinical trial regulations require specific documents to be created for trial conduct. The clinical trial protocol, the investigator's brochure (IB), and informed consent form, are a few of the regulated documents (Chapter 18 The Clinical Trial Protocol and Amendments; Chapter 16 The Investigator's Brochure; Chapter 19 Informed Consent and Other Human Subject Protection). Several other documents, such as a risk management plan, trial operations plan, communication plan, monitoring plan, safety management plan, trial manual, laboratory manual, and the pharmacy manual, as described in this chapter for each activity, may also be created to provide information and instructions to facilitate the conduct of a trial.
- *Human Subject Protection*: All entities and individuals participating in trial conduct will consider the safety, rights, and well-being of the research subject, their first and foremost priority. The sponsor will select qualified investigators for the administration of the investigational product to the subjects and the provision

of medical care for the research subjects. The investigator will ensure that the study has oversight by a duly constituted IRB/IEC, that trained and qualified individuals will be handling and administering the investigational product, administering informed consent to research subjects, carrying out study protocol evaluations on research subjects, identifying and addressing adverse events, and that subject's rights are protected and systems are in place to protect their confidentiality. The sponsor will have systems in place to monitor and assess the risk versus benefit of the implemented trial, for protection of subject confidentiality, for overseeing all trial activities to ensure the overall protection of the research subjects. Amounts and methods for payments to research subjects will be reviewed and approved by the governing IRB/IEC. (Chapter 19 Informed Consent and Other Human Subject Protection)

- *Data Collection and Data Analysis:* Inherent in the definition of a clinical trial is the collection and analysis of data with the object of ascertaining its safety and/or efficacy. Systems for recording, collecting, managing, and analyzing trial data will be set up prior to trial start and may vary within a trial. The investigator will have systems for recording and maintaining source data, for completing, reviewing, and submitting CRFs, and for making corrections to the CRFs. The sponsor will prepare the CRF and have systems for collecting, cleaning, reviewing, and managing study data. Additional systems for data collection and submission to the sponsor (e.g., from central laboratories) should be set up at this time. Systems will also be established for communicating data and/or issues between the sponsor and investigator and other data collection parties as necessary. ALCOAC principles must be applied to all stages of data creation and handling to ensure the integrity and accuracy of the data. All individuals involved in the recording, collection, management, and analysis of trial data must be qualified and trained for their assigned duty(ies).

  If a trial has blinding or randomization properties, procedures, and systems for randomization and blinding must be developed by qualified personnel. Instructions for source documentation and CRF completion, submission, and data corrections, and randomization and blinding as applicable, should be provided and applicable staff trained on the procedures. (Chapter 20 Data Collection and Data Management)

  A statistical analysis plan with methods and instructions for analysis of study data must be prepared *a priori* to trial data analysis. The statistical analysis plan may be prepared prior to trial initiation and updated if the trial analysis plan changes during the course of the conduct of the trial (Chapter 27 Study Design and Data Analysis).

- *Safety Data Collection, Monitoring, and Reporting:* The sponsor and investigator both have obligations for assessing and reporting adverse events identified as a result of administration of the investigational product and the subject's participation in the clinical trial. Investigators will collect, assess, and report safety events to the sponsor and to the IRB/IEC as required. In turn, the sponsor has obligations for reviewing reported safety information from individual sites and in aggregate for the entire trial and for all trials using the same investigational product. Sponsors will report safety events to the regulatory authority(ies) and to investigators using the investigational product, as required per applicable regulatory requirements. Both the sponsor and investigator will establish procedures for the assessment and reporting of adverse events that occur during the course of the trial. A safety management plan with instructions for the identification, assessment, and reporting of safety data should be provided and applicable staff trained on the procedures. (Chapter 21 Safety Monitoring and Reporting).

Independent Data-Monitoring Committee (IDMC) (Data and Safety Monitoring Board, Monitoring Committee, Data Monitoring Committee) may be established by the sponsor to assess at intervals the progress of a clinical trial, the safety data, and the critical efficacy endpoints, and to recommend to the sponsor whether to continue, modify, or stop a trial (ICH E6(R2) 1.25). The membership, responsibilities, timing of data review, and the processes for receiving and reviewing data and for reporting of findings and/or recommendations will be outlined in a Charter for the committee (Chapter 21 Safety Monitoring and Reporting).

- *Clinical Investigator/Institution Selection:* The trial sponsor has responsibility for selecting the investigator and trial site. The sponsor will identify and select qualified physicians or dentists who will perform the role of clinical investigators. The clinics or institutions where the qualified physicians or dentists will administer the test article to trial subjects will also be selected as trial sites. (Chapter 23 Investigator/Institution Selection).
- *Contracting:* The sponsor and the investigator will execute written contractual agreements between them and with others as follows:
  - A written agreement regarding trial obligations and conduct must be in place between the Sponsor and Clinical Investigator prior to the start of the trial.
  - The sponsor will clearly and completely describe trial-related duties that are transferred to CRO(s). CROs have complete regulatory responsibility for any trial-related duties assigned to them and the sponsor has responsibility for oversight of the CRO(s).
  - The investigator will execute agreements with subcontractors. The investigator maintains overall responsibility for the quality of trial data and the conduct of the trial regardless of outsourcing or delegation of responsibilities.
  - The investigator will also sign agreements regarding regulatory obligations, as applicable.
- *Regulatory and Ethics Submission and Approval:* Prior to initiating a clinical trial, the agency that governs the conduct of clinical trials in a country or region (see Chapter 9 Investigator and Sponsor Roles and Responsibilities) will review trial information submitted by the Sponsor. Additionally, the review board or ethics committee (see Chapter 8 IRB/IEC Roles and Responsibilities) that is

ensuring the protection of the rights, safety, and well-being of human subjects involved in the trial, must receive trial information from the Clinical Investigator and must have given favorable opinion of the trial protocol and other trial documents (see Chapter 8 IRB/IEC Roles and Responsibilities) prior to executing any trial protocol procedures.

- *Clinical Investigator/Institution Initiation:* Investigator/Institution initiation refers to the process of training and reviewing the qualifications of a Clinical Investigator and the trial site prior to permitting consenting of the first research participant in a trial at the trial site. (Chapter 24 Investigator/Institution Initiation).
- *Quality Control and Quality Assurance:* Systems with procedures that assure the quality of every aspect of the trial should be implemented (ICH E6(R2) 2.13).The sponsor and investigator will establish procedures for ensuring quality control and quality assurance, including plans and methods for monitoring and auditing, and for identifying and addressing protocol and study deviations. SOPs to be followed during the trial will be identified and documented. Audit plans describing the timing and scope of trial audits should be prepared prior to trial initiation. (See Chapter 22 Monitoring Overview, Chapter 30 Quality Systems in Clinical Research, Chapter 33 Quality Assurance Components).
- *Sponsor and Clinical Investigator Files Set-up:* As the saying goes, "If it is not documented, it did not happen!" This supports the GCP principle that all clinical trial information should be recorded, handled, and stored in a way that allows its accurate reporting, interpretation, and verification. The trial initiation process, therefore, includes setting up infrastructures to record, handle, and store trial information by all parties involved in the conduct of the trial. Plan(s) describing the structure of the sponsor's trial master file and the investigator trial files, who is responsible for the submission and maintenance of what essential documents, timelines for submitting documents, and requirements for handling and storage of documents should be provided and applicable staff trained on the procedures. (see Chapter 29 Essential Documents).

14.2.2.5.2 The Trial Initiation Process

The initiation process involves several activities, some of which are fixed and some that are variable or optional. The process for the specific activities in this initiation phase include determining the critical quality attributes of the trial, the creation of documents, and carrying out certain procedures to prepare for trial initiation. Some of these activities are required by the regulatory authorities and some are nonregulated best practices that add value to the quality and efficiency of the trial.

Before we can commence any initiation activity, it would be helpful for certain items that form the foundation for trial operations to be in place. Such items that would be *prerequisites for initiation of a specific clinical trial* include,

Quality assurance items:

- SOPs – written procedures for the activities involved in trial conduct (Chapter 32 Standard Operating Procedures). SOPs may be supplemented with study-specific plans and procedures (see Administrative items that are determined by the organization below).
- Trial administrative structure and delegation of responsibilities – assigning who will do what for the trial and determining if any trial-related duties will need to be performed outside of the organization; i.e., outsourced. (Chapter 15 Trial Resourcing and Outsourcing)
- Qualification and training records – evidence that trial personnel are qualified for and have been trained on the tasks they will perform during the trial. (Chapter 30 Quality Systems in Clinical Research)
- Audit plans - Identification of audit scope, and determining entities to be audited, audit schedule, and process for review and reporting of audit findings.

Administrative items that are determined by the organization:

- Trial budget – a budget to cover the expenses for the anticipated trial helps the trial and project managers to allocate resources. (Chapter 15 Trial Resourcing and Outsourcing)
- Trial timelines – the target dates for milestones that are consistent with the general development plan or that meet the business needs.
- Trial resources – Identification of sponsor personnel who will be responsible for managing the trial, medical monitoring, regulatory communication, clinical supplies, and other trial initiation activities. Determining if any trial-related duties will need to be performed outside of the organization; i.e., outsourced. (Chapter 15 Trial Resourcing and Outsourcing)
- Identification of desired clinical trial site locations and regulatory intelligence for conducting a clinical trial in those desired locations. (Chapter 23 Investigator/ Institution Selection)
- Risk and quality management – Identification of risks and determination of risk mitigation, and identification of critical quality attributes – the procedures, systems, and resources needed to attain the desired quality outcomes of the clinical trial. (Chapter 13 Risk Assessment and Quality Management)
- Trial management processes – Tools to track trial timelines, budget, activities, and deliverables (Section 14.2.2.4.1)
- Communication responsibilities and pathways – A written plan describing communication pathways, frequency, and methods for documenting communication of trial information is important to ensure clear responsibilities for the communication of trial information, that the appropriate individuals are

transmitting and receiving information, and that relevant trial communication is documented and maintained as essential documents (Chapter 29 Essential Documents).

An organization will have SOPs in place that govern the conduct of all trials (Chapter 32 Standard Operating Procedures). However, clinical trial staff will need additional guidance on how to carry out the trial requirements that are not standard. For example, it is standard that all trials will be monitored per GCP requirements, but the scope and frequency of monitoring will differ among trials. We, therefore, create plans and systems that are customized for the specific protocol. Where applicable, all nonstandard or trial-specific procedures are documented. Those *additional written plans and procedures or controlled systems* that determine how the trial-specific activities will be performed during the on-study and close-out phases describe:

- Monitoring – a description of the extent and nature of monitoring, and of how, when, by whom, and which monitoring activity is conducted. (Chapter 22 Monitoring Overview)
- Statistical analysis – a detailed description of the statistical methods and design of reports to be used for the trial analysis (Chapter 27 Study Design and Data Analysis)
- Safety reporting – a description of how, when, by whom, and which safety data will be collected, processed, and reported (Chapter 21 Safety Monitoring and Reporting)
- Data collection and processing – a description of how, when, by whom, and which trial data will be collected and processed (Chapter 20 Data Collection and Data Managements)
- Essential documents management – a description of how, when, by whom, and which essential documents will be collected and filed (Chapter 29 Essential Documents).
- Trial communication – a description of how, when, by whom, and which information will be transferred between and among the various functions involved in trial conduct, and how the communication is documented. The communication of the following type of trial information must be documented (Chapter 22 Monitoring Overview):
- Trial progress, e.g., trial subjects screened, administered the test article, or discontinued from the trial (Chapter 22 Monitoring Overview)
- Amendments to the trial protocol, e.g. the addition or removal of trial protocol procedures (Chapter 18 The Clinical Trial Protocol and Amendments)
- New information regarding the investigational article, e.g., new safety information (Chapter 16 The Investigator's Brochure)
- Changes to trial processes, e.g., how laboratory samples are shipped (Chapter 19 Informed Consent and Other Human Subject Protection)

- CRO/vendor management – a description of how, when, by whom, and which CRO/vendor activities will be evaluated and tracked. (Chapter 15 Trial Resourcing and Outsourcing)
- Specific instructions for clinical trial site personnel (Chapter 22 Monitoring Overview) – additional detailed instructions, which may be included in a single or topic-specific manual, for clinical trial site personnel regarding trial protocol procedures that are not described in the trial protocol; e.g.,
  - subject recruitment and screening instructions (Chapter 19 Informed Consent and Other Human Subject Protection)
  - pharmacy instructions for receiving, storing, preparing, and returning or destroying the investigational article (Chapter 17 The Investigational Product (Clinical Supplies))
  - laboratory instructions for collecting, processing, and shipping clinical specimens
  - case report form (CRF) instructions for completing the CRF, submitting data to the sponsor, and making corrections to trial data (Chapter 20 Data Collection and Data Management)
  - safety data reporting instructions (Chapter 21 Safety Monitoring and Reporting)
  - source data documentation – instructions, which may include templates, for trial staff at the investigator clinical site to record trial data that are collected contemporaneously with the trial protocol procedure (Chapter 20 Data Collection and Data Management)
- Training – a description of when training or re-training will take place and how the training will be documented (Chapter 32 Standard Operating Procedures; Chapter 15 Trial Resourcing and Outsourcing).
- Issue management – a description of how, when, by whom, and which issues will be addressed.
- Quality audit – a description of how, when, and by whom, which aspects of trial conduct will be systematically and independently examined (Chapter 33 Quality Assurance Components).
- Risk management – a description of anticipated risks and how, when, by whom, and which risk will be addressed (Chapter 13 Risk Assessment and Quality Management).

Regulatory items:

- We also note that GCP requires the availability of nonclinical data – data from biomedical studies performed on animals or in a laboratory setting and which support the proposed investigation in humans (see Chapter 16 The Investigator's Brochure). The creation of documents required *for submissions to* the regulatory authorities (see Chapter 5 Regulatory affairs) and/or to an ethics committee (see Chapter 24 Investigator/Institution Initiation) to support the clinical investigation include:

- IB – a compilation of the clinical and nonclinical data on the investigational product(s) that is relevant to the study of the investigational product(s) in human subjects (ICH E6(R2) 1.36). (Chapter 16 The Investigator's Brochure).
- Protocol– the document that describes the objective(s), design, methodology, statistical considerations, and organization of a trial (ICH E6(R2) 1.44). (Chapter 18 The Clinical Trial Protocol and Amendments)
- Informed consent forms – informed consent forms and other materials, including advertising, used to inform a potential study volunteer of all aspects of the trial that are relevant to the volunteer's decision to participate in the trial (ICH E6(R2) 1.28.) (Chapter 19 Informed Consent and Other Human Subject Protection)
- Other clinical, nonclinical, and CMC documents and information necessary for the regulatory authority(ies) application(s).

Clinical supplies (investigational and comparator product(s)):

- Manufacturing, packaging, labeling, and release of adequate supplies of the investigational product(s) and procurement of the comparator product(s) that conform to the specifications of the protocol and regulatory requirements (Chapter 17 The Investigational Product (Clinical Supplies))

Once the above prerequisites are in place, activities that are necessary to bring the trial to initiation may commence. The *GCP activities* that must be carried out prior to the initiation of a clinical trial are:

- Regulatory authority submission of notification/application of the intent to conduct a trial on humans with an investigational product (Chapter 5 Regulatory affairs)
- If necessary, the acquisition of import/export licenses, if necessary, for transportation of investigational product across borders (Chapter 17 The Investigational Product (Clinical Supplies))
- Trial personnel training on SOPs and trial protocol procedures and plans that are relevant to their function for executing the trial (Chapter 32 Standard Operating Procedures)
- CRO/vendor selection, contracting, qualification, and training (Chapter 15 Trial Resourcing and Outsourcing)
- Investigator/institution selection, contracting, and training (Chapter 23 Investigator/Institution Selection)
- Ethics committee submission of required trial documents and approval or favorable opinion of the trial (Chapter 8 IRB/IEC Roles and Responsibilities)

14.2.2.5.3 On-study Activities

Once the trial is initiated, focus is turned to those activities that involve executing the trial protocol procedures and ensuring that those procedures are conducted as per the protocol, GCP, applicable regulatory requirement(s), SOPs, and all trial-specific plans and procedures. On-study usually refers to the period between the consent of the first trial participant and the last visit of the last trial participant. The *activities* that occur during the trial are:

- *Trial Management:* Study leads continue to ensure the coordination and control of the trial resources, budget, and timelines. Change control will be implemented as necessary to continue to meet the protocol, GCP, regulatory, and business objectives of the trial. Study leads and those involved in making decisions for trial design and conduct should be mindful that changes to any single process are likely to have consequential effects on other processes. Consequential effects should be anticipated, considered, and controlled to ensure desirable outcomes. The trial operations plan, including plans for trial communication, should be updated as necessary and applicable staff trained on the procedures.
- *Resourcing:* All human and technical resources must continue to meet qualification requirements for the trial. Expired licensing and certifications must be renewed for staff, facilities, and equipment must be maintained. If any of these resources must change, potential replacements of CROs, trial staff, facilities, or equipment must be evaluated for qualification and suitability for compliance with trial, GCP, and regulatory requirements. (Chapter 15 Trial Resourcing and Outsourcing)
- *Training:* All new trial personnel who will be involved in trial conduct must be trained to perform his or her respective task(s). Retraining should also be conducted as necessary when there are changes to study processes or protocol procedures and/or when signals of noncompliance to required processes are evident. (see Chapter 33 Quality Assurance Components) Study manual(s) with instructions for study conduct should be updated as necessary and applicable staff trained on the procedures.
- *Clinical Supplies* (investigational and comparator product(s)): Adequate investigational product(s) and other clinical supplies will be shipped and/or made available to the investigator. The investigator will administer the investigational product(s) per the protocol and account for all used and used product(s). Pharmacy manual(s) with instructions for the storage, handling, preparation, administration, destruction, and return of used and unused supplies of investigational product(s) should be updated as necessary and applicable staff trained on the procedures. (Chapter 17 The Investigational Product (Clinical Supplies))
- *Laboratory Testing and Supplies:* Laboratories that will perform centralized testing or analysis of biological specimen or other laboratory testing media will be monitored for continued compliance with the protocol, GCP, and applicable regulatory and health requirements. Necessary collection and shipping supplies must be procured and provided to the investigator. Systems for tracking and reviewing laboratory samples and test results should also be monitored.

Laboratory manual(s) with instructions for the collection, preparation, storage, and shipping of specimen and media should be updated and applicable staff trained on the procedures. (Chapter19 Informed Consent and Other Human Subject Protection).

- *Key Trial Documents:* The clinical trial protocol, the IB, and informed consent form, and other regulatory documents must be updated as needed during the course of the trial to ensure that the design of the study and study procedures will meet study objectives, and new safety and other study information are appropriately communicated to investigators/institutions, regulatory authority(ies), IRBs/IECs, and research subjects. (Chapter 18 The Clinical Trial Protocol and Amendment; Chapter 16 The Investigator's Brochure; Chapter 19 Informed Consent and Other Human Subject Protection). Other trial procedure documents, such as a monitoring plan, safety management plan, and trial manual, laboratory manual, and the pharmacy manual, as described in this chapter for each activity, must be updated as necessary to provide current information and instructions to facilitate the conduct of a trial.

- *Human Subject Protection*: All entities and individuals participating in trial conduct will consider the safety, rights, and well-being of the research subject their first and foremost priority. The sponsor will select qualified investigators for the administration of the investigational product to the subjects and the provision of medical care for the research subjects. The investigator will ensure that the study has oversight by a duly constituted IRB/IEC, that trained and qualified individuals are handling and administering the investigational product, administering informed consent to research subjects, carrying out study protocol evaluations on research subjects, identifying and addressing adverse events, that subject rights are protected and their confidentiality is maintained. The sponsor is also responsible for continuous assessment of the risk versus benefit of the implemented trial, for protection of subject confidentiality, for overseeing all trial activities to ensure the overall protection of the research subjects. Research subjects will receive payments for study participation according to amounts and methods approved by the governing IRB/IEC. (Chapter 19 Informed Consent and Other Human Subject Protection),

- *Data Collection and Data Analysis:* The sponsor and investigator will collect and maintain trial data via validated systems with access control and audit trails and the data will be recorded and processed by qualified individuals. The investigator/institution will record study data to be maintained as source documentation and complete the sponsor's CRFs based on the source data. The sponsor will appropriately review and verify CRF data against the investigator's source documents and submit queries of incomplete or inaccurate data to the investigator for resolution. All changes to trial data must be traceable for who changed what data, and when, and why the data were changed. All persons handling trial data must follow ALCOAC principles to ensure the integrity and accuracy of the data.

If a trial has blinding or randomization properties, these procedures for randomization and blinding must be maintained to ensure integrity of the data. Instructions for source documentation and CRF completion, submission, and data corrections, and randomization and blinding as applicable, should be provided and applicable staff trained on the procedures. (Chapter 20 Data Collection and Data Management)

The statistical analysis plan should be updated if the trial analysis plan changes during the course of the conduct of the trial, e.g., as a result of changes to the study design in a protocol amendment. The statistical analysis plan must be finalized *a priori* to trial analysis. (Chapter 27 Study Design and Data Analysis).

- *Safety Data Collection, Monitoring, and Reporting:* The sponsor and investigator will comply with established procedures for the assessment and reporting of adverse events that occur during the course of the trial. The sponsor and investigator both have obligations for assessing and reporting adverse events identified as a result of administration of the investigational product and the subject's participation in the clinical trial. Investigators will collect, assess, and report safety events to the sponsor and to the IRB/IEC as required. In turn, the sponsor has obligations for reviewing reported safety information from individual sites and in aggregate for the entire trial and for all trials using the same investigational product. Sponsors will report safety events to the regulatory authority(ies) and to investigators using the investigational product, as required per applicable regulatory requirements. The safety management plan with instructions for the identification, assessment, and reporting of safety data should be updated as needed and applicable staff trained on the procedures. (Chapter 21 Safety Monitoring and Reporting).

  If an IDMC (Data and Safety Monitoring Board, Monitoring Committee, Data Monitoring Committee) is employed, trial management will ensure the convening of the Committee, provision of data to the Committee, and review of data and reporting of findings and/or recommendations by the Committee according to the Committee's Charter. The Charter may be updated as necessary during the study (Chapter 21 Safety Monitoring and Reporting).

- *Interim Monitoring:* The trial Sponsor has responsibility for overseeing the progress of a clinical trial, and of ensuring that it is conducted, recorded, and reported in accordance with the protocol, SOPs, GCP, and the applicable regulatory requirement(s). Qualified monitors will be engaged to perform the investigation on and/or off-site monitoring and the sponsor may also conduct centralized monitoring of the progress of the trial. The monitoring plan to guide the processes for monitoring of the specific trial may be updated as needed during the study (Chapter 25 Investigator/Institution Interim Monitoring), (ICH E6(R2) 5).

- *New Clinical Investigator/Institution Selection and Activation:* The sponsor may identify a need to select and add new investigators/institutions after the trial has commenced. At times, sponsors will select additional investigators/institutions prior to trial initiation as back-ups if additional sites are needed for the trial. Any investigator/institution that will be initiated once the trial has started must have been duly selected and initiated per the sponsor's SOPs (Chapter 23 Investigator/Institution Selection; Chapter 24 Investigator/Institution Initiation).

- *Site Contracting:* The sponsor and the investigator will update written contractual agreements between them and with others as needed. Written agreements must be executed for any new parties (investigators/institutions, CROs, and sub-contractors) that are introduced during trial conduct to perform trial-related duties or functions. (see Chapter 15 Trial Resourcing and Outsourcing).

- *Regulatory and Ethics Submission and Approval:* During the trial, changes to the scope of trial and updates on trial conduct will be submitted to the regulatory authority(ies) and to IRB/IECs by the sponsor and investigator, as applicable. An amended trial protocol may be implemented only after it has been approved by or has the favorable opinion of the governing IRB/IEC. Additionally, the review board or ethics committee will review the progress of the investigation based on information that the investigator is required to submit (see Chapter 8 IRB/IEC Roles and Responsibilities) to assess the risk versus benefit of the on-going investigation.

- *Quality Control and Quality Assurance:* The sponsor and investigator will follow established plans and procedures for monitoring and auditing the trial for ensuring quality control and quality assurance. All identified study conduct and protocol deviations will be addressed with corrective and preventive actions as applicable. SOPs to be followed during the trial will be identified and documented. Audit plans describing the timing and scope of trial audits will be updated as necessary during the trial. (see Chapter 25 Investigator/Institution Interim Monitoring, Chapter 33 Quality Assurance Components).

- *Sponsor and Clinical Investigator Files Maintenance:* As the saying goes, "If it is not documented, it did not happen!" All parties involved in trial conduct will follow established procedures for the collection and maintenance of trial essential documents. The sponsor will be maintaining the Trial Master File and the investigator/institution will maintain files at the clinical site. Trial essential documents may be transferred off-site for storage but must be readily available for trial monitoring, auditing, and inspections. The plan(s) describing the structure of the sponsor's trial master file and the investigator trial files, who is responsible for the submission and maintenance of what essential documents, timelines for submitting documents, and requirements for handling and storage of documents should be updated as necessary and applicable staff trained on the procedures. (see Chapter 29 Essential Documents)

14.2.2.5.4   The On-study Process

The on-study general *process* includes the following summary of activities:

- Recruit, consent, and retain trial participants (Chapter 19 Informed Consent and Other Human Subject Protection)
- Conduct routine monitoring (Chapter 22 Monitoring Overview)
- Collect, review, and verify data on the CRFs (Chapter 20 Data Collection and Data Managements)
- Collect, review, and verify data that are not collected via the CRFs but are required for reporting trial results (Chapter 20 Data Collection and Data Managements)
- Control and account for the investigational article (Chapter 22 Monitoring Overview, and Chapter 30 Quality Systems in Clinical Research; Chapter 17 The Investigational Product (Clinical Supplies))
- Report on trial progress (Chapter 5 Regulatory affairs; Chapter 8 IRB/IEC Roles and Responsibilities)
- Report safety events (Chapter 21 Safety Monitoring and Reporting)
- Manage CROs/vendors (Chapter 15 Trial Resourcing and Outsourcing)
- Provide new trial information to trial personnel and trial participants (Chapter 15 Trial Resourcing and Outsourcing)
- Control trial conduct and implement changes to trial conduct, as necessary (Chapter 22 Monitoring Overview; Chapter 30 Quality Systems in Clinical Research)
- Train new trial personnel/retrain trial personnel as needed (Chapter 30 Quality Systems in Clinical Research)
- Collect and maintain essential documents (Chapter 29 Essential Documents)
- Make payments to investigators, CRO's and other vendors (Chapter 15 Trial Resourcing and Outsourcing)
- Conduct quality oversight (Chapter 33 Quality Assurance Components)
- Manage issues and risks (Chapter 13 Risk Assessment and Quality Management)

14.2.2.5.5   End-study and Study Closeout Activities

After all trial data have been collected, focus is turned to those activities that involve ensuring that all trial processes and procedures are completed and all the documentation that reflect trial conduct are in place. Following up on our introductory analogy, the party is over. The guests are leaving, ensuring they have all their belongings, and the host is cleaning and tidying the venue, perhaps putting away the gifts, paying the bills, and sending thank-you notes or sharing pictures with guests. Similarly for a clinical trial, the investigators/institutions as guests are being closed out, ensuring all their files are in order, and the sponsor as the host cleans the trial data, ensures its files are in order, and submits a report of the trial to regulatory authority(ies) as applicable.

End-study usually refers to the period between the last visit or contact for the last subject who enrolled in the study (i.e., when all protocol trial data have been collected for the last enrolled subject in the study) and archiving of the trial. Investigator/ institution closeout usually refers to the final reconciliation of study activities and compilation and archiving of essential documents at the investigator's site and study closeout usually refers to the final reconciliation of study activities and compilation and archiving of the essential documents at all participating locations for the entire trial. Key milestone activities that occur during the end-study period include the collection of the last study data, locking the database, writing the CSR, and archiving essential trial documents. The activities that occur during the end-study phase are:

- *Trial Management:* Study leads will coordinate end-study and study closeout activities, ensuring completion per business objectives and compliance with GCP, the protocol, and applicable regulatory requirements.
- *Resourcing:* Documentation of the final administrative structure for the trial along with documentation of the change history will be retained with the essential documents for the trial. Qualification records for all staff, facilities, and equipment must be retained. Final reconciliation of finances and payments will be made to CROs and investigators/institutions and contracts will be terminated. (Chapter 15 Trial Resourcing and Outsourcing)
- *Training:* Training records for all trial personnel will be retained with the essential documents for the trial. Additionally, copies of training materials and/or descriptions of training content will be retained.(see Chapter 30 Quality Systems in Clinical Research)
- *Clinical Supplies* (investigational and comparator product(s)): All investigational product will have to be accounted for and reconciled for investigator and study closeout. For the investigator, we will be accounting for product received, used (administered or destroyed) and unused at the clinical site. The sponsor will be accounting for product shipped to investigator sites and returned to the sponsor. The full supply chain for investigational product, from shipment to sites through use at the sites and return to the sponsor should be reconciled. All final versions of the Pharmacy manual(s) with instructions for the storage, handling, preparation, administration, destruction, and return of used and unused supplies of investigational product(s) will be retained. (Chapter 17 The Investigational Product (Clinical Supplies))
- *Laboratory Testing and Supplies:* Laboratories that conducted centralized testing or analysis of biological specimen or other laboratory testing media will submit final testing results to the sponsor. Unused laboratory testing supplies should be destroyed as appropriate. Systems for tracking laboratory samples should also be reconciled and documentation retained in the essential documents. If laboratory samples must be traced for future use, then a system for their monitoring and maintenance must remain in place. Laboratory manual(s)

with instructions for the collection, preparation, storage, and shipping of speci-men and media will be retained. (Chapter 19 Informed Consent and Other Human Subject Protection).

- *Key Trial Documents:* All final versions of the clinical trial protocol, the IB, and informed consent form, and other regulatory documents must be retained in the essential documents. (Chapter 18 The Clinical Trial Protocol and Amendments; Chapter 16 The Investigator's Brochure; Chapter 19 Informed Consent and Other Human Subject Protection). Other trial procedure documents, such as a monitoring plan, safety management plan, and trial manual, laboratory manual, and the phar-macy manual, as described in this chapter for each activity, must also be retained.
- *Human Subject Protection*: All evidence of human subject protection, including administration of appropriate informed consent, protection of subject confidenti-ality, identification, assessment and reporting of adverse events, provision of nec-essary medical care, and any other evidence of communication with any research subject or with anyone on their behalf must be retained. Final payments to research subjects for study participation will be made and documentation of payments retained. (Chapter 19 Informed Consent and Other Human Subject Protection)
- *Data Collection and Data Analysis:* The end-study phase includes several activi-ties for preparing the data for presentation and analysis in the CSR. Once the sponsor has collected all CRF data and other annexed study data (such as labora-tory results) have been transferred to the sponsor, final review and queries occur to ensure the data are complete and accurate as verified by source documenta-tion. All data queries are addressed and the investigator and appropriate sponsor representatives will confirm in writing that the data are complete and accurate as collected. The database is then "locked" and data must not be changed there-after unless the change is absolutely necessary and justified. The data are then analyzed per the statistical analysis plan and data reports are used to prepare the CSR. All changes to trial data must be traceable for who changed what data, and when, and why the data were changed. All persons handling trial data must fol-low ALCOAC principles to ensure the integrity and accuracy of the data.

If a trial has blinding or randomization properties, unblinding of trial data will occur per the methods described in the statistical analysis plan and the proto-col. All documentation of treatment allocation and decoding will be maintained. Instructions for source documentation and CRF completion, submission, and data corrections, and randomization and blinding as applicable, will be retained as essential documents. (Chapter 20 Data Collection and Data Management)

The statistical analysis plan should have been final by the time of database lock. It will be used to analyze trial data. Any deviations from the plan will be noted in the CSR. Statistical reports (TFLs) will be produced for the analysis and presentation of the data in the CSR. (Chapter 27 Study Design and Data Analysis).

- *Safety Data Collection, Monitoring, and Reporting:* The sponsor and investigator will comply with established procedures for the assessment and reporting of adverse events that occur during the course of the trial. Safety data reported by the investigator (to the sponsor) and the sponsor (to the regulatory authorities) will be reconciled to ensure that all safety data are captured in the trial database. The investigator will be responsible for any outstanding follow-up of safety events beyond investigator/institution closeout. Events that are unresolved at the end of the trial will be noted as such; however, follow-up will continue as is necessary. The safety management plan with instructions for the identification, assessment, and reporting of safety data will be retained with essential documents. (Chapter 21 Safety Monitoring and Reporting).

  If an IDMC (Data and Safety Monitoring Board, Monitoring Committee, Data Monitoring Committee) is employed, the minutes of meetings and/or reports of data review will be retained along with the Charter with essential documents (Chapter 21 Safety Monitoring and Reporting).

- *Investigator/Institution Close-out:* All interim monitoring would have been completed by the time of database lock. The reports of interim and close-out monitoring and the monitoring plan will be retained as essential documents. (Chapter 22 Monitoring Overview, Chapter 25 Investigator/Institution Interim Monitoring, Chapter 26 Investigator/Institution Close-out).
- *New Clinical Investigator/Institution Selection and Activation:* The reports of investigator/institution selection and activation will be retained as essential documents. (Chapter 23 Investigator/Institution Selection; Chapter 24 Investigator/Institution Initiation).
- *Site Contracting:* The sponsor and the investigator will terminate all contracts, ensuring that provisions are made for post-study obligations. (see Chapter 15 Trial Resourcing and Outsourcing).
- *Regulatory and Ethics Submission and Approval:* Investigators will submit reports of final study status to the IRB/IECs and the sponsor will inform applicable regulatory authority(ies) of the same when the trial is completed. (see Chapter 8 IRB/IEC Roles and Responsibilities; Chapter 5 Regulatory Affairs).
- *Quality Control and Quality Assurance:* All CAPAs for protocol deviations and trial audits should be resolved and closed by the end of the trial. Protocol deviations and the outcomes of audits will be reported in the CSR. Audit certificates, and records of SOPs that were in effect for the entire trial and of personnel training will be retained as essential documents. (see Chapter 26 Investigator/Institution Close-out; Chapter 33 Quality Assurance Components).
- *Sponsor and Clinical Investigator Files Maintenance:* As the saying goes, "If it is not documented, it did not happen!" All essential documents will be retained per GCP and applicable regulatory requirements as evidence of study conduct. (see Chapter 29 Essential Documents)

14.2.2.6 The Study Close-Out Process

14.2.2.6.1 Purpose of Study Closeout

The goal of study closeout is to ensure the availability of evidence of the application of GCP principles and applicable regulations:

- **Subjects** were fully informed and that their rights and well-being were protected.
- The **data** to be submitted in support of the safety and effectiveness of a test article are appropriately recorded, verified, accurate, and complete
- **Compliance** with the protocol, regulations, and GCP principles.

14.2.2.6.2 Timing of Study Closeout

Study closeout occurs when:

- Study has met its enrollment goals and follow-up is complete
- All investigators/institutions participation have been closed
- The CSR is completed
- Notifications of study closure have been provided to IRB/IECs and regulatory authority(ies) as required
- The sponsor prematurely terminates the study for reasons such as:
  - Lack of enrollment
  - The results from an interim analysis:
    - The study has met its endpoints (e.g., achieved significant efficacy and safety results)
    - Lack of efficacy
    - Safety concerns
    - IMP manufacturing issues
    - Business or financial reasons
  - Other ethical or safety concerns
  - Other business reasons

Per ICH E6(R2) 8 Essential Documents, a final close-out of a trial can only be done when the monitor has:

- reviewed both investigator/institution and sponsor files
- confirmed that all necessary documents are in the appropriate files

End-study activities will start after the last visit or contact with the last trial participant. These activities are meant to prepare the data for analysis and reporting, and to ensure that all the evidence of trial conduct is available and archived. In practice, the general process for study closeout includes:

1) Clean data and prepare the database for data analysis (Chapter 20 Data Collection and Data Management)
2) Close clinical investigator sites (Chapter 26 Investigator/Institution Close-out)
3) Perform statistical analysis and generate reports of trial data (Chapter 27 Study Design and Data Analysis)

4) Write the CSR (Chapter 28 The Clinical Study Report)
5) Closeout the trial (See Section 14.2.2.6)
6) Archive trial records (Chapter 29 Essential Documents)

14.2.2.6.3 *Study Closeout Checklist*
The trial closeout checklist to be followed by the trial management and the trial conduct team includes the following (Plate 17 Study Closeout):

1) **Investigational Product**
   - All study drug from site returned or destroyed
   - All study drug are accounted for
   - Unused drug and study supplies are disposed, unless storage of samples required
2) **Investigators**
   - All sites are closed
   - All investigator obligations met, e.g. IRB/IEC reporting
   - All financial disclosures received
   - All sponsor audits completed
   - All final payments made to sites
3) **Data**
   - All CRFs are retrieved
   - All data are have been recorded
   - All queries have been resolved
   - All data are cleaned
   - All other data, e.g. lab data, received, and cleaned
   - All safety data are reconciled
   - All deviations are resolved/closed
   - The database is locked
4) All treatments are **unblinded** and sent to investigators
5) Perform **statistical analysis**
6) **Study Reports**
   - Data tables, figures, and listings are generated
   - Prepare and submit CSR
   - Note: All interim study reports and periodic reports, e.g. annual report, submitted
7) **Vendors**
   - All audits completed and any CAPAs are completed
   - All finances are reconciled and final payments are made
8) All biological specimens are accounted for and, if applicable, a system has been implemented system to track **biological specimen** for future use
9) **QA records**
   - Qualification of all personnel and vendors and training records are complete
   - Audits are completed and any CAPAs resolved
   - SOPs that governed the trial conduct are retained

10) Conduct **pre-inspection readiness** of sponsor and investigator essential documents
11) Host and respond to **regulatory inspections**
12) **Archive data and documents**
    - Sponsor's Trial Master File
    - Investigator's Site Files
    - Electronic systems documentation
13) Create or update information databases, e.g. contacts, regulatory intelligence
14) Evaluate "lessons learned"
15) Get ready for the next trial!

Note: The checklist is similar to Site Close-out (Plate 16 Investigator/Institution Closeout), except for the review of signed ICFs and source documents that must remain at the investigator to protect subject confidentiality.

14.2.2.6.4 *Archiving Essential Documents*
ICH E6(R2) 8 Essential Documents has specific requirements for the maintenance and retention of essential documents:

- The sponsor and investigator/institution should maintain a record of the **location(s)** of their respective essential documents
- The **storage** system (irrespective of the media used) should provide for document identification, search, and retrieval
- The sponsor should ensure that the **investigator has control of and continuous access to**
    - The **CRF data** reported to the sponsor. The sponsor should not have exclusive control of those data.
    - All **essential documents** and records generated by the investigator/institution before, during and after the trial.
    - Any or all of the documents may be subject to, and should be available for, audit by the sponsor's auditor and inspection by the regulatory authority(ies).

- Essential documents should be retained **until at least 2 years** after the last approval of a marketing application in an ICH region and until there are no pending or contemplated marketing applications . . . or at least 2 years have elapsed since the formal discontinuation of clinical development of the investigational product (ICH E6(R2) 4.9.5 (**Investigator**) Records and Reports)
- It is the responsibility of the sponsor to inform the investigator/institution as to when these documents no longer need to be retained (ICH E6(R2) 5.5.12).

14.2.3 Typical Issues in Trial Management

The issues that plague trial management are similar to those that plague the management of any project: finite time, finances, and pool of qualified personnel; the domino effect of implementing changes; and quality and compliance management.

Firms typically have business objectives for the timing of a new clinical trial, and if, done well, the initiation process of a trial takes time, lots of time. The time varies; however, depending largely on the trial phase, complexity of the protocol, trial site locations, and administrative processes. Metrics generated from data collected from past experience help in determining measures for duration; for example, earlier phase studies take less time to start up than later phase studies; clinical trial protocols requiring few routine and simple clinic procedures take less time to prepare for trial initiation than those that require numerous and more complex procedures; single-site trials take less time to get to first subject consent than multicenter trials; central or commercial ethics committees take less time than institutional ethics committees to review and provide feedback on a clinical trial submission; and so on. It is sensible, therefore, for trial Sponsors to know the expected duration for the initiation process for their trial and plan accordingly. Clinical trials with aggressive and unrealistic timelines typically suffer from poor quality outcomes and excessive consumption of time and resources.

Study leads are faced with the challenges of juggling time and resources while ensuring compliance with the protocol, regulatory requirements, GCP and the organization's SOPs. Also, given the nature of a clinical trial, i.e., a controlled experiment on human beings in real life setting versus, e.g., assembling a car in a manufacturing plant, changes in the process are inevitable and the domino effect of implementing a single change is a sneaky stealer of time and resources. The challenge is also to identify all the areas that are affected by the change. For example, if during a trial it was found that there is a need to reduce the drug to a new dose volume, this change could require reformulation and/or repackaging of the investigational article (Chapter 17 The Investigational Product (Clinical Supplies)), an amendment to the protocol (Chapter 18 The Clinical Trial Protocol and Amendments) and revisions to the IB and subject informed consent form (Chapter 16 The Investigator's Brochure; Chapter 19 Informed Consent and Other Human Subject Protection) with ethics and regulatory submissions and approval, updates to the pharmacy manual (Chapter 17 The Investigational Product (Clinical Supplies)), and possibly CRF, data collection, and query programming (Chapter 20 Data Collection and Data Management). In addition, all affected trial personnel would have to be notified of and/or be trained on the change. Such a change would require the study lead to track this subset of activities to ensure that they are all completed within the specified time that is determined by the organization as well as regulatory requirements. For any suggested change, consideration should be given to the domino effect the change has on key documents, study plans, personnel resources, timelines, and budget.

Quality and compliance management are essential for clinical trials. A sponsor is required to implement a system to manage quality throughout all stages of a trial process (ICH E6(R2) 5.0) (Chapter 13 Risk Assessment and Quality Management;

Chapter 31 Quality Responsibilities), and implement quality assurance and quality control systems with written SOPs to ensure that trials are conducted and data are generated, documented, (recorded), and reported in compliance with the protocol, GCP and the applicable regulatory requirement(s) (ICH E6(R2) 5.1.1). As many functions are involved in the design and conduct of a clinical trial, the study lead and other members of the cross-functional teams will face many occasions for decision-making for unanticipated scenarios that do not have associated written procedures for guidance. In such instances, decisions for trial conduct should always prioritize the safety, rights, and well-being of clinical research subjects above all other considerations for a clinical trial. Any considerations for regulatory, scientific, business, or other objectives are secondary. If there is a potential for harm to any research subject as a result of a decision to comply with regulatory requirements (e.g., complying with requirements of the protocol), other scientific, or business objectives (e.g., saving time or money), the decision should be modified in order to protect the research subject even if it means unfavorable consequences for regulatory compliance (e.g., a protocol deviation), or scientific or business objectives (e.g., losing time or money). The trial oversight and execution team will therefore always be mindful that *lack of time and resources is not an acceptable reason for lack of compliance.*

14.3 Summary

Competent and effective trial management is key to ensuring a compliant trial that meets business objectives. All personnel, facilities, and equipment used for a trial will be qualified for trial conduct. It is important to set up procedures and select qualified clinical trial personnel and facilities in the planning process to ensure high quality trial and cost-effective outcomes. The study lead will plan, organize, and control resources, ensuring effective and timely communication through the duration of the trial. A variety of functions and personnel are involved, numerous activities occur, and changes with multiple effects are likely to intervene. All functional representatives will be trained on trial procedures and be informed of any changes to the trial. Any outsourced trial activities must be supervised by the study lead or designee.

All of these factors must be managed to meet the business goals of the organization and regulatory and procedural requirements while always be mindful that *Lack of time and resources is not an acceptable reason for lack of compliance.*

Trial conduct can be divided into three stages:

- Trial initiation refers to the process between the decision to carry out a trial and the start of the trial as defined by the clinical trial protocol. The initiation process involves several activities, some of which are fixed and some that are variable or optional, and some of which are governed by regulatory requirements. The duration of the initiation process for clinical trials varies depending on the nature and location(s) of the trial and the administrative processes. Careful consideration should be given to the design of trial to ensure that it is scientifically and practically feasible. As the saying goes, *Nothing messes up a good plan on paper like putting people in it.* The most homework done at the outset, i.e., during the initiation process, will lay the foundation for an investigational plan and processes to best withstand or adapt to the inevitable breakdowns, failures, or glitches that are inherent to implementing a clinical trial.

- On-study refers to the process between trial initiation and the last visit for the last subject enrolled in the trial. Trial monitoring and oversight are the most important trial management activity during this stage of the trial.
- End-study and study closeout refer to the process between data cleaning and essential documents archiving. The objective during this phase is to ensure that all data are complete and accurately reflect trial results, to account for all trial materials and clinical supplies, and to complete business transactions, and to ensure that complete and accurate documentation of trial conduct are reflected in the essential documents.

The astute study lead may note that clinical trial activities are driven by investigator and sponsor responsibilities. To the responsibilities of these parties, we add the requirements of the study protocol. The sponsor's and investigator's qualifications and the qualification of their staff and equipment and facilities will be reviewed for their adequacy to carry out the responsibilities for the specific protocol. The executed results of these responsibilities are those which are reviewed for preparedness, which are monitored while they are being executed, and which are reviewed for completeness at the end of the trial. The final trial report is presenting the conduct of the trial and the results of the data analyses. The essential documents are the evidence of trial conduct, and without their existence, there was no trial.

Knowledge Check Questions

1) What is the GCP key point to trial management?
2) What are some of the sponsor functions involved in the conduct of a trial?
3) What are some of the investigator functions involved in the conduct of a trial?
4) What are the key milestones for a typical trial?
5) What is the purpose of trial management?
6) What are the key initiation activities for a clinical trial?
7) What are the key on-study activities for a clinical trial?
8) What are the key end-study activities for a clinical trial?

9) Overheard:

I am a Study lead. I do not need to track when the next Investigator's Brochure is due to the regulatory authority.

Comment and discuss:

a) Which function may responsible for tracking the due date for updates to the Investigator's Brochure (IB)?

b) What are some advantages to the study lead knowing when the next IB is due?

Reference

1 International Council for Harmonisation of Technical Requirements for Pharmaceuticals for Human Use (ICH), Integrated Addendum to ICH E6(R1):Guideline for Good Clinical Practice, E6(R2) (2016). Current Step 4 version dated 9 November 2016. https://www.ich.org/page/efficacy-guidelines

15

Trial Resourcing and Outsourcing

Karen A. Henry

GCP Key Point
Each individual involved in conducting a trial should be qualified by education, training, and experience to perform his or her respective task(s). (ICH E6(R2) 2.8) [1]

15.1   Introduction

When sponsors and investigators consider conducting a clinical trial, they first have to determine how they will resource the personnel and facilities that they will need. These resources must also be qualified to comply with the clinical trial protocol, GCP, and applicable regulatory requirements.

The sponsor's Trial Administrative Structure names the individuals and establishments that carry out trial procedures (Chapter 28 The Clinical Study Report). The sponsor may choose to use only employees and its own systems to perform all sponsor-related activities or outsource some or all activities to one or more Contract Research Organizations (CROs). A CRO is a person or an organization (commercial, academic, or other) contracted by the sponsor to perform one or more of a sponsor's trial-related duties and functions (ICH E6(R2) 1.20). The CRO will assume all regulatory responsibility(ies) for the contracted activity(ies), while the sponsor maintains responsibility for oversight of CRO activities to ensure overall protection of the research subjects, data quality, and compliance.

The investigator will maintain a list of appropriately qualified persons to whom the investigator has delegated significant trial-related duties; e.g., Signature Sheet/ Delegation of Responsibility Log (Chapter 9 Investigator and Sponsor Roles and Responsibilities). The investigator may have sub-investigators and other staff

The Fundamentals of Clinical Research: A Universal Guide for Implementing Good Clinical Practice, First Edition. P. Michael Dubinsky and Karen A. Henry.
Companion website: www.wiley.com/go/dubinsky/clinicalresearch

members who are performing different types of study assessments at the clinical site. Additionally, the investigator may subcontract trial activities (e.g., to a local laboratory), and the investigator may also engage "satellite" clinical sites; i.e., more than one location where subjects are treated and trial-related activities are actually conducted. Unlike the sponsor, the named principal investigator maintains full regulatory responsibilities for all trial activities across all satellite site locations and subcontractors.

Both sponsors and investigators will ensure that all individuals involved in performing activities for a clinical trial must be qualified by education, training, and experience to perform his or her respective task(s). Furthermore, all systems and facilities (e.g., electronic systems, CROs, laboratories, and pharmacies) must also be qualified and certified per protocol, GCP, and applicable regulatory requirements.

In this chapter, we will review considerations, responsibilities, and processes involved in resourcing and outsourcing trial-related activities.

15.2 Objectives

The objectives of this chapter are:

1) Describe general considerations for resourcing and outsourcing trial activities
2) Define sponsor responsibilities for resourcing a clinical trial
3) Define investigator responsibilities for resourcing a clinical trial
4) Describe processes for CRO selection
5) Describe processes for CRO contracting
6) Describe processes for CRO management
7) Describe Quality by Design Considerations for resourcing and outsourcing

15.2.1 General Considerations for Resourcing and Outsourcing Trial Activities

Several factors may be considered when a sponsor or investigator is determining whether to outsource any trial-related activity(ies). Among the factors for a sponsor or investigator to consider are:

1) Location of trial-related activities based on their role:
   - The sponsor's role in a clinical trial is to take responsibility for the initiation, management, and/or financing of a clinical trial (ICH E6(R2) 1.53). Due to the nature of the sponsor's role, trial-related activities may be conducted from multiple and varied locations, given the communication advantages provided by technology. For example, a trial manager, sponsor medical monitor, data managers and systems for data management, the biostatistician, an individual

responsible for communication with the regulatory authorities, central laboratories, etc. may all be in different locations. The sponsor may therefore outsource up to all of its trial-related responsibilities.

- The investigator's role in a clinical trial is to recruit the appropriate study subjects to whom the investigator will administer the investigational product and to provide medical care to the study subjects. The investigator is responsible for the conduct of the clinical trial at a trial site (ICH E6(R2) 1.34). Due to the nature of the investigator's role in the clinical trial, trial-related activities are generally centered around the research subject being seen at a clinical site. It may be impractical and potentially unsafe for the subject to be consented, administered investigational product, monitored, and undergo study testing at multiple and varied locations. The investigator may therefore outsource some to none of their trial-related activities, depending on the ability to safely and validly carry out study procedures away from the investigator clinical site.

2) Requirements for qualifications of personnel and facilities:
Careful consideration will have to be given for the qualification of personnel and facilities used to execute trial activities. The sponsor or investigator will assign trial-related duties to only those individuals who are qualified by education, training, and experience and to facilities that are qualified and certified to meet protocol, GCP, and other applicable regulatory requirements.

3) Business objectives:
Subject safety, data integrity, and compliance are the foremost concerns for all involved in planning, initiating, and managing a clinical trial. However, factors of financing and timelines to meet business objectives are realistic constraints. The sponsor will generally be financing the cost of the clinical trial while both the sponsor and investigator will be concerned with meeting timeline goals.

4) Control of quality:
Those evaluating the pros and cons of resourcing and outsourcing should also consider the degree of control that is enabled by the spectrum of no to full outsourcing. Any outsourcing of sponsor responsibilities or of investigator study activities will ensure subject safety, data integrity, and compliance. Resources, e.g., technology, may allow for outsourcing of a variety of trial activities. When activities are outsourced, resources are needed for communication and oversight to ensure compliance as logistical issues may alter the effectiveness of communication and oversight.

When trial-related activities are in multiple and varied locations, the complexity and financial, time, and quality costs for communication and movement of persons and materials should be considered when deciding on the infrastructure for trial conduct. It is expected that additional human and other resources would enhance communication, collaboration, access, oversight, and overall quality for a clinical trial.

15.2.2 Sponsor Responsibilities for Resourcing a Clinical Trial

The sponsor may use all inhouse resources or choose to outsource all its trial-related duties. A sponsor's key responsibilities regarding identifying resources for a clinical trial are:

1) The sponsor should utilize appropriately qualified individuals to supervise the overall conduct of the trial, to handle the data, to verify the data, to conduct the statistical analyses, and to prepare the trial reports (ICH E6(R2) 5.5.1).
2) A sponsor may transfer any or all of the sponsor's trial-related duties and functions to a CRO, but the ultimate responsibility for the quality and integrity of the trial data always resides with the sponsor (ICH E6(R2) 5.2.1).
3) Any trial-related duty and function that is transferred to and assumed by a CRO should be specified in writing (ICH E6(R2) 5.2.2). Note that any trial-related duty or function that is not specified in writing with a CRO is presumed to be the responsibility of the sponsor (ICH E6(R2) 5.2.3).
   a) The CRO should implement quality assurance and quality control for its assumed trial-related functions and duties (ICH E6(R2) 5.2.1; (Chapter 31 Quality Responsibilities).
   b) The CRO will follow all GCP and regulatory requirements that apply to a sponsor to the extent that a CRO has assumed the trial related duties and functions of a sponsor (ICH E6(R2) 5.2.4).
4) The sponsor should ensure oversight of any trial-related duties and functions carried out on its behalf, including trial-related duties and functions that are subcontracted to another party by the sponsor's contracted CRO(s) (ICH E6(R2) 5.2.2).

15.2.3 Investigator Responsibilities for Resourcing a Clinical Trial

An investigator's key obligations regarding identifying resources for a clinical trial are:

1) The investigator(s) should be qualified by education, training, and experience to assume responsibility for the proper conduct of the trial, should meet all the qualifications specified by the applicable regulatory requirement(s), and should provide evidence of such qualifications through up-to-date curriculum vitae and/or other relevant documentation requested by the sponsor, the IRB/IEC, and/or the regulatory authority(ies) (ICH E6(R2) 4.1.1).
2) The investigator should be thoroughly familiar with the appropriate use of the investigational product(s), as described in the protocol, in the current Investigator's Brochure, in the product information, and in other information sources provided by the sponsor. (ICH E6(R2) 4.1.2).
3) The investigator should be aware of, and should comply with, GCP and the applicable regulatory requirements. (ICH E6(R2) 4.1.3).

4) The investigator/institution should permit monitoring and auditing by the sponsor, and inspection by the appropriate regulatory authority(ies). (ICH E6(R2) 4.1.4).

5) The investigator should maintain a list of appropriately qualified persons to whom the investigator has delegated significant trial-related duties. (ICH E6(R2) 4.2.4).

6) The investigator should ensure that all persons assisting with the trial are adequately informed about the protocol, the investigational product(s), and their trial-related duties and functions. (ICH E6(R2) 4.1.5).

7) The investigator should be able to demonstrate (e.g., based on retrospective data) a potential for recruiting the required number of suitable subjects within the agreed recruitment period. (ICH E6(R2) 4.2.1).

8) The investigator should have sufficient time to properly conduct and complete the trial within the agreed trial period. (ICH E6(R2) 4.2.2).

9) The investigator should have available, an adequate number of qualified staff and adequate facilities for the foreseen duration of the trial to conduct the trial properly and safely. (ICH E6(R2) 4.2.3).

10) The investigator should ensure that all persons assisting with the trial are adequately informed about the protocol, the investigational product(s), and their trial-related duties and functions. (ICH E6(R2) 4.2.4).

11) The investigator is responsible for supervising any individual or party to whom the investigator delegates trial-related duties and functions conducted at the trial site. (ICH E6(R2) 4.2.5).

12) A qualified physician (or dentist, when appropriate), who is an investigator or a sub-investigator for the trial, should be responsible for all trial-related medical (or dental) decisions. (ICH E6(R2) 4.2.6).

13) If the investigator/institution retains the services of any individual or party to perform trial-related duties and functions, the investigator/institution should ensure that this individual or party is qualified to perform those trial-related duties and functions and should implement procedures to ensure the integrity of the trial-related duties and functions performed and any data generated. (ICH E6(R2) 4.3.1).

The investigator/institution and the sponsor will ensure that the investigator/institution/subcontractor(s) meets all of the above requirements.

15.2.4   Processes for CRO Selection

As mentioned above, a CRO is a person or an organization (commercial, academic, or other) contracted by the sponsor to perform one or more of a sponsor's trial-related duties and functions (ICH E6(R2) 1.20). Vendors that are used to supply materials or services that are not regulated; i.e., the materials or services do affect trial data or the safety of research subjects, are usually not considered CROs. For example, the sponsor may purchase data-entry systems from a vendor, but the sponsor is responsible for ensuring that the systems meet GCP and regulatory requirements for data entry, processing, and storage.

The process for CRO selection in practice is similar to selection of a clinical trial site. The general steps are:

1) Determine a set of criteria that the **CRO** must meet to be selected.
   The selection criteria are based on:
   a) Trial protocol requirements.
      Will the CRO be able to perform the contracted duty per the study protocol? For example, for a CRO who will monitor the trial, are the monitors qualified by training and experience to review the site activities that are specific to the study protocol? For example, do they have GCP training, are they familiar with the therapeutic area under study? Are they able to adequately communicate (i.e., common language, no logistical hindrances) with the site personnel?
   b) GCP and regulatory requirements.
      Will the CRO be able to perform the contracted duty per GCP and applicable regulatory requirements? For example, does the CRO performing data management use electronic data processing systems that comply with requirements for electronic systems and electronic signatures (ICH E6(R2) 5.5.3)?
   c) Business objectives.
      Will the CRO be able to perform the contracted duty to meet the budget, timelines, and other business objectives?

   The sponsor may evaluate the details for each of the above criteria as needed.

2) Identify potentially appropriate CROs to narrow the pool to a few to request bids.
   The sponsor will use the specified criteria to identify potentially appropriate CROs. Referrals for CROs may come from previous experience, networking, public searches, or other means.
3) Provide the few potential CROs with study information and specifications for the outsourced activity in a Request for Proposal (RFP) in order to obtain their bids.
   The sponsor will prepare an RFP to submit to the CRO. The RFP will contain study information and specifications for the activity(ies) to be contracted so the sponsor should ensure that an agreement of confidentiality is in place between the sponsor and the CRO before providing study information to the CRO.
   The CRO will complete the RFP, including a description of their procedures and systems for completing the activity(ies), number and qualifications of personnel to be assigned to the activity(ies), and estimated timelines and cost for the contracted activity(ies). The CRO will also describe the above for any duties or functions that will they will subcontract to a third party. CRO representatives

may also meet with the sponsor to present their processes and procedures and describe how they may accomplish the potentially contracted activity(ies).

4) Review the bids to identify candidates for on-site review/audit.

The sponsor will review all information collected from and about the CROs and identify 1 or 2 for on-site review or audit of the CRO's personnel, systems, operating procedures, and facilities, as applicable. The on-site review or audit (sometimes referred to as a qualification audit) may be completed by sponsor personnel or independent contractors, who will visit the CRO and any other subcontractors.

5) Select a final CRO based on the set of selection criteria.

The sponsor will select a CRO for final contracting.

15.2.5 Processes for CRO Contracting

It is best practice for the sponsor to create a matrix of responsibilities that identifies all trial activities and the responsible party(ies) for each trial activity based on the sponsor's functions (Plate 4 Individual Clinical Trial – Overview of Investigator and Sponsor Responsibilities; Chapter 14 Trial Management; Start-up, On-Study, and Close-Out). This Trial Matrix of Responsibilities may be used as the basis for developing the contract for each outsourced activity. The sponsor's written contract with an individual CRO will include:

1) A scope of work that specifies any trial-related duty and function that is transferred to and assumed by a CRO and any subcontractors (ICH E6(R2) 5.2.2). We note that any trial-related duty or function that is not specified in writing with a CRO is presumed to be the responsibility of the sponsor (ICH E6(R2) 5.2.3) so the descriptions of transferred duties and functions should be detailed enough such that there is no ambiguity of the ownership of tasks.

2) Requirements for access to study data and other study information. The sponsor is responsible for securing agreement from all involved parties to ensure direct access to all trial related sites, source data/documents, and reports for the purpose of monitoring and auditing by the sponsor, and inspection by domestic and foreign regulatory authorities (ICH E6(R2) 5.1.2).

3) Matrix of responsibilities for each type of activity. The matrix will present the deliverables for the scope of work and the responsible party for each identified deliverable; for example, for outsourced data management, the CRO may draft the CRF, but the sponsor reviews and approves it. The deliverable in this case is a final CRF. Deliverables will most often be an essential document; for example, the final interim monitoring report for a site visit if this activity is outsourced (Chapter 29 Essential Documents; Chapter 25 Investigator/Institution Interim Monitoring).

4) Timelines for deliverables. The due date or milestone for each deliverable should be specified.

5) Conditions for deliverables. The sponsor and the CRO should agree on the status or conditions of each deliverable; for example, draft or final version, or accepted final version of the deliverable.

6) Financial arrangements include a schedule of when, how, and how much will be paid for deliverables; for example, payment will be made upon the sponsor's acceptance of a final interim monitoring report.

7) Determination of standard operating procedures (SOPs) to be followed for the trial. The sponsor and the CRO will review SOPs that pertain to the contracted activity(ies) across both parties to determine which SOPs will be followed for the contracted activity(ies). The parties may choose to follow the CRO's SOPs, the sponsor's SOPs, or a combination selected from both. The final set of SOPs, and any revisions to the selection of SOPs or to the individual SOPs, will be documented, shared as necessary, and trained on by applicable personnel.

8) Changes to scope of work; i.e., how changes to the agreed scope of work, including changes in personnel, systems, and facilities, will be notified and handled.

9) Other instructions and contractual requirements as needed.

15.2.6 Processes for CRO Management

The sponsor should ensure oversight of any trial-related duties and functions carried out on its behalf by contracted CRO(s), including trial-related duties and functions that are subcontracted to another party by the sponsor's contracted CRO(s) (ICH E6(R2) 5.2.2). This oversight means constant and careful monitoring of CRO activities and deliverables.

To enable clear communication and expectations for oversight, it is helpful practice to prepare and follow an SOP and/or plan for managing CRO(s). An SOP may outline instructions for managing any CRO and a trial-specific CRO Management/Oversight Plan may contain information that applies to the specific trial. The Trial Matrix of Responsibilities mentioned above may be used as the basis for developing the CRO Management/Oversight Plan. In addition to the Matrix, the Plan will include contact lists and methods and flow of communication for e.g., timing and hosting team meetings, reporting study status, criteria, and procedures for issue escalation.

15.2.7 Quality by Design Considerations for Resourcing and Outsourcing

A number of principles and operational considerations that promote GCP, quality, and compliance may facilitate subject compliance with the trial requirements. Sponsors should focus on trial activities essential to ensure human subject protection and the reliability of trial results. Quality management includes the design of efficient clinical trial protocols and tools and procedures for data collection and processing, as well as the collection of information that is essential to decision-making. (ICH E6(R2) 5.0). Study protocol design and trial operations considerations to foster trial resourcing and outsourcing by the sponsor and investigator include ensuring that:

- A trial protocol is scientifically sound and financially and logistically feasible without having the potential to compromise resources for ensuring the protection of research subjects, data integrity, and compliance with the protocol, GCP, and applicable regulatory requirements
- Resources are reviewed for qualification prior to trial start up and throughout the course of the trial
- All requirements for outsourced activity(ies) are outlined in a written agreement
- Resources are available and plans/instructions are established to oversee any outsourced activity

A sponsor or investigator should not undertake the responsibilities for sponsoring and/or investigating a clinical trial if it cannot assure having adequate resources for the entire planning, duration, and closeout of a trial. Trials are sometimes terminated or suffer from chronic noncompliance due to shortage or exhaustion of resources. These circumstances may endanger subject safety and may also result in unethical termination of potentially effective treatment for the subjects in the trial. A trial should therefore be initiated and continued only if the anticipated benefits justify the risks, including considerations for resourcing the trial's execution.

15.3   Summary

The success of a clinical trial depends not only on the scientific design of the protocol but also on the resources that are attributed to the trial by both the sponsor and investigator(s). Due to the nature of their respective roles, a sponsor may outsource up to all of its trial-related functions and duties but an investigator retains up to all of its trial-related functions and duties. The sponsor will transfer its GCP and regulatory obligations in a written agreement to CRO(s) that assume trial-related functions and duties from a sponsor but the sponsor maintains GCP and regulatory responsibility for oversight of the CRO(s) to ensure human subject protection and the reliability of trial results. The investigator, on the other hand, maintains oversight and full GCP and regulatory responsibility for all trial-related functions and duties that are delegated to other individuals or party(ies) and will document the roles and names of individuals or party(ies) and their assigned responsibilities. All parties will ensure that they have adequate and qualified resources to ensure the protection of subjects rights, safety, well-being, data integrity, and trial compliance with the protocol, GCP, and applicable regulatory requirements.

Knowledge Check Questions

1) What are some general considerations for resourcing and outsourcing trial activities?
2) What are the responsibilities of a sponsor for trial resourcing?
3) What are the responsibilities of an investigator for trial resourcing?
4) What are some of the differences between the responsibilities of the sponsor and the investigator for resourcing their trial-related duties and functions?
5) What are the elements in a contract between a sponsor and CRO?
6) What are the procedures for managing a CRO?
7) What are some quality-by-design principles that apply to trial resourcing?
8) Overheard:

The CRO will not provide a copy of the trial master file structure because they said it is their proprietary information.

Manager for the Trial Master File (TMF) at a sponsor when asked for a copy of the TMF structure during an audit by an independent auditor engaged by the sponsor. The sponsor had outsourced the maintenance of the TMF to a CRO. Comment and discuss:

a) What GCP requirement is violated in this scenario?
b) What are potential issues with the sponsor's contracting terms with the CRO?
c) How may the sponsor resolve and prevent the issues with the CRO?

Reference

1 International Council for Harmonisation of Technical Requirements for Pharmaceuticals for Human Use (ICH), Integrated Addendum to ICH E6(R1):Guideline for Good Clinical Practice, E6(R2) (2016). Current Step 4 version dated 9 November 2016. https://www.ich.org/page/efficacy-guidelines

16

The Investigator's Brochure

Karen A. Henry

GCP Key Point

Before a trial is initiated, foreseeable risks and inconveniences should be weighed against the anticipated benefit for the individual trial subject and society. A trial should be initiated and continued only if the anticipated benefits justify the risks. (Source: ICH E6(R2) 2.2 [1])

16.1   Introduction

The investigator's brochure (IB) is the precursor to the product label: Everything that is known about the investigational product to date to justify the use of the investigational product in humans and to provide the investigator with sufficient information to make decisions about administration of the product and medical care for research subjects is in the IB. Regulatory authorities require that the user of any medicinal product, investigational or approved, be provided with some minimal information for safe and effective use of the product.

You may be familiar with a label that accompanies a medicinal product that has been approved by the health regulatory authority for marketing or distribution to the public. This label, whether for a product that requires a prescription from an authorized health-care provider or for an over-the-counter product that can be obtained without a prescription, contains some minimal information about the product, such as, active ingredients, inactive ingredients, for what it is indicated, its dosage and dosage form, what precautions should be taken before or during its use, and what side effects are possible.

The Fundamentals of Clinical Research: A Universal Guide for Implementing Good Clinical Practice, First Edition. P. Michael Dubinsky and Karen A. Henry.
Companion website: www.wiley.com/go/dubinsky/clinicalresearch

However, prior to the approval of a product, a brochure will be the repository for such information for the product while it is in its investigational stage for use in clinical trials. This IB will contain similar information based on what is known of the product properties and results of all pertinent non-clinical and clinical studies accumulated up to any point in time. The IB will provide the clinical investigator or investigative health care provider the information they need to maximize safe, and if known, effective, use of the investigational product in clinical research participants. This information may also be used by the sponsor and others involved in the design and development of a protocol and subject informed consent documents.

16.2   Objectives

The objectives of this chapter are:

1) Define an IB
2) Describe the purpose of an IB
3) Describe the context of an IB in a clinical trial and in clinical development
4) Describe the contents of an IB
5) Describe the process for developing an IB
6) To discuss updates to an IB
7) Describe quality-by-design considerations for an IB

16.2.1   Definition of an Investigator's Brochure

The investigator's brochure (IB) is a compilation of the clinical and nonclinical data on the investigational product(s) that is relevant to the study of the investigational product(s) in human subjects (ICH E6(R2) 1.36).

In a case where formal preparation of an IB is impractical, the sponsor should provide, as a substitute, an expanded background information section in the trial protocol that contains the minimum current information (ICH E6(R2) 7.1). A sponsor may refer to an approved product label instead of an IB for use of a product in a clinical trial per its approved product label (e.g., for a comparator product).

16.2.2   Purpose of an Investigator's Brochure

The purpose of an IB is to provide investigators and others involved in the trial with information to facilitate their understanding of the rationale for, and their compliance with, many key features of the protocol, such as the dose, dose frequency/interval, methods of administration, and safety monitoring procedures. The IB also provides insight to support the clinical management of the study subjects during the course of the clinical trial. (ICH E6(R2) 7.1).

Although known as the "investigator's" brochure, the IB will be used by many involved in the design and conduct of a clinical trial:

- Regulatory authority(ies) and ethics committees will review the IB prior to the initiation of a trial to assess the benefit-risk for the use of the investigational product in human subjects
- Regulatory authority(ies) and ethics committees will review updated IBs to continuously assess the benefit-risk for the continued use of the investigational product in human subjects
- Clinical trial investigator(s) will also use the IB for the benefit-risk assessment of the investigational product. Furthermore, the investigator(s) will use the IB as their source for learning of the CMC properties, and safety and efficacy profiles of the investigational product for application during a clinical trial and to guide their handling and administration of the investigational product to trial subjects and for making medical care decisions in the event of adverse events.
- The sponsor will use information contained in the IB as the basis for the rationale for the new or continued development of the investigational product in new or amended study protocols. The IB will help guide the design of new studies or changes to studies.
- The IB is used as a source by those involved in trial conduct and review for the development and evaluation of other trial documents and procedures; e.g., informed consent documents, budgets, pharmacy procedures.

16.2.3   Context for an Investigator's Brochure in a Clinical Trial and in Clinical Development

The following concepts apply to the context of an IB in clinical research:

1) The IB is essentially the pre-cursor to an approved product label.
   The goal of the development program for an investigational product is to collect data to allow the evaluation of the safety and efficacy of the product for approval for marketing the product. The IB and an approved product label serve similar purposes: to provide the clinician and others using the product for the specified indication(s) with relevant CMC, safety, and efficacy information. As the sponsor conducts individual trials in the development program according to its target product profile, CMC, clinical, and non-clinical information build and accumulate in the IB that will be used for the generation of the product label. An IB is the document with this information while the product is investigational and a product label is the document once the product is approved. The information in an IB is selected and organized with this goal in mind.

2) The IB applies to multiple trials for at least one indication.

Unlike a clinical trial protocol that is created for each trial in a development program, a single IB is created to support several trials in the program and it contains integrated and cumulative information for the multiple trials in the program.

The sponsor will create the first IB (usually for a specific product and for one indication) to include CMC, available non-clinical information, and available clinical information (perhaps of the class of product) that are relevant to and that support the investigational product's use in the first clinical trial in the clinical development program of the product. The IB will then be updated as new relevant information become available during the course of the first trial and at the end of the first trial, and similarly for subsequent trials conducted in the clinical development of the product.

3) The IB may contain multiple indications.

Information for new indications with the same investigational product may be presented in a single IB. As the IB is the precursor to the approved label for a product, it is advisable to group indications that have similar clinical characteristics or are in the same therapeutic area. For example, separate IBs would be created for a product that is used to treat asthma and lung cancer; however, a single IB may contain information for a product that is used to treat lung cancer, melanoma, and other cancers. As the IB will summarize safety and efficacy information for each trial and for all trials combined, the grouping should be logical for the integration and evaluation of safety and efficacy data within the IB and for the eventual purposes of the approved product label.

4) The IB is used by a variety of players for several types of product evaluation.

Information in the IB is used by regulatory authority(ies), ethics committees, investigator(s), and sponsors to evaluate the benefit-risk use of an investigational product in a proposed trial, for continued assessment during a trial, and for oversight of the entire development program. The investigator also uses the IB as a guide for handling and administration of the investigational product and for clinical management of the subject who is receives the investigational product. An IB user will receive all information relevant to the use of the investigational product covered by the IB. If an IB user is not privy to all IBs for an investigational product, they should also be informed of events that may be relevant across multiple IBs for the same investigational product. For example, safety events that occur in a trial for one indication covered by the IB (let's say, melanoma) will be assessed for its relevance to all subjects within the trial, as well as to subjects receiving the investigational product for another indication covered by the same IB (let's say, lung cancer). Events for an investigational product that is used across multiple unrelated indications (let's say, asthma and lung cancer, for which there are separate IBs) should also be considered for their relevance across the various IBs.

5) The IB should be reviewed at least annually.

   The IB must be reviewed at least annually to ensure that information is current (ICH E6(R2) 7.1). The sponsor will ensure that the IB contains the most currently available data that support the clinical research use of the product for specified indication(s). The current information in the IB must support the current application of the investigational product in human subjects.

   The IB is a live document that is updated as new and relevant information about the investigational product for the studied indication(s) becomes available, depending on the stage of development and the generation of relevant new information.

   The sponsor will collect and update the IB with relevant:

   - Information from all clinical investigators using the product
   - Non-clinical trial information that is relevant to human subject application
   - Published information about the product or its class
   - Chemistry, manufacturing, and controls (CMC) properties of the product

   Important safety information for an investigational product that is known prior to its inclusion in an updated IB must be immediately provided to regulatory authority(ies), ethics committees, and investigators to ensure that they have the most currently available information (Chapter 21 Safety Monitoring and Reporting). This information will be added to the next IB update.

   Completed and ongoing studies will be identified as such. When data from studies are preliminary and have not yet been verified, such status of the data will be explained in the IB. Data from ongoing blinded studies will be included only if the data are informative to determine benefit-risk and patient management since the association with the investigational product is unknown.

6) IB information will align with other documents.

   Many regulatory and clinical trial documents contain information that are repeated or presented in alternative formats across the documents, depending on the purpose of the document and its audience. IB information should not contradict, although it may have more or less, information in other regulatory and clinical trial documents:

   - The clinical trial protocol (Chapter 18 The Clinical Trial Protocol and Amendments) will summarize necessary information from the IB and refer the reader to the IB for details; e.g., for details of CMC and results of toxicology studies.
   - The informed consent form (Chapter 19 Informed Consent and Other Human Subject Protection) will contain summarized risks and benefits in language understandable to the trial volunteer.
   - Regulatory submissions that summarize benefits and risks, CMC, and clinical and non-clinical information must align with data in the IB, or be explained
   - The IB should not contradict data in summary data safety data sheets, marketing approvals, unless they are explained

7) The IB must contain unbiased information.

Information in the IB must be factual and complete, and may not convey scientifically or statistically unsubstantiated claims regarding the safety and/or efficacy of the investigational product. The sponsor will present favorable and unfavorable results for all relevant trials for the covered indication(s).

16.2.4   Contents of an Investigator's Brochure

The IB contains a variety of information about the investigational product. The type and degree of details for the different types of information contained in the IB will depend on the stage of the development of the investigational product; for example,

a) During early phase development (phase 1 and early phase 2), less is known about the product's stability properties, more is known about the product's non-clinical profile, less may be known of its clinical safety, and perhaps none known of its efficacy profile.

b) During later phase development (later phase 2 and phase 3), more is known about the product's stability properties, substantially more should be known of its safety profile, and at least preliminary efficacy information should be available.

c) For use of the product in phase 4 studies, an approved product label is available so the label may be referenced in lieu of the IB.

NOTE: An up-to-date IB must be provided when the product is used for investigational purposes in a clinical trial; i.e., for any use that has not been approved by the regulatory authority governing the location of use. The IB will contain supporting non-clinical and clinical information to enable a benefit-risk assessment of the appropriateness of the proposed investigational use(s) of the product in humans.

The information should be presented in a concise, simple, and objective, balanced, and nonpromotional form that enables a clinician, or potential investigator to understand it and make his/her own unbiased benefit-risk assessment of the appropriateness of the proposed trial (ICH E6(R2) 7.1).

The ICH E6(R2) 7 outlays minimum information that should be included in an IB and provides suggestions for the format of the IB. Although the section numbering is provided as a guidance, it is used as much as possible so that investigators and other IB users may readily access information that they need, sometimes with urgency. The suggested format and structure are as follows (Plate 9 Investigator's Brochure – Contents):

16.2.4.1   Title Page

The title page will allow the users of the IB to identify the investigational product and indication(s) so that they may readily access it for the relevant clinical trial(s).

The specific topics per ICH E6(R2) 7.4 to include on the title page are:

- **Sponsor's Name:**
  This is the name of the individual, company, institution, or organization that takes responsibility for the initiation, management, and/or financing of the clinical trial(s).
- **Product:**
  This is the name given to the investigational product. If the product is approved, then the approved product name can be used.
- **Research Number:**
  This is typically the identification of the filing with the regulatory authority. If the product is being studied at clinical trial site locations in multiple regulatory regions, the filing identification for each governing regulatory authority is displayed.
- **Name(s):**
  This is the chemical name or, if an approved product, its generic name.
- **Trade Name(s):**
  The registered product name may be displayed if legally permissible and desired by the sponsor.
- **Edition Number:**
  Since an IB will constantly be updated, it is important to maintain version identification, which is typically a consecutive numbering for the edition with a date of the edition. This edition number will identify the current version of the IB.
- **Release Date:**
  This is the date that accompanies the edition number.
- **Replaces Previous Edition Number(s):**
  The title page will include at least the identification of the last edition that is replaced by the current edition or a log of the previous editions of the IB.
- **Date:**
  This is the date that accompanies the edition number for the previous edition(s).

16.2.4.2 Sections Within the Investigator's Brochure

The numbering of the sections for the various information in the IB is standardized via ICH E6(R2) 7 so that investigators and other IB users may readily access information that they need, sometimes with urgency.

The specific topics per ICH E6(R2) 7.3 to include in the IB with the following section numbering are:

- **Confidentiality Statement (optional)**
  This is a statement that instructs the IB user to regard the IB and its contents as confidential and proprietary and the IB and its contents may be used solely for

its intended purpose (ICH E6(R2) 7.2.2). The statement of confidentiality may appear on the Title Page.

- **Signature Page (optional)**
  The signature page holds the name(s) and signature(s) of the sponsor's representative(s) who are attesting to the sponsor's ownership of the document.
- **Section 1. The Table of Contents**
  The table of contents (TOC) will show the section numbers for the various types of information that are included in the IB, and the page number where the information is located. The TOC will include all the required sections and appendices per ICH (ICH E6(R2) 7.3.1).
- **Section 2. Summary**
  This is a brief summary (preferably not exceeding two pages) that highlights the significant physical, chemical, pharmaceutical, pharmacological, toxicological, pharmacokinetic, metabolic, and clinical information available that is relevant to the stage of clinical development of the investigational product (ICH E6(R2) 7.3.2).
- **Section 3. Introduction**
  The introduction orients the IB user to the product, the rationale for the research, the anticipated indication(s), and the general approach that will be employed to evaluate the investigational product. Specific information for this section is (ICH E6(R2) 7.3.3):
  - **Name(s) of drug product (chemical name and, if applicable, generic and trade name(s)**
  - **Active ingredients**
  - **Pharmacological class**
  - **Rationale for performing research with the investigational product**
  - **Proposed indication(s)**
  - **General approach for evaluating the investigational product**
- **Section 4. Physical, Chemical, and Pharmaceutical Properties and Formulation**
  This section provides the following information about the investigational product (ICH E6(R2) 7.3.4):
  - **Description of the product substance(s), including the chemical and/ or structural formula(e),**
  - **Summary of the relevant physical, chemical, and pharmaceutical properties**
  - **Description of the formulation(s) to be used, including excipients, and justification for their clinical application**
  - **Structural similarities to other known compounds**
  - **Instructions for the storage and handling of the dosage form(s)**
- **Section 5. Nonclinical Studies**
  This section will include summarized methodology and results (favorable and unfavorable) from nonclinical pharmacology, pharmacokinetic and product

metabolism, and toxicology studies that are relevant to the clinical investigations for the proposed indications in humans. The discussions in this section will include the most important findings regarding (ICH E6(R2) 7.3.5):
- The dose response of observed effects
- The relevance to humans
- Any aspects to be studied in humans.
- If applicable, the therapeutic index, with a comparison of the effective and nontoxic dose findings in the same animal species
- Comparisons in terms of blood/tissue levels rather than on a mg/kg basis

Results from the following nonclinical testing are provided:
- **Nonclinical pharmacology**
  This is a summary of the pharmacological aspects of the investigational products and, where appropriate, its significant metabolites studied in animals. The summary should incorporate studies that assess potential therapeutic activity (e.g. efficacy models, receptor binding, and specificity) and those that assess safety (e.g., special studies to assess pharmacological actions other than the intended therapeutic effect(s)).
- **Pharmacokinetic and product metabolism in animals**
  This is a summary of the pharmacokinetics and biological transformation and disposition of the investigational product in all species studied. The discussion should address the absorption and the local and systemic bioavailability of the investigational product and its metabolites, and their relationship to the pharmacological and toxicological findings in animal species.
- **Toxicology**
  This is a summary of the toxicological effects found in relevant studies conducted in different animal species to evaluate, where appropriate:
  o Single dose
  o Repeated dose
  o Carcinogenicity
  o Special studies (e.g. irritancy and sensitization)
  o Reproductive toxicity
  o Genotoxicity (mutagenicity)

The reports of nonclinical testing (preferably in tabular format/listings whenever possible) will include the following, as appropriate, if known/available:
- Species tested
- Number and sex of animals in each group
- Unit dose (e.g., milligram/kilogram (mg/kg))
- Dose interval
- Route of administration
- Duration of dosing
- Information on systemic distribution
- Duration of post-exposure follow-up

– Results, including the following aspects:
  o Nature and frequency of pharmacological or toxic effects
  o Severity or intensity of pharmacological or toxic effects
  o Time to onset of effects
  o Reversibility of effects
  o Duration of effects
  o Dose response

Voluminous tabular/listing reports of nonclinical testing may be placed in an appendix to the IB while the summary discussions remain in the main body. This format may be appropriate especially if the investigational product is in later phase development and the IB audience is already familiar with the non-clinical information or more pertinent clinical information is available.

• **Section 6. Effects in Humans**

This section will include a thorough discussion of the known effects (favorable and unfavorable) of the investigational product from each completed clinical trial on healthy volunteers and patients, from any use other than in clinical trials, and, if applicable, from use of the approved product during marketing.

The completed study reports should be sources for data to be compiled in the IB. When studies are ongoing, however, available partial data may be analyzed and presented. The cut-off dates for the collection of the partial data and a notation that the data are preliminary should be stated in the IB and tracked for the next version of the IB. The sponsor should consider if it is practical and informative to present data from blinded and randomized trials where the control arm is different from the investigational product (other active drug or placebo) and the study treatment assignments for subjects are unknown.

Consideration for relevancy and meaning should be applied when pooling data from different formulations of the investigational product. The product formulation may morph from early to late phases of clinical development as, for example, open capsules become coated tablets or lyophilized powder for solutions.

Known effects from the following clinical testing are provided:

– **Pharmacokinetics and product metabolism in humans (ICH E6(R2) 7.3.6.a):**
  o Pharmacokinetics (including metabolism, as appropriate, and absorption, plasma protein binding, distribution, and elimination)
  o Bioavailability of the investigational product (absolute, where possible, and/or relative) using a reference dosage form
  o Population subgroups (e.g., gender, age, and impaired organ function)
  o Interactions (e.g., product-product interactions and effects of food)
  o Other pharmacokinetic data (e.g., results of population studies performed within clinical trial(s)

– **Safety and Efficacy (ICH E6(R2) 7.3.6.b):**

Clinical safety and efficacy information build and coalesce as development of the investigational product progresses through the clinical phases. Tables may be restructured to add accruing trial data and analyses and discussions may evolve to apply the expanding data base. These summaries of safety and efficacy help to provide the reader with information to determine benefit-risk of the investigational product based on prior clinical experience.

– **Safety**

   o Tabular summaries of adverse drug reactions for all the clinical trials (including those for all the studied indications) would be useful. Important differences in adverse drug reaction patterns/incidences across indications or subgroups should be discussed.

   o A description of the possible risks and adverse drug reactions to be anticipated on the basis of prior experiences with the product under investigation and with related products.

   o A description should also be provided of the precautions or special monitoring to be done as part of the investigational use of the product(s)

   o As much as possible, considering differences in indications, the safety data should be pooled and analyzed

   o Note: All relevant safety information must be included in the IB and the IB must be updated at least annually or earlier if new relevant safety information become available (ICH E6(R2) 7.1).

– **Efficacy**

Efficacy results should be presented from relevant studies. The sponsor should consider what is practical and meaningful when combining data results from studies with different designs and different study populations. Additionally, the sponsor may prudently choose to include only efficacy results that have been publicized (e.g., published or presented at scientific meetings) in order to protect proprietary information.

Tabulations, descriptions, and discussions of the available efficacy results for each clinical trial. When efficacy in its true sense cannot be measured, then the effectiveness of the investigational product may be presented with surrogate markers. The discussion in the IB will inform the reader of the measures used to determine efficacy and the outcomes of those measures. Efficacy and the alternative effectiveness data speak to the benefits of the use of the investigational product.

– **Pharmacodynamics and dose response**

The results of pharmacodynamic and dose response trials will be summarized. The implications for safety and efficacy of these results may also be discussed.

Individual study and pooled results should be presented for clinical testing of the biochemical, physiologic, and molecular effects of the investigational product on the body and the mechanism of its action. Both favorable and unfavorable effects should be presented; that is, evaluation of what is expected and what is not expected. For example, in the case of a treatment for multiple sclerosis, if the favored mechanism of a drug is to reduce the ability of inflammatory immune cells to pass through the blood-brain barrier preventing their attack on the myelin sheath of brain cells, then all possible unfavorable consequences of this action on the body, e.g., preventing normal immune surveillance and suppression of opportunistic organisms, should also be presented, evaluated, and discussed.

– **Marketing Experience:**

It is important for the IB "audience" to know and understand the use of the product, not only in the investigational controlled clinical trial setting, but also from public use if the product has been approved. Any significant data reported from marketed use should be included. Information about the formulations, dosages (e.g., overdosing), routes of administration, adverse reactions (e.g., any not listed on the approved label), or any associated device issues (e.g., the nebulizer for an inhaled drug) should be summarized from post-marketing surveillance studies, reports to the sponsor, published in literature, submissions to regulatory authorities, or other safety data reporting and mining sources. The IB will therefore (ICH E6(R2) 7.3.6.c):

o Identify countries where the investigational product has been marketed or approved.

o Identify all the countries where the investigational product did not receive approval/registration for marketing or was withdrawn from marketing/ registration.

o Summarize any significant information arising from the marketed use (e.g., formulations, dosages, routes of administration, and adverse product reactions).

Safety data from marketing experience may be from different sources:

o Systems are typically established for the public to report significant safety information such as adverse reactions, overdosing, issues with formulations and outcomes of pregnancies for women who received the approved product

o Regulatory authority(ies) may require the sponsor to conduct post-approval studies to evaluate long-term effects or preliminary but unconfirmed effects of the investigational product from pivotal trials that did not preclude marketing authorization

o The sponsor may conduct trials with the product in accordance with its approved specifications to assess, e.g. quality of life, interactions with other treatments, safety and/or efficacy against competing products

Additionally, unintended favorable effects may be reported (e.g., an antihypertensive medication may promote hair and nail growth), providing the sponsor with additional development opportunities.

• **Section 7. Summary of Data and Guidance for the Investigator**

Information in this section are summary tabulations, descriptions, and discussions of the available and integrated (where appropriate) physical, chemical, pharmaceutical, pharmacological, toxicological, and clinical information on the investigational product(s). The information should provide the investigator with:

- The most informative interpretation of the available data
- A clear understanding of the specific tests, observations, and precautions that may be needed for a clinical trial
- A clear understanding of the possible risks and adverse reactions

The summarized safety profile will include identifications and descriptions of risks based on previous human experience. This information helps the investigator to identify which events are expected (i.e., listed in the IB) or not expected and to therefore determine the causality of events experienced by a research subject or the research subjects at the investigator's clinical site. The sponsor will also assess causality of the event from a broader perspective, given their access to all information from all clinical studies and sites.

- The recognition and treatment of possible overdose and adverse drug reactions that is based on previous human experience and on the pharmacology of the investigational product.
- Published reports on related products (i.e., products in the same class) to anticipate adverse drug reactions or other problems in clinical trials
- An assessment of the implications of the information for future clinical trials

- **References**

  This section will contain literature references for IB information where appropriate. During early clinical development phases where less is known of the safety and efficacy profile of the investigational product, literature may be cited to support characteristics of the class of similar products, theorized mechanism of action, and other rationales to justify the initiation or use of the investigational product in humans.

- **Appendices** (if any)

  Appendices for the IB are helpful to organize lengthy tables or reports that are summarized within the IB. The objective is to ensure that the IB is organized in a manner that enable its users to quickly identify and access information in sometimes urgent situations. Quality review should be applied to ensure that information across sections are not contradictory, incomplete, or inaccurate.

The sponsor should refer to regulatory authority requirements for additional specific contents and/or formats for IBs.

16.2.5 Process for Developing an Investigational Brochure

As seen from the prescribed contents of the IB, as is for the protocol, the information to be included are of a wide variety and, in product development, these information are generated by a variety of specialized expertise.

The development process is also similar to that for creating any document: creating an outline, drafting, review, and finalization. In the case of an IB, it is standard practice for the document to also be ascribed formal signature(s) of approval.

16.2.5.1 Defining Roles and Timelines

Per ICH E6(R2) 5.4, the sponsor should utilize qualified individuals (e.g., biostatisticians, clinical pharmacologists, and physicians) as appropriate, throughout all stages of the trial process, from designing the protocol and CRFs and planning the analyses to analyzing and preparing interim and final clinical trial reports. For the collaboration, it will be necessary to identify who is the owner of the document's content and who is the writer for the document (if the individuals are different), who are the reviewers and approvers, and who will make final decisions in the event of conflicting opinions or unresolved issues. At a minimum, a medically qualified person should generally participate in the editing of the IB (ICH E6(R2) 7.1) but the contents of the IB should be approved by the disciplines that generated the described data. Standard operating procedures for the firm may stipulate which roles in the organization are the required reviewers and approvers.

The IB has contributions from various subject matter experts (SMEs), such as the medical monitor, biostatistician, and pharmacovigilance, non-clinical, pharmacology, CMC, and regulatory affairs personnel. Function representatives will collaborate to determine required benefit-risk information to be included in the IB.

To facilitate the collaboration, a meeting may be organized with contributors, reviewers, and approvers to agree on the scope of the data to be included in the IB, development timelines, expected deliverables from contributors, and the scope of review from reviewers and approvers. The timelines will include the anticipated date for delivery of the statistical outputs (tables, figures, and listings) as these are needed to prepare the study results. The IB writer will inform each SME of the specific information needed for IB and establish a system for receiving the information.

16.2.5.2 Investigator Brochure Structure and Content

As described above, the structure and content for the IB are generally already stipulated by the ICH (ICH E6(R2) 7) and applicable regulatory requirements, which may be reflected in standard operating procedures along with additional contents specific to the firm, including writing styles and conventions. IB sections comprise text, in-text tables, figures, and listings, references, and appendices as necessary.

16.2.5.3 Drafting, Reviewing, and Approving the Investigator's Brochure

The IB sections may be drafted and reviewed all at once, or in parts as a time-saving strategy. For example, the writer may circulate prepared non-clinical, CMC sections, and individual study data sections while waiting for integrated data results for the Guidance for the Investigator section.

The typical process for the development of a document is displayed in Plate 19 Typical Process for Document Development. For an IB:

1) The writer uses the contributions from SMEs, the scope as discussed with the SMEs, and other sources of information to draft the IB, ensuring that the minimum elements are included.
2) The drafted document is reviewed by assigned reviewers and approvers, and their comments are adjudicated until there is agreement on the contents. The writer will be keen to maintain version control throughout the development process.
3) To foster quality, the document should be checked for accuracy and compliance with standard operating procedures and regulatory requirements prior to being finalized, for example, a checklist may be used to ensure that all required elements are present.
   - The IB content should be checked against its sources, for internal consistency of information within the document, and for consistency with the appendices.
4) The person(s) who will take responsibility for the content of the IB will lastly document their approval.
5) The IB will be submitted to the regulatory authority(ies) and investigator(s), as applicable.

16.2.6 Updating an Investigator's Brochure

The IB should be reviewed at least annually and revised as necessary in compliance with a sponsor's written procedures. More frequent revision may be appropriate depending on the stage of development and the generation of relevant new information. (ICH E6(R2) 7.1).

The IB will be updated according to the firm's procedures when new nonclinical, clinical, CMC, or other information become available that are needed to adequately describe the risks and benefits of the use of the investigational product for the covered indication(s). For an IB update, the medical monitor, pharmacovigilance and regulatory affairs representative, biostatistician and other SMEs will determine the scope of information to be included in the update and dates for when data will be "cut" for ongoing studies to include them in the IB. The updated IB should include any safety reports that were generated and communicated to regulatory authority(ies) and investigator(s) since the last IB version.

If at the time of an annual review the trial team determines that no update to the IB is necessary, this decision should be documented.

16.2.7   Quality by Design Considerations for the Contents of an Investigator's Brochure

A number of principles and operational considerations that promote GCP, quality, and compliance may guide the planning and contents an IB. Data principles and trial operations considerations to foster quality for the IB include establishing systems to:

- Cross-check alignment of IB content with other documents (see Section 16.2.3)
- Track who needs to receive the IB; i.e., all trial investigator(s) using the investigational product and regulatory authority(ies)/ECs who have oversight of those trials
- Track IB distribution; i.e., who (regulatory authority and investigator) received what version of the IB and when to ensure complete distribution
- Track IB review/acknowledgement of receipt and acceptance by regulatory authority(ies), ECs, and investigators
- Ensure supply of IB information from all sources using the investigational product
- Review potential IB information to determine inclusion in the IB
- Maintain information to be included in the next IB update
- Ensure IB content is adequate to meet its scientific, trial, and GCP objectives
- Ensure IB content is compliant with regulatory requirements
- Track when and what information was included in the IB; e.g., data cutoffs for ongoing trials
- Version control of the document during development
- Track documentation of no annual review

The study team should establish processes that will ensure the accurate and complete reporting of trial data in an IB.

16.3   Summary

The IB is a is a compilation of the clinical and nonclinical data on the investigational product(s) that is relevant to the study of the investigational product(s) in human subjects.

The purpose of an IB is provide investigators and others involved in the trial with the information to facilitate their understanding of the rationale for, and their compliance with, many key features of the protocol, such as the dose, dose frequency/interval, methods of administration, and safety monitoring procedures. The IB also provides insight to support the clinical management of the study subjects during the course of the clinical trial.

The IB is essentially the pre-cursor to an approved product label. It applies to multiple trials for at least one indication, but may contain information that support multiple indications. The IB is used by a variety of players for several types of product evaluation, including benefit-risk of the investigational product and must contain unbiased information. The IB should be reviewed at least annually and the content should align, where necessary and appropriate, with other regulatory and clinical trial documents.

The contents of an IB are prescribed by the ICH E6(R2) 7 Guidance or applicable regulatory requirements. An IB generally contains a variety of information about the investigational product, including nonclinical, clinical, pharmacological, and CMC information. The type and degree of details for the different types of information contained in the IB will depend on the stage of the development of the investigational product. The sponsor will determine which ICH sections are applicable to the type of product and may also add sections as appropriate. All IB information should be supported by sources contained in the essential documents for a trial.

An IB or IB update is developed similarly to other clinical technical documents with assigned owners, writers, reviewers, and approvers. Minimum approvers are stipulated by regulatory requirements. The IB should be reviewed for updates at least annually.

Several considerations to enable quality by design principles can be factored into the preparation of information for an IB CSR to ensure the inclusion of appropriate and correct information that will be distributed to the correct and appropriate parties.

Knowledge Check Questions

1) What is an IB?
2) What is the purpose of an IB?
3) What are the contents of an IB?
4) What are some of the triggers for changing an IB?
5) What are the key quality-by-design considerations for IBs?
6) Overheard:

   Let's not give the same version of the IB to that regulatory authority. They may start questioning the data about this sub-population for which we do not intend to seek marketing authorization approval in that region.

   Clinical development executive referring to adverse events data that were particularly associated with a sub-population in a pivotal study.

   Comment and discuss:

   a) What are advantages and disadvantages of presenting the same data to all regulatory authorities governing the use of an investigational product?
   b) What are advantages and disadvantages of presenting different data to the regulatory authorities governing the use of an investigational product?

Reference

1 International Council for Harmonisation of Technical Requirements for Pharmaceuticals for Human Use (ICH), Integrated Addendum to ICH E6(R1):Guideline for Good Clinical Practice, E6(R2) (2016). Current Step 4 version dated 9 November 2016. https://www.ich. org/page/efficacy-guidelines.

17

The Investigational Product (Clinical Supplies)

P. Michael Dubinsky

GCP Key Point

The nexus between GCP and cGMP must be fully understood and applied to investigational medicinal/drug products. Ensuring the quality and integrity of the investigational product depends on adherence to both.

17.1 Introduction

The title of this chapter – "Clinical Supplies" – might be something of a misnomer. . . The terminology will not be found in the ICH E6(R2) or any set of regulatory requirements for investigational drug products, but it is used by people involved in conducting clinical trials. Another term often used is *test article*. We will use the term *investigational product* (IP) instead.

The terms IP and *investigational medicinal product* (IMP) are used both in GCP and in the controlling regulations of the FDA and EMA. A clinical trial's purpose is to obtain data supporting safety, efficacy, and adequate directions for use of an IP, so the level of control exercised must be thorough. Terms such as *traceability*, *chain of custody*, and *full accountability* come to mind. The responsibility for control over clinical supplies lies primarily with the sponsor; however, once IP reaches the trial site, the control responsibility shifts. That said the level of control must be just as rigorous. The control and oversight requirements remain in place through the final use and/or disposition of the IP. In this chapter, we will examine the fundamentals that are described in the ICH E6(R2), as well as some points about how those fundamentals are best implemented as control of the IP is transferred from sponsor to site to subject.

The Fundamentals of Clinical Research: A Universal Guide for Implementing Good Clinical Practice, First Edition. P. Michael Dubinsky and Karen A. Henry.
© 2022 John Wiley & Sons, Inc. Published 2022 by John Wiley & Sons, Inc.
Companion website: www.wiley.com/go/dubinsky/clinicalresearch

17.2 Objectives

This chapter's objective is to outline the following:

- Manufacturing and labeling requirements
- IP accountability and management
- Factors to consider in the overall trial risk-assessment

17.3 Manufacturing and Labeling Requirements

The information supporting the administration of an IP to humans is submitted as part of an application to conduct a clinical study; it is usually composed of studies in animals and at the laboratory bench via in vitro studies. There may be data from some human use and, if so, that data would also be included.

The sponsor of the trial may or may not be the manufacturer of the IP, but as the sponsor they will be responsible for defining specifications and parameters for the IP. Much of the pertinent information about the IP will be found in the Investigator's Brochure and the Protocol.

In the publication *Guidelines on Clinical Drug Research*, the American Society of Health-System Pharmacists lists the following types of data points which are consistent with ICH E6(R2) Sec 7:

a. *Drug designation and common synonyms.*
b. *Dosage forms and strengths.*
c. *Usual dosage range, including dosage schedule and route of administration.*
d. *Indications pursued in this study.*
e. *Expected therapeutic effect to be studied.*
f. *Expected and potential adverse effects, including symptoms of toxicity and their treatment.*
g. *Drug–drug and drug–food interactions.*
h. *Contraindications.*
i. *Storage requirements.*
j. *Instructions for dosage preparation and administration, including stability and handling guidelines.*
k. *Instructions for disposition of unused doses*
(Source: ASHP Research Guidelines [1], p. 623)

Manufacturing or cGMP requirements do apply to IP; however, the sponsor bears the primary responsibility for meeting those expectations. Unless the clinical trial situation involves a sponsor–investigator, cGMP associated with manufacturing tasks would fall to the sponsor. It is useful to note that the rigor with which conformance to cGMP requirements is assessed does have some wrinkles. For example, in 2008 the US FDA published guidance [2] for the manufacture of IP used in Phase I clinical trials that allowed for the fact that IP at the Phase I stage was not a product being routinely manufactured in a commercial capacity; therefore, some expectations, such as validation of the manufacturing process, would not be enforced. However, not all regulatory authorities have such policy provisions in place. It is useful to mention that the US FDA does not routinely inspect the manufacture of IP as part of its Bioresearch Monitoring (BIMO) inspection programs. However, the EMA member states do visit the manufacturing location and inspect manufacturing of IP.

As with manufacturing, labeling requirements generally fall to the sponsor and are drawn from applicable regulations. Labeling includes the label on the immediate container and any accompanying literature. For the purposes of this text, we are listing the most demanding set of label requirements, which come from the regulations implemented by the EMA. Those requirements are reproduced below, from Annex VI to Regulation EU No. 536/2014 [3]:

LABELLING OF INVESTIGATIONAL MEDICINAL PRODUCTS AND AUXILIARY MEDICINAL PRODUCTS

A. UNAUTHORISED INVESTIGATIONAL MEDICINAL PRODUCTS
*A.1. **General rules***
1. The following particulars shall appear on the immediate and the outer packaging:

> *(a) name, address, and telephone number of the main contact for information on the product, clinical trial and emergency unblinding; this may be the sponsor, contract research organisation or investigator (for the purpose of this Annex this is referred to as the 'main contact');*
>
> *(b) the name of the substance and its strength or potency, and in the case of blind clinical trials the name of the substance is to appear with the name of the comparator or placebo on the packaging of both the unauthorised investigational medicinal product and the comparator or placebo;*
>
> *(c) pharmaceutical form, route of administration, quantity of dosage units;*
>
> *(d) the batch or code number identifying the contents and packaging operation;*
>
> *(e) a clinical trial reference code allowing identification of the trial, site, investigator and sponsor if not given elsewhere;*
>
> *(f) the subject identification number and/or the treatment number and, where relevant, the visit number;*
>
> *(g) the name of the investigator (if not included in (a) or (e));*

(h) *directions for use (reference may be made to a leaflet or other explanatory document intended for the subject or person administering the product);*
(i) *'For clinical trial use only' or similar wording;*
(j) *the storage conditions;*
(k) *period of use (expiry date or re-test date as applicable), in month and year format and in a manner that avoids any ambiguity; and*
(l) *'Keep out of reach of children', except when the product is for use in trials where the product is not taken home by subjects.*

A summary of the key label expectations on an IP might include:

a) Name, address, and telephone number of sponsor, contract research organization (CRO), or investigator
b) Trial reference code
c) Trial subject identification number or treatment number
d) Name of the investigator
e) Directions for use (administration)
f) The phrase "For clinical trial use only"

The US FDA's labeling requirements, found at 21 CFR 312.6, call for a cautionary statement indicating that the drug is intended for investigational use, but they do not list all the expected statements, as the EMA does. In addition, the FDA calls for no false or misleading statements to be made on the labeling.

It is essential to ensure that IP is manufactured in compliance with cGMP and that label/labeling statements meet regulatory requirements; this task will fall to the sponsor, but all sites and the IRB should have knowledge of how compliance is being met in these areas.

In the European Union (EU), regulations require that compliance with cGMP be certified by a "qualified person." The definition of a qualified person is found in EC Directive 2001/83/EC article 49, paragraph 2: *A qualified person shall be in possession of a diploma, certificate or other evidence of formal qualifications awarded on completion of a university course of study, or a course recognized as equivalent by the Member State concerned, extending over a period of at least four years of theoretical and practical study in one of the following scientific disciplines: pharmacy, medicine, veterinary medicine, chemistry, pharmaceutical chemistry and technology, biology* [4]. From a practical standpoint, most qualified persons are pharmacists.

Certificates of analysis (COA) for IP are an expectation as noted in the ICH E6(R2) sections 8.2.16 and 8.3.9. COAs are not mentioned in the US FDA regulations but are now routinely used because they are required in many regions and countries. The preceding paragraph mentions the EU requirement that a qualified person must certify compliance with cGMP. A COA would be part of the information a qualified person would review to make such a determination.

   While this is not specifically linked to GCP on a day-to-day basis, IPs shipped between countries will most likely need to meet specific import and export requirements of the countries from which they are shipped and in which they are received. Import/export requirements are primarily designed to ensure that regulatory authorities know what is leaving and entering their jurisdictions, but in some cases testing requirements may be in place. Of course, if an IP is not permitted entry into a country where a clinical test site is located, the trial will be impacted. Organizing compliance with import/export requirements almost always falls to the sponsor.

17.4   IP Accountability and Management

Regulatory authorities consider the authorization they give to conduct an investigational drug trial to be a serious and significant decision. After all, they are permitting a drug that does not yet have adequate directions for use to be shipped interstate and administered to humans. They authorize the use of the IP under the terms of a specific protocol, and they recognize that they may be asked to answer for that decision if issues arise. They do not expect the IP to be used in any manner that differs from the stipulations in the protocol. This mind-set is reinforced when one reviews the inspectional guidance the US FDA gives its investigators in chapter 48 of Program 7348.811 in its *Compliance Program Manual*, titled "Bioresearch Monitoring: Clinical Investigators and Sponsor-Investigators" [5]. These instructions, which concern the review of drug accountability records during inspections, read as follows:

> *L. CONTROL OF INVESTIGATIONAL PRODUCT*
>
> 1. *Review records that document shipment, receipt, disposition, return, and destruction of investigational product. Review any written procedures for investigational product accountability and evaluate investigational product accountability to determine compliance with applicable regulations (i.e. 21 CFR 312.62(a) and 21 CFR 812.140(a)(2)).*
>   *Compare the amount of investigational product shipped, received, used, and returned or destroyed and obtain the information below.*
> 2. *Determine how the investigational product arrived at the clinical site, and whether shipping records documented shipment dates, batch or lot numbers, and method of shipment to allow for adequate tracking of investigational product batches, shipping conditions (e.g., specific temperature controls), and accountability. Determine who received/accepted the shipment, and whether the shipment package was immediately inspected.*

3. *Determine how the investigational product was stored upon arrival to the clinical site, and whether the investigational product was stored under appropriate conditions.*
4. *Determine if the clinical investigator and/or study personnel were to be blinded to the contents of the investigational product, and if so, determine if blinding procedures were appropriately followed.*
5. *Determine if the investigational product requires preparation (e.g., specific reconstitution fluids and procedures, protection from light) before administration, where the preparation was performed, by whom and how this was documented. For studies involving animals, refer to Part III Section P (Food Animal and Laboratory Effectiveness Studies) of this CP.*
6. *Determine who is authorized to dispense or administer the investigational product.*
7. *Determine whether the investigational product was supplied to a person not authorized to receive it.*
8. *Determine whether the investigational product requires specific conditions for administration and whether such conditions were adhered to (e.g., specific device for infusion, infusion rate or times).*
9. *Compare the amount of investigational product shipped, received, dispensed, used, and returned or destroyed. Verify the following:*
   a. *Receipt date(s), quantity received, and the condition upon receipt;*
   b. *Date(s), subject number, and quantity dispensed;*
   c. *Date(s) and quantity returned to sponsor; and*
   d. *If not returned to sponsor, determine if the protocol or study documents outline destruction/disposition of the investigational product and describe the disposition of the investigational product.*

As with all of the records that are expected to be in place pursuant to ICH E6(R2) sections 8.2.15, 8.3.8, 8.3.23, 8.4.1, and 8.4.2, documentation of the receipt, shipping, storage, and dispensing of IP calls for records of IP shipping, receipt, storage, return, and destruction/disposition to be maintained and available. The structure of the record-keeping system may differ from site to site and sponsor to sponsor, but the records must reflect the chain of custody of the IP. The records will be the evidence that accountability was complete.

Institutions that are routinely engaged in clinical trials, such as academic medical centers, will be routinely receiving IPs from a variety of sponsors for several different clinical trials. In order to accurately process the incoming IP, such institutions establish Investigational Drug Service (IDS) units staffed by pharmacists who are specially trained in handling IP, be it drug, biologic, or biotech product. IDS units will have written procedures and policies in place, as well as record-keeping systems, that can stand up to inspectional scrutiny by regulatory authorities. Section 4.6 of the ICH E6(R2) speaks directly to assigning responsibility for IP to a pharmacist.

17.5   Factors to Consider in the Overall Trial Risk-Assessment

The topic of clinical supplies, or IP, brings up several factors that provide fuel for the overall trial risk-assessment process. One must keep in mind that the integrity of the IP represents an aspect of the trial that is critical in terms of quality. If there is some compromise of the IP due to inappropriate storage, dispensing, disposition, or any aspect related to accountability, the quality of the data supporting safety and efficacy can be adversely affected. It is also useful to note that in terms of remote monitoring, the accountability and management of the IP is not usually one of the parameters for which tolerances are established. Examination of the physical control steps that surround the IP must be assessed firsthand.

Satisfactory storage of the IP considers parameters such as access, temperature, and equipment. In terms of access, the number of people who are granted or have access to the IP should generally be limited to those who need access. All types of storage containers – whether a room, a refrigerator, or a cabinet – ought to be locked. If the site has IDS, then controls over these aspects of storage are likely to be in place, but if not, establishing who has access and how access is documented is important and doable. Take into consideration the fact that people become ill, take vacations, or could be in training. Will there be an alternate individual available to ensure IP is dispensed when necessary? How will the alternate gain the needed access? What are the alternate's qualifications? Such questions should be asked and answered before IP is delivered to the site.

The sponsor will have defined the IP's storage temperature requirements, and this information should be listed on the label as well as in the protocol and IB. Temperature records are notorious for being fabricated. This is not always done for a nefarious purpose rather; it is done because it is easy and not often considered to be a serious issue. In more than one inspection, I have found evidence that temperature records were fabricated. Once, a handwritten temperature record was already filled in for many days into the future. When asked, the person responsible explained that since the temperature for the equipment (in this case a refrigerator) was always the same (or close to the same) and never went out of range, there seemed to be no reason not to fill in the information ahead of time. In addition, the equipment had a temperature recorder installed, so a chart/graph was available. Perhaps there was only a minimal chance of a temperature aberration occurring, but the fact that the record was fabricated called into question all other records for which the person had responsibility. Such issues are not trivial when uncovered during an inspection.

Disposition of IP may involve returning unused quantities to the sponsor or their designee, or destroying it at the trial site. Never assume that IP will be handled as expected or per SOP when it is sent for processing as biohazardous waste at a medical facility. I recall a situation when, during an inspection, an investigator traveled to the unit responsible for disposal of biohazardous waste, such as unused IP, and found that no records showing that the IP had been destroyed were available. The inquiry eventually revealed that the IP was being sold on the black market along with other valuable drugs. It is not a situation you would expect to encounter, but it is wise to expect the unexpected.

From the standpoint of risk assessment, these types of situations may be unlikely to occur, but when they do, the consequences are serious. A program of internal audits in the area of IP controls is worth considering as a mitigation step. Internal audits are cost-effective and keep all parties on their best behavior.

It is also appropriate to mention that, while all the QA/QC building blocks apply to clinical supplies oversight (see Chapter 30 Quality Systems in Clinical Research, Section 30.1.3), record-keeping and documentation, written procedures, and training and qualification of personnel should be the focus.

17.6 Summary

Clinical supplies, or IP, are an aspect of clinical trials that must be considered critical to quality. For instance, if IP is stored improperly, its purity, strength, or identity may be somehow compromised. Data from subjects who were administered a compromised IP may be unusable or questionable at a minimum. The steps necessary to exercise control over the IP, thereby ensuring accountability, are all drawn from the QA/QC building blocks and are well entrenched in GCP culture. That said, there are aspects of record-keeping, storage, and control that seem to elude many players in the clinical trial endeavor. Being savvy about compliance in this area is both desirable and doable.

Knowledge Check Questions
1) The sponsor shares the responsibility for cGMP requirements with the pharmacist at the clinical trial site. True or False?
2) Both the US FDA's and the EMA's IP labeling requirements include a provision for a label statement such as "For Investigational Use Only" to appear on IP. *True* or False?
3) Records documenting _____ of IP, _____ of IP, _____ of IP, and _____ of IP are required. [receipt, storage, dispensing, disposition]
4) In assessing overall trial risks, the control over IP should be included. True or False?
5) IDS stands for Investigational Device Suitability. Yes or No

References

1 American Society of Health-System Pharmacists (1998). Guidelines on clinical drug research. https://www.ashp.org/-/media/assets/policy-guidelines/docs/guidelines/clinical-drug-research.ashx?la=en&hash=8973560F661752ABFE1F66 EC65D7DD6D4EC03B15 03 (accessed 17 December 2019).

2 Food and Drug Administration (2008). Guidance for industry: CGMP for Phase I investigational drugs. https://www.fda.gov/downloads/Drugs/GuidanceCompliance RegulatoryInformation/Guidances/UCM070273.pdf (accessed 17 December 2019).

3 Regulation (EU) No. 536/2014 of the European Parliament and the Council (16 April 2014). Clinical trials of medicinal products for humans for human use. *Official Journal of the European Union.* https://ec.europa.eu/health/human-use/clinical-trials/regulation_en (accessed 19 February 2019).

4 Directive 2001/83/EC of the European Parliament and of the Council (6 November 2001). https://eur-lex.europa.eu/LexUriServ/LexUriServ.do?uri=OJ:L:2001:311:006 7:0128:en:PDF (accessed 19 February 2019).

5 Food and Drug Administration (2008). Program 7348.811, chapter 48, "Bioresearch Monitoring: Clinical Investigators and Sponsor-Investigators." https://www.fda.gov/media/75927/download (accessed 16 August 2021).

18

The Clinical Trial Protocol and Amendments

Karen A. Henry

GCP Key Point
Design and implement to meet the target product profile and Good Clinical Practice objectives

18.1   Introduction

A clinical trial, broadly, is a scientific experiment on human subjects. Specifically, it is any investigation in human subjects intended to discover or verify the clinical, pharmacological and/or other pharmacodynamic effects of an investigational product(s), and/or to identify any adverse reactions to an investigational product(s), and/or to study absorption, distribution, metabolism, and excretion of an investigational product(s) with the object of ascertaining its safety and/or efficacy. The terms clinical trial and clinical study are synonymous. (ICH E6(R2) 1.12).

A protocol may be defined as a system of rules that explain the correct conduct and procedures to be followed in a situation, a plan for a scientific experiment or medical treatment, or a description of the details of a treaty or formal agreement between countries [1]. It is generally a written design and methods for the experiment on humans.

In an oversimplified manner, we can also think of the protocol as the recipe to conduct the experiment. A recipe has a desired outcome; ingredients or inputs, equipment, methods, and principles are required for its execution; and the results of the outcome are measured by specified characteristics. In this context, the:

- Desired outcome are the trial objectives
- Inputs are human subjects and the investigational product

The Fundamentals of Clinical Research: A Universal Guide for Implementing Good Clinical Practice, First Edition. P. Michael Dubinsky and Karen A. Henry.

- Methods are recruiting the subjects, conducting the visit procedures, administering the investigational product, monitoring the health of the subjects, and collecting and analyzing the data to determine the safety and effectiveness of their treatment.
- Principles are GCP, regulatory requirements, and best practices
- Results are measured by the trial endpoints

In this chapter, we will focus on the contents of and the operational activities involved in developing a clinical trial protocol to meet the regulatory requirements. This chapter does not describe trial design (Chapter 27 Study Design and Data Analysis). In this chapter, "protocol" refers to a clinical trial protocol.

18.2   Objectives

The objectives of this chapter are:

1) Define a protocol
2) Describe the context for a protocol in clinical development
3) Describe the purpose of a protocol in a clinical trial
4) Describe the contents of a protocol
5) Describe the process for developing a protocol
6) Discuss changes to a protocol
7) Describe the principles for implementing a protocol or amended protocol
8) Quality-by-Design Considerations for the Contents of a Protocol

18.2.1   Definition of a Protocol

A clinical trial protocol (protocol) is a document that describes the objective(s), design, methodology, statistical considerations, and organization of a trial. The protocol usually also gives the background and rationale for the trial, but these could be provided in other protocol referenced documents. Throughout the ICH GCP Guideline the term protocol refers to protocol and protocol amendments. (ICH E6(R2).1.44) [2]. The clinical trial protocol is the investigational plan for the trial. The plan is carefully designed to safeguard the health of the participants as well as answer-specific research questions. To ensure highest quality, undesirable results are anticipated and controls are put in place to prevent or mitigate them.

18.2.2   Context for a Protocol in Clinical Development

Recall that a clinical trial protocol is only one of the set of various protocols that will be executed as part of the general clinical development or investigational plan that supports the target product profile for a product (Chapter 3 GCP in Context; Plate 1 Drug Development Methodology). Therefore, each individual clinical trial protocol is designed to obtain specific information that will enhance knowledge of the safety and efficacy of the use of the product in the target patient population.

Within the context of the overall clinical trial process, the clinical trial protocol is the investigational plan for conducting the trial. In addition, the clinical trial process requires the collection of the data via case report forms (CRFs) to support the trial objectives and endpoints that are described in the protocol, a Statistical Analysis Plan that outlines the details of how the collected data will be analyzed, followed by reporting of the trial results in a Clinical Trial Report that is expected to fully reflect how the trial was conducted. The case report forms (CRFs), clinical database, Statistical Analysis Plan, and the Clinical Study/trial Report are, therefore, closely connected with the protocol in terms of their contents. Given the interrelationship of these components, it is prudent that the protocol writing team considers the logistics for executing the protocol procedures, the capabilities and limitations of the data collection media and process (Chapter 20 Data Collection and Data Management), the principles related to analyzing the data (Chapter 27 Study Design and Data Analysis), the required contents of the Clinical Study Report, and other individual and integrated study results reporting requirements (Chapter 28 The Clinical Study Report) to ensure that they are harmonized. (Plate 1 Drug Development Methodology).

18.2.3 Purpose of a Protocol in a Clinical Trial

A protocol describes the objective(s), design, methodology, statistical considerations, and organization of a trial that will enhance knowledge of the safety and efficacy of the use of the product, while ensuring that the benefits outweigh the risks for volunteers participating in the clinical trial. The regulatory authority(ies), sponsor, investigator(s), and IRB/IEC(s) (Plate 3 Players Roles and Responsibilities: IRB/EC, Investigator, Sponsor/CRO Regulatory Agency) will review and use specific information in the protocol to carry out their regulatory responsibilities. The responsibilities of these key players for a protocol are essentially threefold:

1) Regulatory authority review of the trial:
   a) Due to historical events (e.g., the 1962 Kefauver-Harris Drug Amendments and Nuremberg trials (Chapter 1 History), and the resulting ICH principle (ICH E6(R2) 2.2), a sponsor is required to develop and submit a protocol to the governing regulatory authority for review of safety and scientific quality, and acceptance and/or permission prior to initiating the clinical trial (ICH E6(R2)(R2) 5.10).
2) Ethics committee review of the trial: Prior to initiating the trial,
   a) The sponsor should provide the investigator with the protocol (ICH E6(R2) (R2) 5.6.2)

    b) The investigator will obtain the approval/favorable opinion from an ethics committee before initiating the trial (ICH E6(R2) 4.4.1)

    c) An ethics committee will review that the proposed protocol and/or other document(s) adequately addresses relevant ethical concerns and meets applicable regulatory requirements for such trials, and approve/provide favorable opinion on the trial protocol (ICH E6(R2) 3.1)

    d) The sponsor will confirm that the trial has received the approval/favorable opinion of an ethics committee (ICH E6(R2) 5.11).

3) Investigator and sponsor compliance with the trial requirements:

    a) The investigator and sponsor will agree to the protocol in writing (ICH E6(R2) 4.5.1, 5.1.4, 5.6.3)

    b) The protocol, in addition to other information, will provide the investigator and staff (ICH E6(R2) 4.1.2, 4.2.4), as well as the sponsor and its representatives, the information they need to conduct the clinical investigation (ICH E6(R2) 5.2.1, 5.5).

    c) The investigator will comply with the requirements of the protocol and should not implement any deviation from, or changes of the protocol without agreement by the sponsor and prior review and documented approval/favorable opinion from the IRB/IEC of an amendment, except where necessary to eliminate an immediate hazard(s) to trial subjects, (ICH E6(R2) 4.5.2; Chapter 9 Investigator and Sponsor Roles and Responsibilities)

18.2.4 Contents of a Protocol

Clinical trials should be scientifically sound, and described in a clear, detailed protocol (ICH E6(R2) 2.5). Specific information is required in a protocol to serve the needs of its stakeholders, namely the regulatory authority, the ethics committee, investigator and staff, and the sponsor and its representatives. The topics or elements to be included in a protocol are guided by the principles of GCP (ICH E6(R2) 2) and the ICH (E6(R2) 6) has prescribed topics or elements to be included in a protocol. Protocol developers must also be aware of local regulatory requirements to ensure inclusion of any other required contents, and any additional information or requirements that are specific to the study should also be included if they are necessary to facilitate execution of the study. While a protocol may contain administrative and business contractual elements, in practice, its contents are usually limited to information that describe the scientific and regulatory elements required for its execution in accordance with the protocol objectives, GCP, and applicable regulatory requirements. The administrative and business contractual information may otherwise be contained in a clinical trial agreement (Chapter 15 Trial Resourcing and Outsourcing). The ICH also allows for some scientific and procedural details to be contained in other referenced documents, such as the Investigator's Brochure

(Chapter 16 The Investigator's Brochure), or a pharmacy manual (Chapter 14 Trial Management; Start-up, On-Study, and Close-Out). Comprehensive details of the operations of the trial may be contained in other trial manuals (Chapter 14 Trial Management; Start-up, On-Study, and Close-Out).

Quality management for a clinical trial also includes giving thought to certain aspects of the design and contents of the protocol. For example, critical consideration should be given for the impact of study and operational procedures on human subject protection and the validity and reliability of study results. Additionally, risk mitigation activities may be incorporated in protocol design (ICH E6(R2) 5.0; See Chapter 13 Risk Assessment and Quality Management).

The general topics to be included in a protocol and the functions that will typically provide the information are as follows:

18.2.4.1 General Information

This general information is intended to identify the protocol (its identification number, title, and version), provide the names and contact information for the sponsor or its representatives responsible for medical expertise and signing the protocol (i.e., medical monitor), and monitoring (Chapter 22 Monitoring Overview), and all persons and entities that will influence trial results, e.g., investigators and their staff (Chapter 9 Investigator and Sponsor Roles and Responsibilities), laboratories. (Note that the protocol identification information for an amendment is for the final approved version of a protocol amendment and not for draft versions created during development. Also, in practice, information that is highly likely to change during the course of the trial, e.g., names of investigators, may be provided to the interested stakeholders in another format in order to avoid a formal amendment to the protocol, which is an involved and time-consuming process every time there is a change (See Section 18.2.7). The identification of key responsible trial personnel facilitates contact, as well as transparency of responsibilities and assessment of qualifications.

The specific topics per ICH E6(R2) 6.1, to be included in the section are:

- Protocol title, protocol identifying number, and date of the original protocol and any amendments
- Name and address of the sponsor and monitor (if other than the sponsor).
- Name and title of the person(s) authorized to sign the protocol and the protocol amendment(s) for the sponsor.
- Name, title, address, and telephone number(s) of the sponsor's medical expert (or dentist when appropriate) for the trial.
- Name and title of the investigator(s) who is (are) responsible for conducting the trial, and the address and telephone number(s) of the trial site(s).

- Name, title, address, and telephone number(s) of the qualified physician (or dentist, if applicable) who is responsible for all trial-site-related medical (or dental) decisions (if other than investigator).
- Name(s) and address(es) of the clinical laboratory(ies) and other medical and/or technical department(s) and/or institutions involved in the trial.

18.2.4.2 Background Information

Before a trial is initiated, foreseeable risks and inconveniences should be weighed against the anticipated benefit for the individual trial subject and society. A trial should be initiated and continued only if the anticipated benefits justify the risks. In addition, the available nonclinical and clinical information on an investigational product should be adequate to support the proposed clinical trial (ICH E6(R2) 2.4). The background information is intended to give the audience the justification for exposing humans to the investigational article for the indication under investigation. This section in the protocol, therefore, summarizes the epidemiology of the indication, unmet medical need for the indication, the planned exposure of the trial participants to the investigational article, and the rationale or risk versus benefit assessment of what is known so far about the product to justify the selected exposure. In cases where preparation of a formal IB is impractical, the sponsor–investigator should provide, as a substitute, an expanded background information section in the trial protocol that contains the minimum current information described in this guideline (ICH E6(R2) 7.1 IB).

The specific topics per ICH E6(R2) 6.2, to be included in the section are:

- Name and description of the investigational product(s)
- A summary of findings from nonclinical studies that potentially have clinical significance and from clinical trials that are relevant to the trial.
- Summary of the known and potential risks and benefits, if any, to human subjects.
- Description of and justification for the route of administration, dosage, dosage regimen, and treatment period(s).
- A statement that the trial will be conducted in compliance with the protocol, GCP, and the applicable regulatory requirement(s).
- Description of the population to be studied.
- References to literature and data that are relevant to the trial and that provide background for the trial.

18.2.4.3 Trial Objectives and Purpose

This section is answering the questions: What are you trying to achieve? What are the desired outcomes? For example,

- Phase 1: Determine the pharmacokinetics and safety
- Phase 2: Determine the maximum tolerated dose and safety
- Phase 3: Determine the efficacy of active vs comparator treatment

The individual objectives are typically ranked as primary, secondary, exploratory, etc., depending on the phase of development of the article (Chapter 27 Study Design and Data Analysis).

The specific topic per ICH E6(R2) 6.3, to be included in the section is:

- A detailed description of the objectives and the purpose of the trial.

18.2.4.4 Trial Design

The protocol is designed to meet the objectives of the trial and to ensure collection of data that will facilitate analysis of the endpoints. In addition to trial conduct being compliant with GCP and regulatory requirements, the credibility of the data and the scientific integrity of the trial depend on the trial design. The optimal trial design seeks "to generate statistically and scientifically sound answers to the questions that are being asked and meet the objective(s) of the study" (WHO Handbook for good clinical research practice Principle 2, p 27). This section describes and provides a schematic diagram for the scientific construct of the study, what response variables (endpoints) will be used to measure the objectives, controls for potential confounding factors, and the planned study interventions.

The specific topics per ICH E6(R2) 6.4, to be included in the section are:

- A specific statement of the primary endpoints and the secondary endpoints, if any, to be measured during the trial.
- A description of the type/design of trial to be conducted (e.g., double-blind, placebo-controlled, and parallel design) and a schematic diagram of trial design, procedures and stages.
- A description of the measures taken to minimize/avoid bias, including:
- Randomization.
- Blinding.
- A description of the trial treatment(s) and the dosage and dosage regimen of the investigational product(s). Also include a description of the dosage form, packaging, and labelling of the investigational product(s).
- The expected duration of subject participation, and a description of the sequence and duration of all trial periods, including follow-up, if any.
- A description of the "stopping rules" or "discontinuation criteria" for individual subjects, parts of trial and entire trial.
- Accountability procedures for the investigational product(s), including the placebo(s) and comparator(s), if any.
- Maintenance of trial treatment randomization codes and procedures for breaking codes. The investigator should follow the trial's randomization procedures, if any, and should ensure that the code is broken only in accordance with the protocol. If the trial is blinded, the investigator should promptly document and explain to the sponsor any premature unblinding (e.g., accidental unblinding,

unblinding due to a serious adverse event (SAE)) of the investigational product(s) (ICH E6(R2) 4.7).

- The identification of any data to be recorded directly on the CRFs (i.e. no prior written or electronic record of data), and to be considered to be source data.

18.2.4.5 Selection and Withdrawal of Subjects

This section defines the criteria that determine who is eligible to participate in the trial, the criteria for discontinuing their trial treatment or withdrawing them from the trial, and the expected safety management of subjects who withdraw. The "inclusion criteria" answer the question, what type of subject is being studied for this indication? They list, for example, the trial population's sex, age, and indicated diagnosis, and that the participant must provide informed consent to participate in the trial. Conversely, the exclusion criteria answer the question, what excludes the included subject from the study? These are criteria that have the potential to confound trial data results or render it unsafe or contraindicated for the participant to be exposed to the trial treatments (investigational, approved, or placebo) or procedures. Such criteria may include clinical testing parameters (e.g., labs, serology, pregnancy, substance use, and psychological testing), allergies and anticipated drug interactions and contraindications, concomitant medications, and participation in other trials with investigational articles. The inclusion and exclusion criteria should not simply list the opposite of each other. Consideration should be given to the phase of the study to ensure criteria are appropriately specific or appropriately vague to ensure that they are not too strict to unnecessarily limit enrollment nor too vague to reduce the specificity of the subject population.

The specific topics per ICH E6(R2) 6.5, to be included in the section are:

- Subject inclusion criteria.
- Subject exclusion criteria.
- Subject withdrawal criteria (i.e. terminating investigational product treatment/ trial treatment) and procedures specifying:
  a) When and how to withdraw subjects from the trial/ investigational product treatment.
  b) The type and timing of the data to be collected for withdrawn subjects.
  c) Whether and how subjects are to be replaced.
  d) The follow-up for subjects withdrawn from investigational product treatment/ trial treatment.

18.2.4.6 Treatment of Subjects

The trial participant's exposure to the investigational product, i.e., how much they receive over the course of the trial, is a critical factor for assessing the scientific objectives of the trial. This section describes the trial participant's exposure to what product(s), for how long, how much of the product(s), and how the product(s) will be administered. It must be clearly stated which product(s) are of an investigational nature. In addition, it presents how it will be assured that participants receive the trial treatments as prescribed; for example, if qualified clinic staff will administer trial treatments and document such administration, or if drug concentration testing will be used to monitor treatment compliance if participants will be self-administering the trial treatments without direct supervision by the clinic staff. The protocol will also prescribe that the investigational product(s) are used only in accordance with the approved protocol (ICH E6(R2) 4.6.5).

The specific topics per ICH E6(R2) 6.6, to be included in the section are:

- The treatment(s) to be administered, including the name(s) of all the product(s), the dose(s), the dosing schedule(s), the route/mode(s) of administration, and the treatment period(s), including the follow-up period(s) for subjects for each investigational product treatment/trial treatment group/arm of the trial.
- Medication(s)/treatment(s) permitted (including rescue medication) and not permitted before and/or during the trial.
- Procedures for monitoring subject compliance.

18.2.4.7 Assessment of Safety and Efficacy

The endpoints for a trial are inherently critical scientific measures of the trial objectives (see Chapter 27 Study Design and Data Analysis) and the endpoints will use the results of the trial assessments that the trial participants will undergo. This section describes the methods and timing of the clinical assessments and laboratory tests that trial participants will undergo and how the results will be recorded and reported. All SAEs should be reported immediately to the sponsor except for those SAEs that the protocol or other document (e.g., Investigator's Brochure) identifies as not needing immediate reporting (ICH E6(R2) 4.11.1). Adverse events (AEs) and/or laboratory abnormalities identified in the protocol as critical to safety evaluations should be reported to the sponsor according to the reporting requirements and within the time periods specified by the sponsor in the protocol (ICH E6(R2) 4.11.2).

The specific topics per ICH E6(R2) 6.7, 6.8, to be included in the section are:

- Assessment of Efficacy
  - Specification of the efficacy parameters.
  - Methods and timing for assessing, recording, and analyzing of efficacy parameters.
- Assessment of Safety
  - Specification of safety parameters.
  - The methods and timing for assessing, recording, and analyzing safety parameters.

- Procedures for eliciting reports of and for recording and reporting AE and intercurrent illnesses.
- The type and duration of the follow-up of subjects after AEs.

18.2.4.8 Medical Care of Trial Subjects

A qualified physician (or dentist, when appropriate), who is an investigator or a subinvestigator for the trial, should be responsible for all trial-related medical (or dental) decisions. During and following a subject's participation in a trial, the investigator/institution should ensure that adequate medical care is provided to a subject for any AEs, including clinically significant laboratory values, related to the trial. The investigator/institution should inform a subject when medical care is needed for intercurrent illness(es) of which the investigator becomes aware. It is recommended that the investigator inform the subject's primary physician about the subject's participation in the trial if the subject has a primary physician and if the subject agrees to the primary physician being informed. Although a subject is not obliged to give his/her reason(s) for withdrawing prematurely from a trial, the investigator should make a reasonable effort to ascertain the reason(s), while fully respecting the subject's rights (ICH E6(R2) 4.3).

18.2.4.9 Statistics

This section describes the statistical assumptions used to estimate the trial sample size and the methods that will be used to analyze the data in support of the trial objectives (see Chapter 27 Study Design and Data Analysis).

The specific topics per ICH E6(R2) 6.9, to be included in the section are:

- A description of the statistical methods to be employed, including timing of any planned interim analysis(es).
- The number of subjects planned to be enrolled. In multicentre trials, the numbers of enrolled subjects projected for each trial site should be specified. Reason for choice of sample size, including reflections on (or calculations of) the power of the trial and clinical justification.
- The level of significance to be used.
- Criteria for the termination of the trial.
- Procedure for accounting for missing, unused, and spurious data.
- Procedures for reporting any deviation(s) from the original statistical plan (any deviation(s) from the original statistical plan should be described and justified in protocol and/or in the final report, as appropriate).
- The selection of subjects to be included in the analyses (e.g., all randomized subjects, all dosed subjects, all eligible subjects, and evaluable subjects).

18.2.4.10   Direct Access to Source Data/Documents

As described in Chapter 9 Investigator and Sponsor Roles and Responsibilities; Chapter 22 Monitoring Overview; Chapter 25 Investigator/Institution Interim Monitoring; Chapter 8 IRB/IEC Roles and Responsibilities; Chapter 33 Quality Assurance Components; Chapter 34 Regulatory Authority Inspections, the sponsor is required to monitor the investigation (ICH E6(R2) 5.18) and the sponsor, IRB/IEC, or regulatory authorities may audit the investigator's conduct of the trial (ICH E6(R2) 5.19). The investigator must, therefore, allow these various parties to access the trial data at the site, which includes the source documents that reflect trial conduct (ICH E6(R2) 5.15) (Chapter 20 Data Collection and Data Management).

The specific topics per ICH E6(R2) 6.10, to be included in the section are:

- The sponsor should ensure that it is specified in the protocol or other written agreement that the investigator(s)/institution(s) will permit trial-related monitoring, audits, IRB/IEC review, and regulatory inspection(s), providing direct access to source data/documents.

18.2.4.11   Quality Control and Quality Assurance

This section includes a declaration of the regulations that apply to the trial conduct and a summary of the procedures that will be used to assure and control the quality of the trial. Such procedures include, for example, assurance of the qualifications of clinical investigators, staff, and facilities prior to trial initiation; and trial monitoring and auditing.

The ICH E6(R2) 6.11 does not specify items to be included under this topic.

18.2.4.12   Ethics

In accordance with the ICH principle ICH E6(R2) 2.3, "The rights, safety, and well-being of the trial subjects are the most important considerations and should prevail over interests of science and society." In this section, the procedures that concern ethical treatment of trial participants are outlined; e.g., IRB/IEC review, informed consent, and maintenance of the confidentiality of records that contain personal identification of trial participants.

The specific topic per ICH E6(R2) 6.12, to be included in the section is:

- Description of ethical considerations relating to the trial.

18.2.4.13   Data Handling and Recordkeeping

A brief summary describing how the trial data will be collected, stored, and managed to meet the applicable regulatory requirements is in this section. The data to be analyzed will be collected via CRFs, which should specifically record all of the protocol required information to be reported to the sponsor on each trial subject (ICH E6(R2) 1.11). Consideration should be given for trial data starting with informed consent, demographics, then screening outcomes, eligibility, randomization, study treatment, on-study procedures, follow-up, AEs, concomitant medications, and through end-of-study procedures. Additionally, this section can include the requirement to state which data will be recorded directly onto CRFs and not on source documents, i.e., will not have documentation on a source against which the data in the CRF can be verified. If all data for all subjects will not be collected in the same manner, then it is important to explain what data will be collected for which subset of subjects, keeping in mind that data should be collected to support all the endpoint measures and operational procedures described in the protocol. See Chapter 20 Data Collection and Data Management for additional information. This section may also include a description of the requirements for maintaining an audit trial to track who, when, and why source data were changed, regardless of the medium used to collect and maintain the data.

The ICH E6(R2) 6.13 does not specify items to be included under this topic.

18.2.4.14 Financing and Insurance

The definition of a contract per ICH E6(R2) 1.17 is a "written, dated, and signed agreement between two or more involved parties that sets out any arrangements on delegation and distribution of tasks and obligations and, if appropriate, on financial matters. The protocol may serve as the basis of a contract." Additionally, ICH E6(R2) 5.1.4 recommends that agreements, made by the sponsor with the investigator/institution and any other parties involved with the clinical trial, should be in writing, as part of the protocol or in a separate agreement. However, often in practice, the protocol will describe the general delegation and distribution of tasks and obligations (e.g., those of the investigator, sponsor, or CRO) that are relevant to the trial procedures, but specific financial arrangements are outlined in separate agreements. This separation is practical as the requirements relevant to the trial procedures generally apply to all parties involved in trial conduct but the financial details would be individualized to a site or CRO and may also be considered confidential. See Chapter 15 Trial Resourcing and Outsourcing for further information.

The specific topic per ICH E6(R2) 6.14, to be included in the section is:

- Financing and insurance, if not addressed in a separate agreement.

18.2.4.15 Publication Policy

An avenue to inform the scientific community and the general public of trial results is publications. Both trial sponsors and investigators have an interest in publishing but sponsors prefer to control the timing of the release of trial results to protect their proprietary, product development, and business interests. This section is used for sponsors to state the publication policy regarding who may publish what and when. As stated in the ICH E6(R2) GCP Guideline, this policy may also be addressed in a separate agreement.

The specific topic per ICH E6(R2) 6.15, to include in the section is:

- Publication policy, if not addressed in a separate agreement.

18.2.4.16 Supplements

Supplemental information to the protocol would be those items that must be provided to the investigator but do not fit any of the standard sections. Typically, supplements or appendices include, for example, a tabular representation of the trial safety and efficacy assessments or procedures (Appendix: see Protocol Synopsis, Example of Trial Activities Template), clinical rating scales or indices (note that published rating scales may have copyright limitations).

The ICH E6(R2) 6.16 does not specify items to be included under this topic.

18.2.5   Process for Developing a Protocol

As seen from the prescribed contents of the protocol, the information to be included are of a wide variety and, in product development, these information are generated by a wide variety of specialized experts. The development process for a protocol is therefore a collaboration among various subject matter experts (SMEs) and the dynamics are like any other collaboration: it requires leadership, coordination, sharing knowledge, negotiations, and building consensus to realize shared goals. The development process is also similar to that for creating any document: creating an outline, drafting, review, and finalization. In the case of a clinical trial protocol, it is standard procedure for the document to also be ascribed formal signature(s) of approval.

18.2.5.1   Defining Roles and Timelines

Per ICH E6(R2) 5.4, the sponsor should utilize qualified individuals (e.g., biostatisticians, clinical pharmacologists, and physicians) as appropriate, throughout all stages of the trial process, from designing the protocol and CRFs and planning the analyses to analyzing and preparing interim and final clinical trial reports. For the collaboration, it will be necessary to define the roles regarding document content owner and document writer (if different from the owner), reviewers, approvers, and who will be designated to make final decisions in the event of conflicting opinions or unresolved issues. Standard operating procedures for the firm may stipulate which roles in the organization are the required reviewers and approvers. To facilitate the collaboration, a meeting may be organized with contributors, reviewers, and approvers to agree on timelines and expected deliverables from contributors and scope of review from reviewers and approvers.

18.2.6   Protocol Structure and Content

The outline for the protocol is generally already stipulated by GCP (ICH E6(R2) 6; Plate 10 Study Protocol – Contents) and applicable regulatory requirements. The required outline may be reflected in standard operating procedures along with additional contents specific to the firm, including writing styles and conventions.

It is common practice for clinical trial protocols to include a Synopsis or Summary that displays conceptual information for the protocol, such as the trial title, phase, interventions, study population, duration, design, study objectives and endpoints, and methods (Appendix: Protocol Synopsis, Example of Trial Activities Template).

18.2.6.1 Creating the Protocol Synopsis or Summary

The protocol Synopsis or Summary is useful for the firm to organize and document the general concepts of the trial before development of the full protocol commences. This is usually achieved through a team of contributors that will include those who are responsible for clinical study design, the clinical safety of the trial participants, statistical analysis, investigational product supplies, non-clinical information that supports the advancement of the use of the investigational product in humans, and oversight of the use of the intellectual property. All contributors are considering a scientifically sound trial design that is conducive to achieving the firm's clinical development objectives while ensuring that the anticipated benefits justify the risks for the trial participants (Chapter 27 Study Design and Data Analysis). It is recommended that at least one clinical physician expert, who is currently practicing in the clinic in the therapeutic area being studied, also be consulted to ensure that the protocol design and procedures are feasible in the clinic setting and are conducive to achieving the trial objectives.

To complement the documented trial concepts, it is helpful to encourage an early thoughtful construct of which trial assessments and activities (e.g., informed consent, vital signs, laboratory testing, imaging assessments, and AEs evaluation), will be performed and when they will be performed (Appendix: Protocol Synopsis, Example of Trial Activities Template). The protocol Synopsis or Summary, along with the Schedule of Activities, are often used for budgeting (Chapter 15 Trial Resourcing and Outsourcing), investigator (Chapter 23 Investigator/Institution Selection) or CRO selection (Chapter 15 Trial Resourcing and Outsourcing), or informed consent documents development (Chapter 19 Informed Consent and Other Human Subject Protection).

18.2.6.2 Drafting, Reviewing, and Approving the Protocol

The typical process for the development of a document is displayed in Plate 19 Typical Document Development Process. For a protocol:

1) The writer starts development of the full protocol using information from the Synopsis or Summary and Schedule of Activities, contributions from SMEs, and ensuring that the required elements are included.
2) The drafted document is reviewed by assigned reviewers and approvers, and their comments are adjudicated until there is agreement on the protocol

contents. The writer will be keen to maintain version control throughout the development process.

3) To foster quality, the document should be checked for accuracy and compliance with standard operating procedures and regulatory requirements prior to being finalized, for example, a checklist may be used to ensure that all required elements are present.

4) The person(s) who will take responsibility for the content of the protocol will lastly document their approval.

18.2.7 Changes to a Protocol

A protocol amendment is a written description of a change(s) to or formal clarification of a protocol (ICH E6(R2) 1.45). The protocol may be formally amended if it is found that it no longer adequately or accurately describes the desired design or procedures or displays accurate administrative information. Causes for amendments may be identified as a result of acquiring new information on the safety and efficacy of the investigational product, alternative available treatments, the characteristics of the study population, regulatory requirements, investigational product manufacturing or availability, protocol administration or implementation logistics, or business development. For example, to modify the dosing volume of the investigational article, to modify subject eligibility requirements, to add or remove trial assessments, or change safety reporting procedures, may require a formal amendment or clarification.

When deciding on changes to a protocol, the same considerations for the context of an original protocol in clinical development, quality and risk management, and the impact on subject health and data quality outcomes apply. The typical process for the development of the amended protocol may be similar to developing a full protocol (Plate 19 Typical Document Development Process). Any substantive change to a protocol, i.e., those that affect subject safety or data integrity, must have the approval of a qualified IRB/IEC prior to its implementation at the clinical site. Other local regulatory requirements may apply.

18.2.8 Implementing the Protocol or Protocol Amendment

The protocol is the document that describes how the study will be conducted. It will be reviewed by and given favorable opinion by the governing regulatory authority(ies) and ethics committee(s) prior to trial initiation; i.e., prior to any procedure described in the protocol is implemented.

An investigator will sign an agreement to follow the protocol and will ensure that all relevant site staff members are trained on its requirements, and the sponsor will train all relevant staff responsible for execution of the protocol.

Likewise, for protocol amendments, procedures may not be implemented until after approval or favorable opinion from an ethics committee and all persons participating in its execution must be trained on the changes. Local requirements may differ regarding the approval of the amendment by the regulatory authority(ies).

NOTE: It is prudent to confirm that the approval/favorable opinion from the governing ethics committee has indeed formally occurred per the IRB/IEC's procedures and that the documentation is available before implementing protocol or amended protocol procedures.

18.2.9 Quality-by-Design Considerations for the Contents of a Protocol

The statistical principles for the design of a clinical trial are beyond the scope of this book. However, a number of principles and operational considerations that promote GCP, quality, and compliance may guide the contents of a protocol. See also Chapter 31 Quality Responsibilities.

18.2.9.1 Trial Design

18.2.9.1.1 Trial Objectives, Endpoints, and Procedures

Generally, each objective will have a corresponding endpoint, and each endpoint will have appropriate study safety and efficacy assessment(s) or evaluation(s) that will provide the data to be analyzed for the endpoints. Given the linkage between the trial objectives, endpoints, and study assessments, charting them helps the protocol development team to systematically consider and map the:

1) Objectives of the study as they relate to the development program of the product
2) Study endpoints for the Statistical Analysis Plan, how the endpoints align with those in other trials in the development program to facilitate integration of trial data, and if the endpoints are acceptable in the scientific and regulatory community
3) Study procedures that will need to be performed to obtain the data, and if they are standards in the clinical setting

This charting also ensures only necessary statistical analyses and study assessments required for the study are included in the protocol.

An example of these elements for a phase 2 study is in Table 18.1.

18.2.9.2 Sample Sizes

Study sample sizes are based on a statistical equation that includes a certain *power* for a test, given a predetermined Type I error rate α (Chapter 27 Study Design and Data Analysis). The larger the sample size, the more the tendency is toward increased precision for the study results. However, the conduct of clinical trials in

Table 18.1 Example of phase 2 study objectives, endpoints, and study assessments.

Objectives	Endpoints	Study assessment
Primary	Primary	
• Safety of Drug X	• Frequency of Adverse Events and Serious Adverse Events for Drug X vs Drug Y	• Adverse events reporting
Secondary	Secondary	
• Preliminary efficacy of Drug X	• Response rate of Drug X vs Drug Y	• Biomarker testing
Exploratory	Exploratory	
• Quality of life	• Quality of life outcome for Drug X vs Drug Y	• Quality of Life questionnaire administration

the real world assumes limited time and resources because firms may neither have the luxury of time to wait until a large number of subjects have been enrolled, nor have personnel and finances to manage and pay for the cost of enrolling the large number of subjects ideally needed for ultimate precision. Also, a sponsor, especially in early development, may not have sufficient data to reasonably estimate a true response rate or treatment effect. Given these limitations, sponsors will consider the *minimum* number of subjects needed to have sufficient data to ascertain conclusions regarding the safety and/or effectiveness of the investigational article.

It is important for a sponsor to ensure that the sample is sufficiently adequate, however, to ensure that they will have the potential to get meaningful conclusive results (in either a positive or a negative direction) to prevent the need for trial duplication, and ethically, exposing more participants than are necessary to the unapproved product.

How accessible the patient population is for all study groups may be a factor for determining sample sizes. Presumably, smaller sample sizes may be required for participants with rare diseases (i.e., in the United States, it affects fewer than 200 000 persons [3]; however, it may take larger numbers of participants to enroll in the trial to obtain the evaluable population needed for analysis.

18.2.9.3 Randomization and Blinding

Whether a trial needs randomization and/or blinding as measures to control bias will largely depend on its phase in the development process, e.g., exploratory phase 2 versus confirmatory phase 3 (Chapter 3 GCP in Context).

Randomization procedures, such as generating, maintaining, applying the schema, must be performed by qualified personnel or systems (Chapter 27 Study

Design and Data Analysis). In the case of blinding, all efforts should be made to prevent unauthorized breach of treatment codes (Chapter 27 Study Design and Data Analysis). How to operationalize administration of an investigational product that is obviously different from its comparative control in a blinded trial is challenging and can be costly. Whether it is creating an identical-looking placebo, having a participant turn their head so they do not see the color of similar formulations, having blinded efficacy evaluators, having separate blinded and unblinded trial monitoring teams, having sham surgery versus active treatment surgery, or another creative measure, procedures need to be implemented to ensure that the blinding is maintained for all parties at each level of masking.

18.2.9.4 Interim Analyses
If and when interim analyses occur may be statistically or clinically driven. On the advice of the statistician, the sponsor will understand that a loss of *power* occurs with every planned interim analysis, especially for confirmatory trials (Chapter 27 Study Design and Data Analysis). Also, the sponsor may choose to periodically review open-label trial data without "penalty." A sponsor may plan interim review of a confirmatory trial if, e.g., a trial has a long follow-up safety period after the timepoint for collection of data for the primary efficacy endpoint. The sponsor will need to prespecify the procedures for how the data cut, cleaning, and unblinding if necessary, will be implemented.

18.2.9.5 Investigational Products
Many factors should be considered when determining the test and control products to be used in the study. Among the many are:

- How they will be procured. Will the sponsor provide to investigators? Will investigators procure and be reimbursed? Will participants be asked to pay for the product as "standard of care" and is this ethical or allowed per applicable regulatory requirements? How accessible is the product if not manufactured by the sponsor? Will there be shipping and handling concerns? Are import/export licenses necessary?
- Is the desired formulation readily available? Is the available formulation suitable for the study population?
- What are the risks versus benefits for using a matched placebo as a comparative control for the investigational product? Can the control be "standard of care" or must it be a placebo? Is it unethical to withhold available treatment from participants? Are participants willing to volunteer for the study given the probability of their assignment to the tested versus the control product?
- Will there be issues for packaging and labeling? Will the packaging be suitable for use in the clinic or by the participant as required by the protocol? Are ancillary devices required? Can the product be packaged to facilitate control of the blind?

- Will there be issues for storage and handling? Will specialized equipment be necessary? Do investigational sites already have the equipment or will the sponsor need to provide? Can procedures to effectively monitor storage be implemented?
- How will the treatment compliance be monitored if the trial treatments are self-administered by research participants or administered by other health-care or personal-care givers without the supervision of the trial staff?
- How long will initial procurement of trial supplies take? How risk-free is resupply and how long does resupply take?
- What data regarding the use of the investigational product must be collected? What procedures are necessary to account for the full chain of custody of all clinical supplies (Chapter 17 The Investigational Product (Clinical Supplies))?

18.2.9.6 Eligibility Criteria

Knowing the characteristics of the population that is intended for study is fundamental to develop appropriate eligibility criteria for the protocol. If the criteria are too stringent, then enrollment may be unnecessarily stiffled. On the other hand, criteria that are too vague or broad may obscure or confuse the characteristics of the target population, or may produce confounding study results that cannot be confidently attributed to the intended study population.

The characteristics of the population are both clinical and demographic. An under-represented sample from a clinical or demographic subgroup may narrow the possibility for approval of the indication for the under-represented subgroup. Eligibility criteria must therefore be inclusive of the desired target population for approval of the indication, and at the same time, exclusive of a subpopulation that is not intended. For example, if the population for a vaccine is to be "healthy" adults, then the advantages and disadvantages for including the "general" population, which may include very "unhealthy" adults and potentially result in confounding safety findings that are not typical of a "healthy" population, should be thoroughly measured.

18.2.9.7 Informed Consent

Per ICH E6(R2) principle 2.9, freely given informed consent should be obtained from every subject prior to clinical trial participation. While consent is required from all participants prior to undergoing any protocol-related procedure, a parent or legally authorized representative may provide consent, such as in the case of a minor. Other exceptions to consent are allowed as per regulatory requirements (Chapter 19 Informed Consent and Other Human Subject Protection).

An IRB/IEC must review and approve all study documents or materials (e.g., study handouts or devices for data collection) that will be provided to, either directly or indirectly (e.g., via advertising) prior to their use.

Regulatory authorities and or IRB/IECs may also require additional consent for specific procedures, such as biopsies, genetic testing, or for continued treatment with the test product although the participant is not responding to the treatment and a delayed response is theoretically expected due to the nature of the investigational product.

18.2.9.8 Safety Monitoring

Monitoring participants' safety is the foremost responsibility of all players involved in the conduct of a clinical trial. Regulatory requirements impose specific responsibilities on investigators, sponsors, and IRB/IECs (Chapter 7 Players Roles and Responsibilities Overview) to monitor subject safety. Regulatory authorities and IRB/IECs will review a protocol prior to their implementation, and the sponsor and investigator have ongoing reporting obligations to the regulatory authorities and IRB/IECs. However, the best antidote to corrective actions is prevention.

During development of the protocol, the sponsor should consider methods to limit participants' exposure to test products and to risky protocol procedures. Only study procedures that are required to obtain data to evaluate study endpoints and objectives should be included in the protocol. Procedures that are "nice to have" or "may be useful" or "just for curiosity" are highly discouraged because they do not contribute to the planned analysis and may be considered unethical. The following are some factors for consideration:

- Domiciling versus Outpatient Care
  If, for example, the investigational product is being used for the first time in humans, or strict monitoring of concomitant medications and food intake, or continuous blood draws or other procedural testing are required, then it is best to administer the study drug to participants in a setting where they are domiciled. On the other hand, if the investigational product can be self-administered by participants in their own home, then outpatient care may be suitable for the study procedures. Consideration must be given to processes and procedures needed to monitor and account for administration of the investigational product outside of the investigational site, whether it is in the patient's home, or at another facility.
- Safety Reporting Periods in the Protocol
  The collection period (time of onset) for AEs, SAEs, and pregnancies may coincide or may differ in a given protocol. The collection periods will depend on the half-life of the product, the expected AEs profile, and local reporting requirements. For example, instead of AEs, SAEs, and pregnancies collected as of informed consent until 30 days after the end of the study, AEs may be collected after study drug administration until 30 days post the last study drug administration, whereas SAEs may be collected from the time of informed consent (which

means that the collection period includes screening) until 90 days after the end of the study. AEs that occur between informed consent and the first study drug administration may be recorded as medical history. Comparably, the occurrence of pregnancies may be reported up to 120 days after the end of the study.

The follow-up period (how long to follow an event once it has started) for AEs, SAEs, and pregnancies may also differ. For example, the follow-up period for AEs may stop at 60 days after the last study drug administration so that there are 30 days of follow-up after the collection period ends; the follow-up for SAEs may be until they resolve or stabilize, and the follow-up for pregnancies would go until the outcome of the pregnancy is determined.

The sponsor and investigator will set up and implement procedures to enable timely review, evaluation, and reporting of all safety events.

- Contraception

  What, if any, contraception is required of female and male participants and for how long? This will depend on the known or unknown teratogenicity of the investigational product or its product class. Consideration should be given for cultural, religious, or local regulatory requirements for contraception. Also, clear definitions for men and/or women of childbearing potential must be specified in the protocol.

- Sponsor Monitoring of Safety

  For a trial where the sponsor is not blinded, the sponsor may choose to perform all continuous safety review, unless independent review is required for specific type of safety events, e.g., dose limiting toxicities for a dose finding study. For a sponsor-blinded trial, an Independent Data Monitoring Committee (IDMC) must be chartered to perform periodic review of blinded-data and to recommend to the sponsor whether the trial is safe to continue.

  The DMC will also advise, with the sponsor in consultation with the regulatory authority, if a participant's treatment code may be unblinded in a non-emergency situation. In an emergency situation, the investigator is expected to treat the symptoms and withdraw treatment if necessary. Un-blinding may only occur in the event of an immediate emergency situation where knowledge of the assigned study treatment will alter the course of medical care of the participant. Sponsor, investigator, and safety committee personnel must be thoroughly trained on safety monitoring procedures.

  Continuous safety review includes the analysis of individual events from individual participants, events by investigator sites, events by trial, and events reported from all ongoing trials using the investigational product. The sponsor must implement procedures to allow this continuous monitoring and oversight of safety reporting by qualified personnel (Chapter 21 Safety Monitoring and Reporting).

- Withdrawal Criteria and Stopping Rules

  The protocol will specify criteria under which study drug treatment may be discontinued for a trial participant. It is often recommended that a participant is encouraged to continue with a specified subset of or all safety follow-up procedures although they have discontinued receiving the study drug. It should be clear in the Statistical Analysis Plan how the data for these participants will be analyzed (Chapter 27 Study Design and Data Analysis).

The protocol will also specify criteria under which a participant may be discontinued from participating in the study, and if, in addition to participants who do not meet eligibility criteria after screening, the participant may be replaced. It should be clear in the Statistical Analysis Plan how the data for participants who are replaced will be analyzed (Chapter 27 Study Design and Data Analysis).

The reason for study drug treatment discontinuation or study discontinuation must be recorded in the sources documents and collected in the CRFs (Chapter 20 Data Collection and Data Management).

The protocol will also list criteria for withdrawing all participants for trial treatment or for terminating the trial.

18.2.10 Study Assessments

As previously mentioned, the sponsor should consider methods to limit participants' exposure to test products and to risky protocol procedures. The study dose and dosing schedule should be based on previous information obtained from non-clinical testing or previous clinical testing.

- Staggered Dosing
  Since the effect of first initiation of the investigational product in humans is inherently unknown, extreme caution must be taken when scheduling treatment. It is recommended that drug administration to participants be staggered, e.g., for cellular and gene therapy products [4]. The protocol will be designed for there to be a lag of specified time after administering the first dose to each participant and before treating the next participant. Additionally, only a few (usually less than 12) participants will be receiving treatment in the first part of the study. Dose limiting toxicities may be assessed for each participant and a safety committee may have to declare a *safe to proceed* for each participant or for each treatment cohort.
- Order, Number of Assessments, and Logistical Feasibility
  The order and number of study procedures that a participant will undergo in a single day are also to be evaluated for their effect on the participant's safety. If scientifically feasible, it is best to schedule procedures of cognitive testing early on the study visit day and before strenuous procedures. Requiring the presence of a caregiver may be necessary for certain study populations or after certain types of study procedures. The order assessments should be written into the protocol, and participants must consent to the requirement for a caregiver. Likewise, the number of assessments to be performed in a single study

visit day can be potentially exhausting and thereby yield erroneous study data, and/or not logistically feasible for participants nor investigator site personnel. Additionally, are there clinical or logistical restrictions for the completion of an assessment? For example, can the subject go to the clinic to undergo assessments and receive treatment?

- Visit Windows

  Allowance may be given for a "window" around each timepoint for the collection of protocol assessments. These windows help investigator sites to perform study assessments within a reasonable timeframe instead of requiring an on-time assessment which may not be practical. Windows are determined based on what is scientifically acceptable for the spread of the assessment. For example, assessments that are performed daily, may have a window of plus or minus one hour, whereas, windows for visits every six months may be plus or minus seven days.

- Standard of Care Procedures

  Procedures that are considered "standard of care" for the indication being studied may be accepted as protocol procedures. For example, if an imaging scan is part of the standard of care and is required for eligibility assessment, the protocol's eligibility criteria may allow the scan in the study if it meets protocol criteria in terms of specifications and timing. This reduces the number of procedures the participant needs to undergo. The same consideration may be given to clinical laboratory testing, especially with the added advantage of not having to wait for the lab results.

- Data Collection

  All the data that are necessary to document study conduct should be recorded and collected. Data for participants who do not meet eligibility criteria ("screen failures") need to be collected to allow determination of unbiased selection of enrolled (i.e., having received study treatment) participants.

  Simultaneously, consideration should be given to what is the best way to collect the data that are required by the protocol, i.e., simplicity of variable names and data coding, consistency of data coding and variable names across studies to facilitate data integration.

  If a trial has an "adaptive design," the database and CRFs must be designed to adapt to the anticipated modifications.

18.2.11   Subject's Rights and Medical care

Per ICH E6(R2) Principle 2.3, the rights, safety, and well-being of the trial subjects are the most important considerations and should prevail over interests of science and society. In addition to implementing processes and procedures for safety oversight, the investigator and sponsor also have obligations to protect the rights and well-being of the trial participants.

The protection of subject's rights includes not only informed consent, but also protecting their privacy. All study data that identify an individual study participant must remain confidential. The participant will agree on who may see their personal information and how the information may be used via the consent process (Chapter 19 Informed Consent and Other Human Subject Protection). Given this limitation, the sponsor and investigator will have to ensure that procedures are in place to always protect participant's confidentiality, including restricting access to data, and ensuring that the participant's identifying information are redacted as necessary.

The investigator is responsible for ensuring that the participant receives medical care (either from the investigator or from another qualified healthcare provider) for all medical events the participant may sustain, whether the event is deemed associated or not associated with the use of the investigational product. The sponsor must finance the cost of medical care for all events that are deemed associated with the use of the investigational product. The investigator and/or investigator institution will have agreements on how these payments will be made.

The protocol will specify how study data will be used and who will have access to the study data, including the right for the sponsor, IRB/IEC, and regulatory authorities to audit or inspect study documentation. Consideration should be given to the need for tracking tissue samples for future testing. Local regulatory requirements may allow participants to access their sample during the study or after the study has ended. Some authorities will, however, permit the collection of tissue samples without a participant's option to retract if the samples are unidentified and the data are used only in aggregated form.

18.2.12 Protocol Feasibility and Potential for Protocol Deviations

The sponsor should ensure that all aspects of the trial are operationally feasible and should avoid unnecessary complexity, procedures, and data collection (ICH E6(R2) 5.0). To this end, it is recommended that the sponsor consults with experienced investigator site personnel (and Contracted Research Organizations if relevant (Chapter 15 Trial Resourcing and Outsourcing)), to test the feasibility of a protocol and other related study documents before finalizing the protocol. The following are a few of the key factors to be tested for the protocol:

- Appropriateness of the eligibility criteria for the study population
- Ability to recruit the study population
- Ability to store, handle, administer, and account for the investigational product
- Appropriateness of study assessments for measuring the study endpoints
- Appropriateness of the order, number, and logistical feasibility

The following are a few of the key factors to be tested for the CRF:

- Accuracy and completeness of the CRF
- Appropriateness of the order of study assessments
- Appropriateness of the CRF specifications for protocol data collection
- Easiness to complete the CRF
- Easiness to follow the CRF instructions
- Easiness to address data queries

The following are a few of the key factors to be tested and/or confirmed for the informed consent information in the protocol:

- Necessity for consent for specific procedures
- Appropriateness of procedures for procedure-specific consents; e.g., how long may biological samples be retained
- Appropriateness of procedures for protecting subject identification information

All team members should collaborate to anticipate the potential for protocol deviations and ensure controls are put in place to prevent or mitigate them. Evaluating the desired protocol design, study procedures, and study processes for their feasibility with those who are the end users will provide greater confidence for the implementation of a trial with quality outcomes.

18.3 Summary

The clinical trial protocol describes the methods for conducting the trial that will provide further information about the investigational article during its development toward ultimate approval for marketing. The protocol provides the responsible parties the information they need to review to ensure that clinical experiments on human subjects are scientifically sound in design and do not present undue risks that outweigh the benefits of being administered the investigational product. It also provides clear and concise description of the procedures to be followed by the trained and qualified parties responsible for execution of the clinical trial. If changes are necessary to a protocol, those changes should be documented and substantive changes, i.e., those that affect subject safety or data integrity, must have the approval of a qualified IRB/IEC prior to its implementation at the clinical site. A trial subject may not undergo any procedure that is required by the protocol or protocol amendment until the document has been approved or given favorable opinion of an ethics committee. Other local regulatory requirements may apply.

Several considerations to enable quality-by-design principles can be factored into the design and operationalization of a protocol. To ensure human subject protection and the reliability of trial results, undesirable study outcomes are anticipated and controls are put in place to prevent or mitigate them.

Knowledge Check Questions

1) What is a clinical trial protocol?
2) What is the purpose of a clinical trial protocol?
3) What are the contents of a clinical trial protocol?
4) What are the key quality-by-design considerations for creating a clinical trial protocol?
5) What are some of the triggers for changing a protocol?
6) Overheard:

   We can collect [require study assessments to get data] whatever we want, just in case we need it.

   Sponsor medical monitor while designing a clinical trial.

   Comment and discuss:
   a) What might be the motivation for this decision?
   b) What assessments may be required and what data may be collected for a protocol?
   c) What are the risks to study subjects if unnecessary procedures are performed?
   d) What are the risks to the sponsor for collecting unnecessary data?

References

1 Merriam-Webster's Learner's Dictionary. http://www.merriam-webster.com/dictionary/protocol

2 International Conference on Harmonisation of Technical Requirements for Registration of Pharmaceuticals for Human Use, ICH Harmonised Tripartite, Guideline, Guideline for Good Clinical Practice, E6 (R2), dated 9 November 2016. https://www.ich.org/page/efficacy-guidelines

3 U.S. Department of Health and Human Services Food and Drug Administration. Title 21, Chapter I, Subchapter D, Part 316.20. https://www.ecfr.gov/cgi-bin/retrieveECFR?gp=&SID=718f6fcbc20f2755bd1f5a980eb5eecd&mc=true&n=sp21.5.316.c&r=SUBPART&ty=HTML#se21.5.316_120

4 U.S. Department of Health and Human Services Food and Drug Administration. Guidance for Industry Considerations for the Design of Early-Phase Clinical Trials of Cellular and Gene Therapy Products, Center for Biologics Evaluation and Research June 2015. https://www.fda.gov/downloads/BiologicsBloodVaccines/GuidanceComplianceRegulatoryInformation/Guidances/CellularandGeneTherapy/UCM564952.pdf

Appendix

Protocol Synopsis

Title of Study:

Protocol No.:

Protocol Revision History:

Phase:

Sponsor:

Investigational Product(s):

No. of Study Centers:

Study Objectives and Endpoints:

Study Design:
- Schema
- Description

Duration of Subject Participation:

Study Duration:

No. of Subjects Planned:

Target Population:
1) Inclusion criteria
2) Exclusion criteria

Statistical Methods:

Appendix A: Schedule of Activities

Visit:	Screening	Treatment Period					End of Study
Day:	Day -28 to -1	Day 0	Day 7	Day 14	Day 28	Day 42	Day 56
Informed Consent	✓						
Demographics	✓						
Medical and Medication History	✓						
Eligibility Criteria	✓	✓					
Physical Examination	✓	✓		✓			✓
Vital Signs	✓	✓		✓	✓	✓	✓
Haematology/ Biochemistry	✓	✓		✓			✓
Urinalysis	✓	✓		✓			✓
Pregnancy Test (Serum at screening and 'dipstick' at other visits pre-dosing)	✓	✓	✓	✓	✓	✓	
Study Drug Administration		✓	✓	✓	✓	✓	
Pharmacokinetic Blood Sampling		✓	✓	✓	✓	✓	
AEs &Concomitant Medications	← Adverse events (AEs) and Concomitant medications →						

19

Informed Consent and Other Human Subject Protection

Karen A. Henry

GCP Key Point
The protection of human the rights, safety, and well-being of human subjects is the foremost concern in the conduct of clinical trials.

19.1   Introduction

Let us first start with why we have informed consent and the protection of subject's rights, safety, and well-being in clinical research.

Historically, humans have always and continue to experiment with the use of objects and medicinal articles to treat or cure physical and psychological ailments. When the experiments are systematic and when the medicinal articles are administered to humans, the experiments are said to be clinical research. In order to gain more information about the "test article," the "investigator" will administer it to a "sample" of "subjects" (humans who are receiving the experimental article) from the "study population" then make inference about how it will work on the "general population." In the past, some articles or procedures have been administered to humans with dire effects on their safety and well-being. Other noninterventional experiments have also caused irreversible harm, not only to the subject in the experiment, but also to their partners or their children. These experiments were conducted with products and procedures without the research subject's consent in the name of benefit to science and society. In each case, the research subjects were not given any information about the intended experiments, were given false or incomplete information about

The Fundamentals of Clinical Research: A Universal Guide for Implementing Good Clinical Practice, First Edition. P. Michael Dubinsky and Karen A. Henry.
© 2022 John Wiley & Sons, Inc. Published 2022 by John Wiley & Sons, Inc.
Companion website: www.wiley.com/go/dubinsky/clinicalresearch

the study, were forced to undergo the procedures, and/or were not given any opportunity to consent for the procedures. (Chapter 1 History).

Due to public outcry, a number of public policies and international codes of ethics were implemented to provide guidance to those involved in the conduct of clinical research to prevent a repeat of these types of atrocities. These policies and codes include the creation of informed consent guidelines and regulations and ethics boards to oversee the protection of humans participating in research (Chapter 1 History).

Today, administration of an "unapproved" test article on human subjects may be conducted only in a clinical research setting. An unapproved product is said to be "investigational" because the information accumulated to date has not been sufficient for a regulatory or health authority to declare it "safe and effective" for its "indication;" i.e., intended therapeutic use by the general public. The product, therefore, may only be administered to humans under approved (i.e., by an ethics committee) and carefully monitored conditions.

In this Chapter, we will review the principles and measures for protecting human subjects in participating in a trial. ICH E6(R2) refers to subject or trial subject. In practice, other terms such as "volunteer" and "participant" may be used. We will continue to use "subject" in this chapter for consistency with the Guideline.

19.2 Objectives

The objectives of this chapter are to describe:

1) The key GCP principles for human subjects protection
2) The general measures used for protecting human subjects
3) Responsibilities of players
4) Ethics review of study information
5) Procedures for informed consent of study information
   - The process of informed consenting
   - The situations for informed consent
   - Minimum elements of consent
   - Process for developing consent information
   - Study documentation of subject consent
6) Procedures for maintaining confidentiality of subject study information and protection of their identity
   - Procedures for the protection of all biological specimen collected from the research subject
7) Compensation for injury and study participation
8) Ensuring medical care for the treatment of non- and study-related adverse events
9) Ability for the subject to withdraw from the study
10) Summary of study documentation records for human subject protection

19.2.1 Key GCP Principles of Human Subjects Protection

Upon review of the Principles of ICH GCP (ICH E6(R2); Chapter 6 GCP Definition and Principles), four key principles that are specific to the protection of human subjects stand out (Source: ICH [1]):

#2.3 The rights, safety, and well-being of the trial subjects are the most important considerations and should prevail over interest of science and society.

#2.7 The medical care given to, and medical decisions made on behalf of, subjects should always be the responsibility of a qualified physician or, when appropriate, of a qualified dentist.

#2.9 Freely given informed consent should be obtained from every subject prior to clinical trial participation.

#2.11 The confidentiality of records that could identify subjects should be protected, respecting the privacy and confidentiality rules in accordance with the applicable regulatory requirement(s).

These principles point to the major components of protecting the rights, safety, and well-being of the research subjects.

19.2.2 Measures to Protect Human Subjects

Measures to protect the rights, safety, and well-being of human subjects include:

- Ethics (IRB/IEC) review of study information prior to initiation of the study
- Protection of their safety to ensure that the benefits outweigh the risks of participating in the study

- Protection of their right to have:

  a) Fully informed consent and voluntarily participate in a trial without coercion
  b) Confidentiality of their identity and health information
  c) Compensation for trial-related injury and for the time, effort, and expenses for their involvement in the study
  d) Medical care for study-related injury or intercurrent illness(es)
  e) The ability to withdraw from the study at any time

19.2.3 General Responsibilities for Protection of Human Subjects

Avoiding exposure of subjects to unreasonable risks during the course of the study is of primary concern for all individuals involved in the oversight and conduct of the study. The risks associated with the use of the investigational product and study procedures versus the potential benefit to the subject for their participation in the study and/or the potential benefit to science and society should be weighed prior to initiating the trial as well as while the study is ongoing:

- The IRB/IEC is responsible for:
  - Review of the protocol, informed consent information, and study drug information to assess potential study risk and benefit prior to implementation of the protocol
  - Continuing review of new safety information that are generated once the study commences to assess study risk against benefit

- The sponsor is responsible for:
  - Manufacturing the test article per good manufacturing practices (GMPs). The investigational product should be designed and manufactured to optimize its stability, integrity, handling, and storage. It should be easy for the person who is preparing and administering to the patient and have minimum safety risk. (Chapter 17 The Investigational Product (Clinical Supplies)).
  - Submission to regulatory authority(ies) for authorization/approval/notification of the use of an investigational product in humans (Chapter 5 Regulatory affairs).
  - Confirming the qualifications of IRB/EC and all individuals who are involved in the creation of informed consent documents and administration of informed consent (Chapter 14 Trial Management; Start-up, On-Study, and Close-Out; Chapter 22 Monitoring Overview).
  - Verifying that each subject was appropriately consented for the study (Chapter 22 Monitoring Overview).
  - Overseeing the handling, administration, and accountability per the product's requirements and GCP (Chapter 17 The Investigational Product (Clinical Supplies)).
  - Designing and implementing a scientifically sound clinical trial protocol that can be justified by the known clinical and nonclinical risks (Chapter 18 The Clinical Trial Protocol and Amendments).
  - Implementation of procedures to evaluate the safety of the product (Chapter 18 The Clinical Trial Protocol and Amendments) when administered to the subjects.
  - Providing the investigator with decodes for blinded trials (Chapter 24 Investigator/Institution Initiation)
  - Safety monitoring. Study data should be reviewed as they are received during the study to continuously assess the safety risk versus benefit for the continued participation of study subjects. Oversight by an independent safety committee may be necessary for blinded trials. (Chapter 21 Safety Monitoring and Reporting)

- The investigator is responsible for (Chapter 9 Investigator and Sponsor Roles and Responsibilities):
  - Documentation of qualification of IRB/EC
  - Documentation of qualification and delegation of responsibility of those administering consent

- Having written procedures for informed consent
- Having written procedures for maintaining subject confidentiality
- Ensuring that the investigational product is stored, handled, and administered according to the trial protocol
- Immediate and complete evaluation of adverse events that arise during the study
- Medical care of the subject for any study-related physical and mental adverse reactions or other health issues that arise during the study.

• A trial should be immediately discontinued by the IRB/IEC, sponsor, or investigator, if the use of the investigational product and/or associated study procedure(s) (e.g., a device used for administration of the investigational product) pose(s) unreasonable physical or mental risks to subject subjects (Chapter 8 IRB/IEC Roles and Responsibilities; Chapter 9 Investigator and Sponsor Roles & Responsibilities).

19.2.4 Ethics Review of Study Information

Ethics review boards (IRBs/IECs) are charged with safeguarding the rights, safety, and well-being of all trial subjects (ICH E6(R2) 3.1.1).

All study-related information that will be given to or be seen by a potential trial research subject or an on-going subject must be reviewed by and given the favorable opinion of a qualified IRB/IEC (Chapter 8 IRB/IEC Roles and Responsibilities; Chapter 9 Investigator and Sponsor Roles and Responsibilities) (ICH E6(R2) 4.4.1) prior to its dissemination. These include:

• Detailed description of the study protocol procedures
• Description of study risks and information about the investigational article
• Advertising and other recruitment materials
• Ancillary study information, materials (e.g., questionnaires, diary devices, study treatment instructions, or devices) that will be given to the subject
• Information or training materials and equipment that will be shared with the subject during interactions with study personnel
• Monetary or other form of compensation that will be given to the subject

The objectives of the ethics review are to:

a) Prevent the dissemination of any information or implementation of any procedure that may be coercive or that unduly influences a subject's decision to participate or continue participating in the study
b) Review the risk versus benefit of all procedures and equipment related to the study

If the IRB/IEC conditions its approval/favorable opinion upon change(s) in any aspect of the trial, such as modification(s) of the protocol, written informed consent form and any other written information to be provided to subjects, and/or other procedures, the sponsor should obtain from the investigator/institution a copy of the modification(s) made and the date approval/favorable opinion was given by the IRB/IEC. (ICH E6(R2) 5.11.2)

19.2.5 Informed Consent

Clinical research subjects have the right to fully informed consent (i.e., they will receive all available information that may influence their decision to volunteer for the study and to continue participating in the study) and to voluntarily participate in a trial without any form of coercion.

Informed Consent is defined as (ICH E6(R2) 1.28):

- A process by which a subject voluntarily confirms his or her willingness to participate in a particular trial, after having been informed of all aspects of the trial that are relevant to the subject's decision to participate. Informed consent is documented by means of a written, signed, and dated informed consent form.

There are several factors to consider for informed consent. Human research ethical codes provide guidelines for the process of administering consent under different circumstances and what information must be conveyed during consenting.

19.2.5.1 The Process of Consenting

The process of consenting starts before study participation and continues as needed to provide updates to the subject throughout the study. Generally, before undergoing any procedure or activity that is specific for the study, i.e., any procedure or activity that the subject would undergo only because they are in the study, documented consent for the procedure or activity is required from a study subject. In all cases below, the subject may be represented by their legally authorized representative.

The process for consenting includes:

a) Ethics approval (ICH E6(R2) 4.8.1, 4.8.2)
   - All information to be provided to the volunteer must have been reviewed and given the favorable opinion of an IRB/IEC (Section 19.2.4).
b) Administration by qualified individuals (ICH E6(R2) 4.8.5)
   - Consent will be administered by the investigator designed qualified individual(s) who will personally sign and date the consent form.
c) No coercion (ICH E6(R2) 4.8.3)
   - No person or material given to the study subject may coerce them to volunteer for the study or to continue to participate in the study.
   - Consider that group or peer pressure may influence a subject's participation (asking questions or deciding to consent for the study) if more than one subject is administered consent together.
   - Implement procedures to ensure that each subject has private opportunity(ies) for asking questions or discussing the study with the investigator or study staff prior to signing consent and throughout the trial.

Legend:

PLATE 1

Section Reference

Chapter Reference

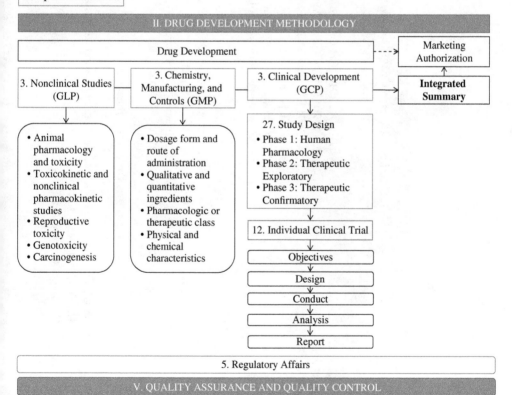

II. DRUG DEVELOPMENT METHODOLOGY

Drug Development → Marketing Authorization

3. Nonclinical Studies (GLP) | 3. Chemistry, Manufacturing, and Controls (GMP) | 3. Clinical Development (GCP) → Integrated Summary

- Animal pharmacology and toxicity
- Toxicokinetic and nonclinical pharmacokinetic studies
- Reproductive toxicity
- Genotoxicity
- Carcinogenesis

- Dosage form and route of administration
- Qualitative and quantitative ingredients
- Pharmacologic or therapeutic class
- Physical and chemical characteristics

27. Study Design
- Phase 1: Human Pharmacology
- Phase 2: Therapeutic Exploratory
- Phase 3: Therapeutic Confirmatory

12. Individual Clinical Trial

Objectives

Design

Conduct

Analysis

Report

5. Regulatory Affairs

V. QUALITY ASSURANCE AND QUALITY CONTROL

PLATE 2

Legend:

| Chapter Reference |

| 1. Significant Dates in GCP History |

.... 2016 ICH Guideline for Good Clinical Practice E6(R2)
.... 2011 ISO GCP for Medical Device
.... 2004 EU Clinical Trial Directive 2001/20/EC
.... 1996 ICH Guideline for Good Clinical Practice E6
.... 1990 ICH established by Japan, USA, and EU
.... 1980's Additional countries established regulatory controls over
                        clinical trials
.... 1979 The Belmont Report
.... 1976 US General Accounting Office Report
.... 1974 US National Research Act
.... 1972 US Public Health Service's Tuskegee Syphilis Study
.... 1965 US National Institutes of Health
.... 1964 The Declaration of Helsinki
.... 1962 Kefauver-Harris Drug Amendments to the FFDCA
.... 1949 The Nuremburg Code
.... 1938 US Congress enacts the Federal Food, Drug and Cosmetic Act
.... 1906 US Food and Drugs Act
.... 1902 US Biologics Control Act

PLATE 3

Legend:

Chapter Reference

7. PLAYERS ROLES AND RESPONSIBILITIES:
IRB/EC, INVESTIGATOR, SPONSOR/CRO, REGULATORY AGENCY

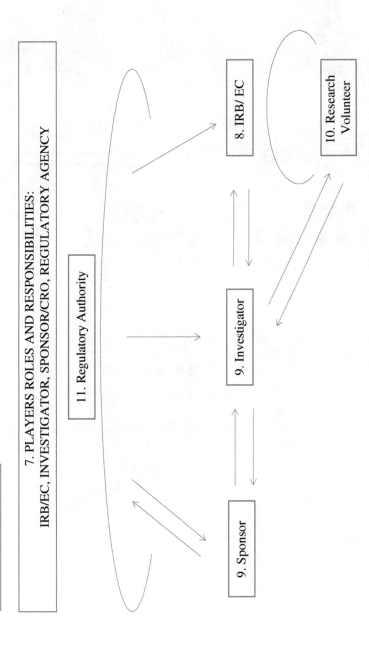

11. Regulatory Authority

8. IRB/ EC

10. Research Volunteer

9. Investigator

9. Sponsor

PLATE 4

Legend:

Chapter Reference	ICH E6(R2): **INVESTIGATOR RESPONSIBILITIES**	**SPONSOR RESPONSIBILITIES**

9. Individual Clinical Trial – Overview of Investigator and Sponsor Responsibilities

TRIAL DESIGN

SUBJECT RIGHTS AND SAFETY

DATA INTEGRITY

TRIAL PROTOCOL	TREATMENT-INVESTIGATIONAL PRODUCT	HUMAN SUBJECT PROTECTION	SAFETY MONITORING AND REPORTING	DATA COLLECTION AND MANAGEMENT	DATA ANALYSIS

18. Study Protocol and Amendments

16. Investigator's Brochure

17. Clinical Supplies

19. Human Subject Protection

19. Safety, Pharmacokinetics, and Pharmacodynamics Laboratory Testing

21. Safety Monitoring and Reporting

20. Data Collection and Data Management

27. Statistics and Data Analysis

4.6 INVESTIGATIONAL PRODUCTS

4.3 MEDICAL CARE OF SUBJECTS

4.11 SAFETY REPORTING

4.7 RANDOMIZATION PROCEDURES AND UNBLINDING

4.9 RECORDS AND REPORTS

5.4 TRIAL DESIGN

5.12 INFORMATION ON INVESTIGATIONAL PRODUCT(S)

5.13 MANUFACTURING, PACKAGING, LABELING, AND CODING INVESTIGATIONAL PRODUCT(S)

5.14 SUPPLYING AND HANDLING INVESTIGATIONAL PRODUCT(S)

4.8 INFORMED CONSENT OF TRIAL SUBJECTS

5.3 MEDICAL EXPERTISE

5.8 COMPENSION TO SUBJECTS AND INVESTIGATORS

5.16 SAFETY INFORMATION

5.17 ADVERSE DRUG REACTION REPORTING

5.0 QUALITY MANAGEMENT

5.5 TRIAL MANAGEMENT, DATA HANDLING, RECORDKEEPING, AND INDEPENDENT DATA MONITORING COMMITTEE

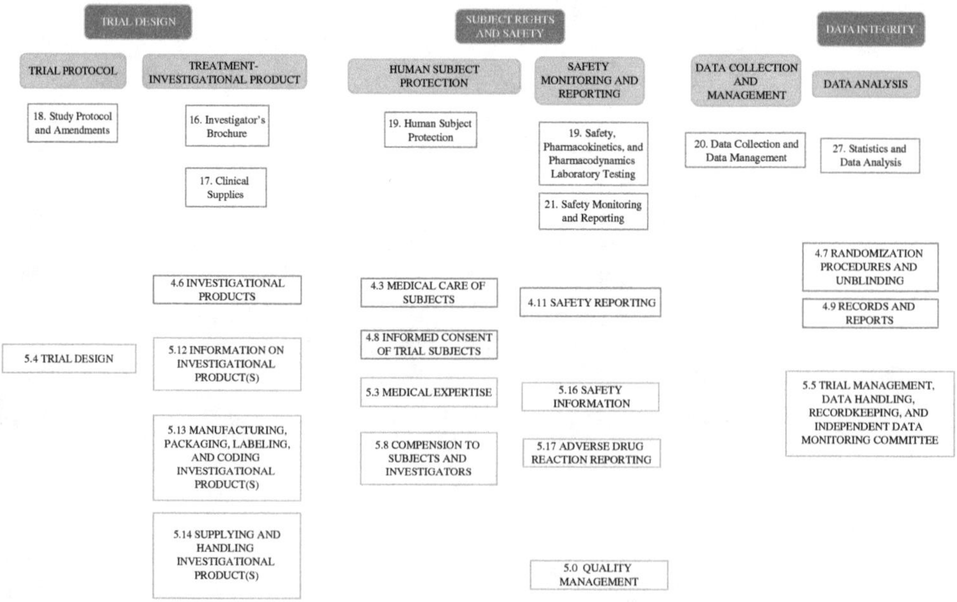

Source: ICH E6(R2) 4, 5.

TRIAL OVERSIGHT
AND COMPLIANCE

REPORTING OF
TRIAL CONDUCT

RECORDS	TRIAL COMPLIANCE	RESOURCING	QUALIFICATIONS AND TRAINING	REPORTING OF TRIAL CONDUCT	
29. Essential Documents	14. Trial Management	15. Resourcing / Outsourcing	23. Investigator and Site Selection	9. IRB / Ethics and Regulatory Authority Communication	28. Clinical Study Report
	33. Audits				
	34. Inspections		24. Trial Initiation		
	25. Interim monitoring				
	26. Investigator sites and study closeout				
	4.5 COMPLIANCE WITH PROTOCOL	4.2 ADEQUATE RESOURCES	4.1 QUALIFICATIONS AND AGREEMENTS		4.4 COMMUNICATION WITH IRB/IEC
					4.10 PROGRESS REPORTS
	5.1 QUALITY ASSURANCE AND QUALITY CONTROL	5.2 CONTRACT RESEARCH ORGANIZATION	5.6 INVESTIGATOR SELECTION	5.10 NOTIFICATION/SUBMISSION TO REGULATORY AUTHORITY(IES)	4.12 PREMATURE TERMINATION OR SUSPENSION OF A TRIAL
	5.15 RECORD ACCESS	5.7 ALLOCATION OF RESPONSIBILITIES			4.13 FINAL REPORTS
	5.18 MONITORING	5.9 FINANCING		5.11 CONFIRMATION OF REVIEW BY IRB/IEC	
	5.19 AUDIT			5.21 PREMATURE TERMINATION OR SUSPENSION OF A TRIAL	
	5.20 NONCOMPLIANCE			5.22 CLINICAL TRIAL/STUDY REPORTS	
	5.23 MULTICENTER TRIALS				

PLATE 5

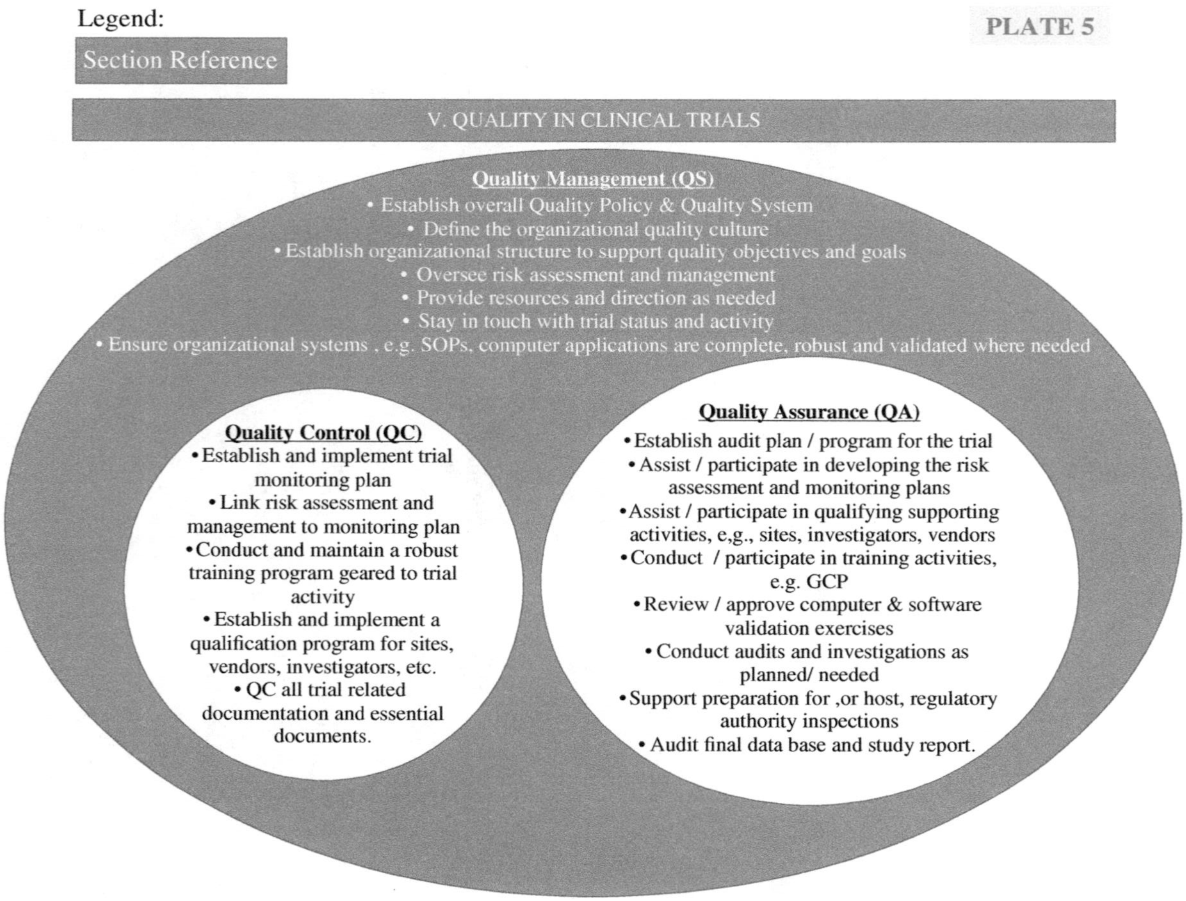

Legend:

V. QUALITY IN CLINICAL TRIALS

Quality Management (QS)
- Establish overall Quality Policy & Quality System
- Define the organizational quality culture
- Establish organizational structure to support quality objectives and goals
- Oversee risk assessment and management
- Provide resources and direction as needed
- Stay in touch with trial status and activity
- Ensure organizational systems , e.g. SOPs, computer applications are complete, robust and validated where needed

Quality Assurance (QA)
- Establish audit plan / program for the trial
- Assist / participate in developing the risk assessment and monitoring plans
- Assist / participate in qualifying supporting activities, e.g., sites, investigators, vendors
- Conduct / participate in training activities, e.g. GCP
- Review / approve computer & software validation exercises
- Conduct audits and investigations as planned/ needed
- Support preparation for ,or host, regulatory authority inspections
- Audit final data base and study report.

Quality Control (QC)
- Establish and implement trial monitoring plan
- Link risk assessment and management to monitoring plan
- Conduct and maintain a robust training program geared to trial activity
- Establish and implement a qualification program for sites, vendors, investigators, etc.
- QC all trial related documentation and essential documents.

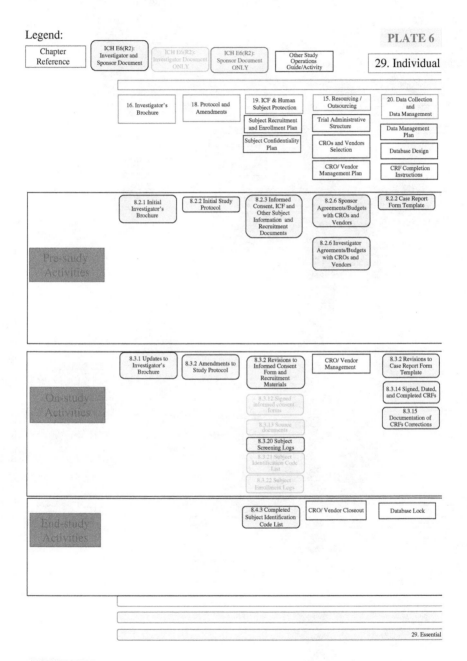

Legend:

| Chapter Reference | ICH E6(R2): Investigator and Sponsor Document | ICH E6(R2): Investigator Document ONLY | ICH E6(R2): Sponsor Document ONLY | Other Study Operations Guide/Activity |

PLATE 6

29. Individual

	16. Investigator's Brochure	18. Protocol and Amendments	19. ICF & Human Subject Protection	15. Resourcing / Outsourcing	20. Data Collection and Data Management
			Subject Recruitment and Enrollment Plan	Trial Administrative Structure	Data Management Plan
			Subject Confidentiality Plan	CROs and Vendors Selection	Database Design
				CRO/ Vendor Management Plan	CRF Completion Instructions

Pre-study Activities

8.2.1 Initial Investigator's Brochure	8.2.2 Initial Study Protocol	8.2.3 Informed Consent, ICF and Other Subject Information and Recruitment Documents	8.2.6 Sponsor Agreements/Budgets with CROs and Vendors	8.2.2 Case Report Form Template
			8.2.6 Investigator Agreements/Budgets with CROs and Vendors	

On-study Activities

8.3.1 Updates to Investigator's Brochure	8.3.2 Amendments to Study Protocol	8.3.2 Revisions to Informed Consent Form and Recruitment Materials	CRO/ Vendor Management	8.3.2 Revisions to Case Report Form Template
		8.3.12 Signed Informed consent forms		8.3.14 Signed, Dated, and Completed CRFs
		8.3.13 Source documents		8.3.15 Documentation of CRFs Corrections
		8.3.20 Subject Screening Logs		
		8.3.21 Subject Identification Code List		
		8.3.22 Subject Enrollment Logs		

End-study Activities

| 8.4.3 Completed Subject Identification Code List | CRO/ Vendor Closeout | Database Lock |

29. Essential

Sources: ICH E6(R2) 8.

Clinical Trial – Essential Documents

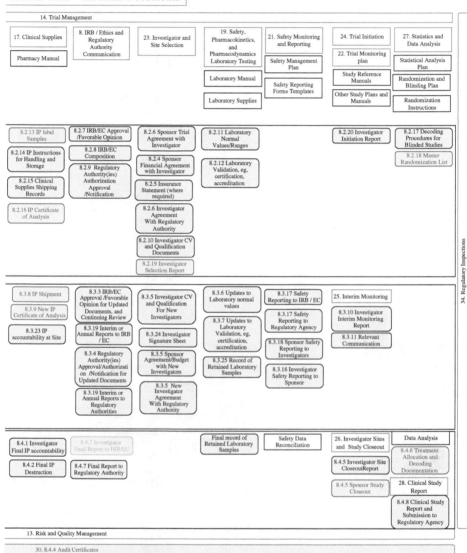

14. Trial Management

17. Clinical Supplies	8. IRB / Ethics and Regulatory Authority Communication	23. Investigator and Site Selection	19. Safety, Pharmacokinetics, and Pharmacodynamics Laboratory Testing	21. Safety Monitoring and Reporting	24. Trial Initiation	27. Statistics and Data Analysis
Pharmacy Manual				Safety Management Plan	22. Trial Monitoring plan	Statistical Analysis Plan
			Laboratory Manual	Safety Reporting Forms Templates	Study Reference Manuals	Randomization and Blinding Plan
			Laboratory Supplies		Other Study Plans and Manuals	Randomization Instructions

8.2.13 IP label Samples	8.2.7 IRB/EC Approval /Favorable Opinion	8.2.6 Sponsor Trial Agreement with Investigator	8.2.11 Laboratory Normal Values/Ranges		8.2.20 Investigator Initiation Report	8.2.17 Decoding Procedures for Blinded Studies
8.2.14 IP Instructions for Handling and Storage	8.2.8 IRB/EC Composition	8.2.4 Sponsor Financial Agreement with Investigator	8.2.12 Laboratory Validation, eg, certification, accreditation			8.2.18 Master Randomization List
8.2.15 Clinical Supplies Shipping Records	8.2.9 Regulatory Authority(ies) Authorization Approval /Notification	8.2.5 Insurance Statement (where required)				
8.2.16 IP Certificate of Analysis		8.2.6 Investigator Agreement With Regulatory Authority				
		8.2.10 Investigator CV and Qualification Documents				
		8.2.19 Investigator Selection Report				

8.3.8 IP Shipment	8.3.3 IRB/EC Approval /Favorable Opinion for Updated Documents, and Continuing Review	8.3.5 Investigator CV and Qualification For New Investigators	8.3.6 Updates to Laboratory normal values	8.3.17 Safety Reporting to IRB / EC	25. Interim Monitoring
8.3.9 New IP Certificate of Analysis	8.3.19 Interim or Annual Reports to IRB / EC	8.3.24 Investigator Signature Sheet	8.3.7 Updates to Laboratory Validation, eg, certification, accreditation	8.3.17 Safety Reporting to Regulatory Agency	8.3.10 Investigator Interim Monitoring Report
8.3.23 IP accountability at Site	8.3.4 Regulatory Authority(ies) Approval/Authorization /Notification for Updated Documents	8.3.5 Sponsor Agreement/Budget with New Investigators	8.3.25 Record of Retained Laboratory Samples	8.3.18 Sponsor Safety Reporting to Investigators	8.3.11 Relevant Communication
	8.3.19 Interim or Annual Reports to Regulatory Authorities	8.3.5 New Investigator Agreement With Regulatory Authority		8.3.16 Investigator Safety Reporting to Sponsor	

8.4.1 Investigator Final IP accountability	8.4.7 Investigator Final Report to IRB/EC		Final record of Retained Laboratory Samples	Safety Data Reconciliation	26. Investigator Sites and Study Closeout	Data Analysis
8.4.2 Final IP Destruction	8.4.7 Final Report to Regulatory Authority				8.4.5 Investigator Site CloseoutReport	8.4.6 Treatment Allocation and Decoding Documentation
					8.4.5 Sponsor Study Closeout	28. Clinical Study Report
						8.4.8 Clinical Study Report and Submission to Regulatory Agency

13. Risk and Quality Management

30. 8.4.4 Audit Certificates

Documents: Plans, Maintenance, Reconciliation, and Closeouts

34. Regulatory Inspections

PLATE 7

Legend:

Chapter Reference

22. Monitoring

ICH E6(R2) 5.18.2 Selection and Qualifications of Monitors

ICH E6(R2) 5.18.3 Extent and Nature of Monitoring

ICH E6(R2) 5.18.4 Monitor's Responsibilities

ICH E6(R2) 5.18.5 Monitoring Procedures

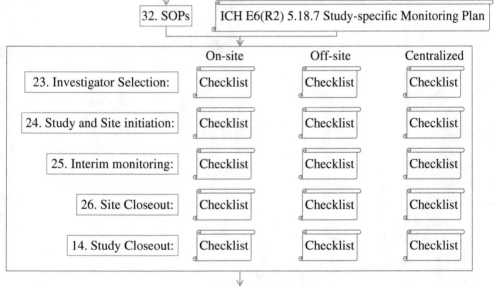

32. SOPs   ICH E6(R2) 5.18.7 Study-specific Monitoring Plan

	On-site	Off-site	Centralized
23. Investigator Selection:	Checklist	Checklist	Checklist
24. Study and Site initiation:	Checklist	Checklist	Checklist
25. Interim monitoring:	Checklist	Checklist	Checklist
26. Site Closeout:	Checklist	Checklist	Checklist
14. Study Closeout:	Checklist	Checklist	Checklist

5.18.6 Monitoring Report

Source: ICH E6(R2) 5.18

PLATE 8

Legend:

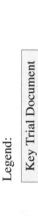

Key Trial Document

Chapter Reference

Individual Study - Data Framework/Information Flow Among Key Trial Documents

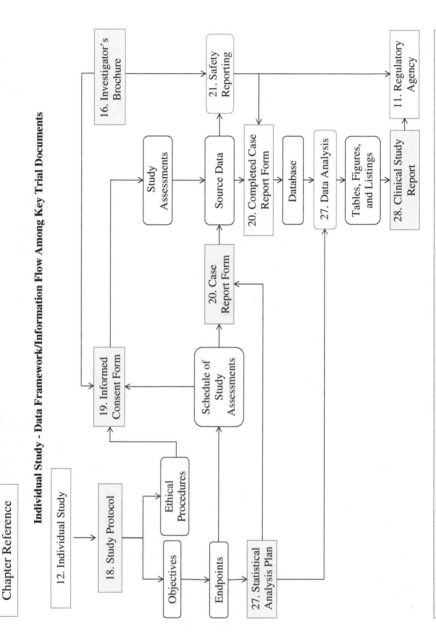

32. Standard Operating Procedures and Other Written Procedural Guidelines

PLATE 9

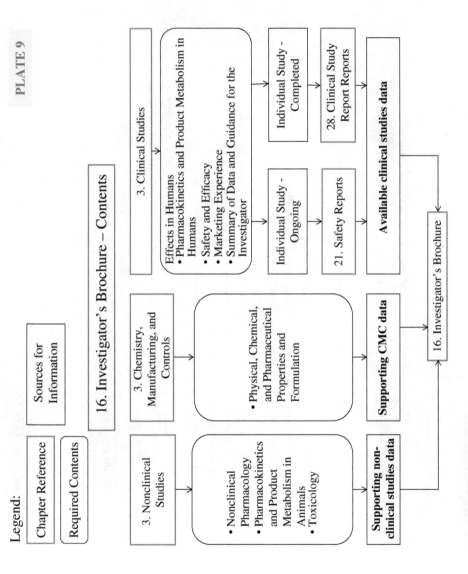

Legend:

Chapter Reference

Sources for Information

Required Contents

16. Investigator's Brochure – Contents

3. Nonclinical Studies

- Nonclinical Pharmacology
- Pharmacokinetics and Product Metabolism in Animals
- Toxicology

Supporting non-clinical studies data

3. Chemistry, Manufacturing, and Controls

- Physical, Chemical, and Pharmaceutical Properties and Formulation

Supporting CMC data

16. Investigator's Brochure

3. Clinical Studies

Effects in Humans
- Pharmacokinetics and Product Metabolism in Humans
- Safety and Efficacy
- Marketing Experience
- Summary of Data and Guidance for the Investigator

Individual Study - Ongoing

21. Safety Reports

Available clinical studies data

Individual Study - Completed

28. Clinical Study Report Reports

Source: ICH E6(R2) 7.

PLATE 10

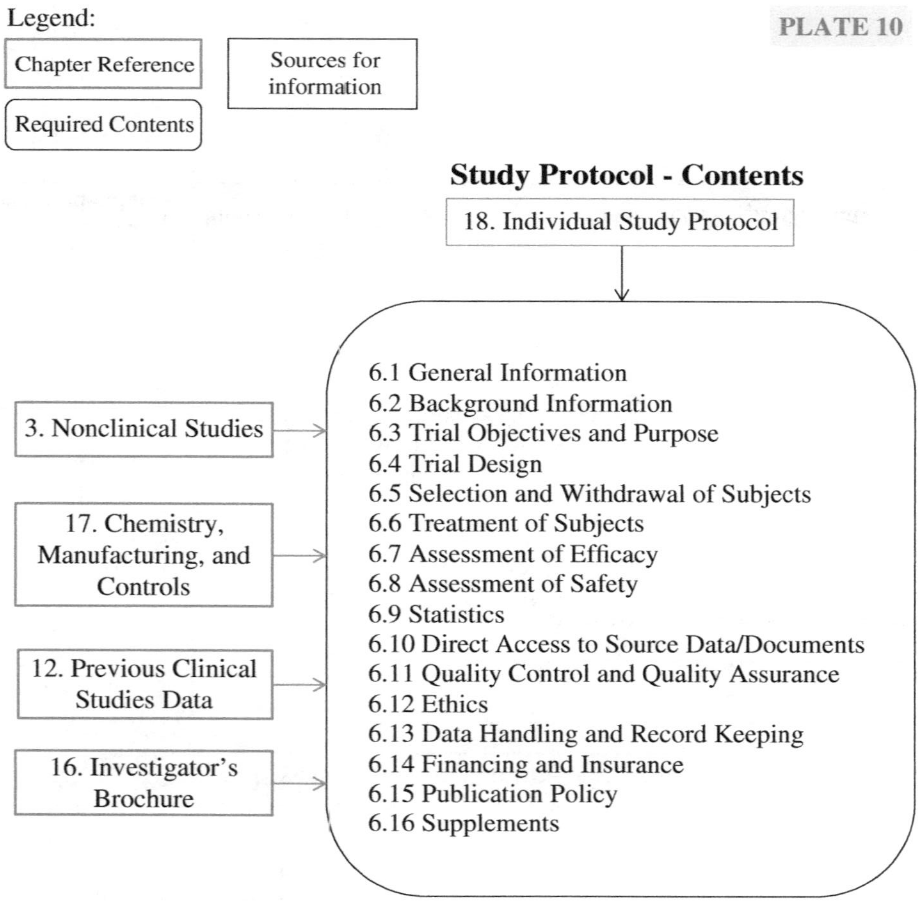

Legend:

Chapter Reference

Required Contents

Sources for information

Study Protocol - Contents

18. Individual Study Protocol

6.1 General Information
6.2 Background Information
6.3 Trial Objectives and Purpose
6.4 Trial Design
6.5 Selection and Withdrawal of Subjects
6.6 Treatment of Subjects
6.7 Assessment of Efficacy
6.8 Assessment of Safety
6.9 Statistics
6.10 Direct Access to Source Data/Documents
6.11 Quality Control and Quality Assurance
6.12 Ethics
6.13 Data Handling and Record Keeping
6.14 Financing and Insurance
6.15 Publication Policy
6.16 Supplements

3. Nonclinical Studies

17. Chemistry, Manufacturing, and Controls

12. Previous Clinical Studies Data

16. Investigator's Brochure

Source: ICH E6(R2) 6.

PLATE 11

Legend:

| Chapter Reference |

| Required Contents |

Informed Consent Form – Contents

| 19. Informed Consent Form |

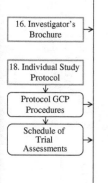

| 16. Investigator's Brochure |

| 18. Individual Study Protocol |

| Protocol GCP Procedures |

| Schedule of Trial Assessments |

(a) That the trial involves research.

(b) The purpose of the trial.

(c) The trial treatment(s) and the probability for random assignment to each treatment.

(d) The trial procedures to be followed, including all invasive procedures.

(e) The subject's responsibilities.

(f) Those aspects of the trial that are experimental. The reasonably foreseeable risks or inconveniences to the subject and, when applicable, to an embryo, fetus, or nursing infant.

(h) The reasonably expected benefits. When there is no intended clinical benefit to the subject, the subject should be made aware of this.

(i) The alternative procedure(s) or course(s) of treatment that may be available to the subject, and their important potential benefits and risks.

(j) The compensation and/or treatment available to the subject in the event of trial-related injury.

(k) The anticipated prorated payment, if any, to the subject for participating in the trial.

(l) The anticipated expenses, if any, to the subject for participating in the trial.

(m) That the subject's participation in the trial is voluntary and that the subject may refuse to participate or withdraw from the trial, at any time, without penalty or loss of benefits to which the subject is otherwise entitled.

(n) That the monitor(s), the auditor(s), the IRB/IEC, and the regulatory authority(ies) will be granted direct access to the subject's original medical records for verification of clinical trial procedures and/or data, without violating the confidentiality of the subject, to the extent permitted by the applicable laws and regulations and that, by signing a written informed consent form, the subject or the subject's legally acceptable representative is authorizing such access.

(o) That records identifying the subject will be kept confidential and, to the extent permitted by the applicable laws and/or regulations, will not be made publicly available. If the results of the trial are published, the subject's identity will remain confidential.

(p) That the subject or the subject's legally acceptable representative will be informed in a timely manner if information becomes available that may be relevant to the subject's willingness to continue participation in the trial.

(q) The person(s) to contact for further information regarding the trial and the rights of trial subjects, and whom to contact in the event of trial-related injury.

(r) The foreseeable circumstances and/or reasons under which the subject's participation in the trial may be terminated.

(s) The expected duration of the subject's participation in the trial.

(t) The approximate number of subjects involved in the trial.

Source: ICH E6(R2) 4.8.

PLATE 12

Legend:

Chapter Reference

Required Contents

Sources for
information

Statistical Analysis Plan - Contents

27. Statistical Analysis Plan

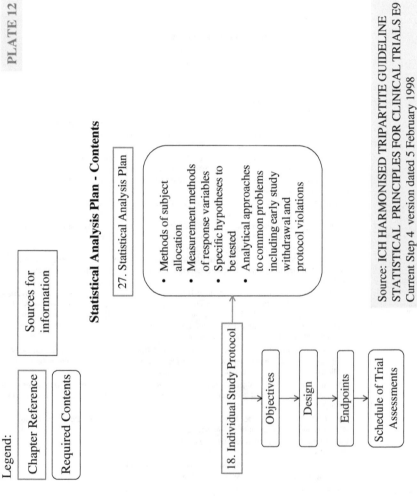

- Methods of subject allocation
- Measurement methods of response variables
- Specific hypotheses to be tested
- Analytical approaches to common problems including early study withdrawal and protocol violations

18. Individual Study Protocol

Objectives

Design

Endpoints

Schedule of Trial Assessments

Source: ICH HARMONISED TRIPARTITE GUIDELINE
STATISTICAL PRINCIPLES FOR CLINICAL TRIALS E9
Current Step 4 version dated 5 February 1998

PLATE 13

Legend:

| Chapter Reference |

| Sources for information |

(Required Contents)

Case Report Form - Contents

| 20. Case Report Form |

CONTENTS
- Informed consent date and time
- Subject demographics
- Eligibility
  - Inclusion criteria
  - Exclusion criteria
- Medical history
- Medication history
- Investigational product administration
- Safety assessments
- Efficacy assessments
- Adverse events
- Concomitant medications
- Reason for end of treatment/end of study

| 18. Individual Study Protocol |

- Eligibility Criteria
- Safety Assessments
- Efficacy Assessments
- Schedule of Trial Assessments
- Ethical procedures

DESIGN
- Variable names
- Data definitions

| 27. Statistical Analysis Plan |

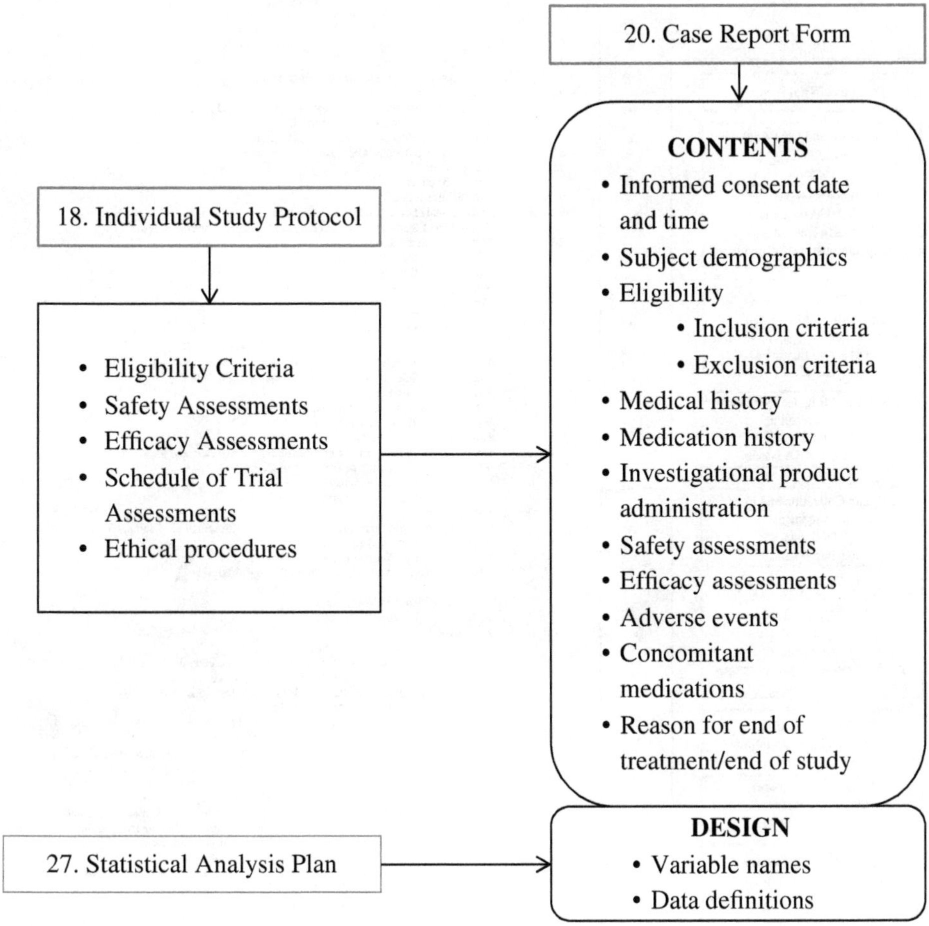

PLATE 14

Legend:

| Chapter reference |

| Sources for information |

| Required Contents |

| 18. Clinical Trial Protocol |

| 27. Statistics and Data Analysis
Methods
Reports |

| 14. Trial Management
Study conduct
Study administrative structure |

| 17. Clinical Supplies
Identity and batch (es)
Subject allocation (randomization
and actual treatment) |

| 9. IRB/IEC and Regulatory Authority
Communication
IRB/IECs used
IRB/IECs or RA Issues |

| 20. Data Collection and Data
Management
Trial data
CRF templates |

| 19. Laboratory Testing
Testing procedures
Testing results
Standardization of normal ranges |

| 22. Trial Monitoring
Protocol and trial deviations |

| 33. Quality Assurance
Quality procedures
Audits and findings |

| 34. Regulatory Inspections
Inspections and findings |

| Publication(s) of study results |

1.0	Title Page
2.0	Synopsis
3.0	Table of Contents
4.0	List of Abbreviations and Definitions of Terms
5.0	Ethics
5.1	Institutional Review Board (IRB) or Ethics Committee (EC)
5.2	Ethical Conduct of the Study
5.3	Subject Information and Consent
6.0	Investigators and Study Administrative Structure
7.0	Introduction
8.0	Study Objectives
9.0	Investigational Plan
9.1	Overall Study Design and Plan Description
9.2	Discussion of Study Design, Including the Choice of Control Groups
9.3	Selection of Study Population
9.3.1	Inclusion Criteria
9.3.2	Exclusion Criteria
9.3.3	Removal of Subjects from Therapy or Assessment
9.4	Treatments
9.4.1	Treatments Administered
9.4.2	Identification of Investigational Products
9.4.3	Method of Assigning Subjects to Treatment Groups
9.4.4	Selection of Doses in the Study
9.4.5	Selection and Timing of Dose for Each Patient
9.4.6	Blinding
9.4.7	Prior and Concomitant Therapy
9.4.8	Treatment Compliance
9.5	Efficacy and Safety Variables
9.5.1	Efficacy and Safety Measurements Assessed and Flow Chart
9.5.2	Appropriateness of Measurements
9.5.3	Primary Efficacy Variables
9.5.4	Drug Concentration Measurements
9.6	Data Quality Assurance
9.7	Statistical Methods Planned in the Protocol and Determination of Sample Size
9.7.1	Statistical and Analytical Plans
9.7.2	Determination of Sample Size
9.8	Changes in the Conduct of the Study or Planned Analyses
10.0	Study Subjects
10.1	Disposition of Subjects
10.2	Protocol Deviations
11.0	Efficacy Evaluation
11.1	Data Sets Analyzed
11.2	Demographic and Other Baseline Characteristics
11.3	Measurements of Treatment Compliance
11.4	Efficacy Results and Tabulations of Individual Patient Data
11.4.1	Analysis of Efficacy
11.4.2	Statistical/Analytical Issues
11.4.2.1	Adjustments for Covariates
11.4.2.2	Handling of Dropouts or Missing Data
11.4.2.3	Interim Analyses and Data Monitoring
11.4.2.4	Multicenter Studies
11.4.2.5	Multiple Comparisons/Multiplicity
11.4.2.6	Use of and "Efficacy Subset" of Subjects
11.4.2.7	ActiveControl Studies Intended to Show Equivalence
11.4.2.8	Examination of Subgroups
11.4.3	Tabulation of Individual Response Data
11.4.4	Drug Dose, Drug Concentration, and Relationships to Response
11.4.5	DrugDrug and DrugDisease Interactions
11.4.6	ByPatient Displays
11.4.7	Efficacy Conclusions

Source: ICH E3 STRUCTURE AND CONTENT OF CLINICAL
Current Step 4 version dated 30 November 1995

Clinical Study Report - Contents

28. Clinical Study Report

STRUCTURE AND CONTENT

STUDY REPORTS

PLATE 15

Legend:

Chapter Reference

22. Monitoring Overview

22. Investigator Selection, Initiation, Interim Monitoring, and Closeout

30. QA incl. audits, incl. SOPs, audits, sponsor staff & CRO qualification and training

9. Regulatory Authority & IRB/IEC Reporting, communication, and approval

13. Study Oversight and Risk Management

19. Laboratory specimen collection, processing, storage, testing, results assessment and tracking

17. IMP GMP, shipping, accountability & disposition (and storage)

27. Randomization and Blinding

10. Human Subject Protection, Recruitment, Informed consent, subject eligibility, medical care, & subject confidentiality

27. Data analysis & TFL reports and clinical Study Reports

29. Investigator, CRO/Vendor, & Sponsor Trial File maintenance and archiving

22. Study and Protocol Deviations and CAPAs

20. Source Documentation, CRFs and Queries completion

21. Adverse events Assessment, reporting, and follow up

14. Study Closeout

30. Audits & Inspection CAPAs

15. Subject, Investigator, CRO/Vendor Payments

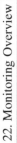

➤ *Oversight of the study -investigator and sponsor responsibilities*

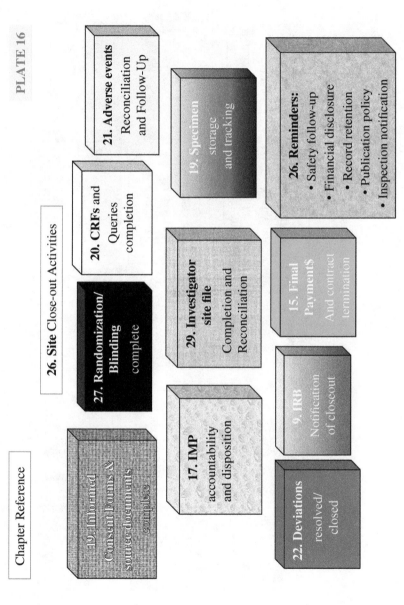

PLATE 16

Legend:

Chapter Reference

26. Site Close-out Activities

21. Adverse events
Reconciliation
and Follow-Up

20. CRFs and
Queries
completion

19. Specimen
storage
and tracking

26. Reminders:
• Safety follow-up
• Financial disclosure
• Record retention
• Publication policy
• Inspection notification

27. Randomization/
Blinding
complete

29. Investigator
site file
Completion and
Reconciliation

15. Final
Payment$
And contract
termination

19. Informed
Consent Forms &
source documents
complete

17. IMP
accountability
and disposition

9. IRB
Notification
of closeout

22. Deviations
resolved/
closed

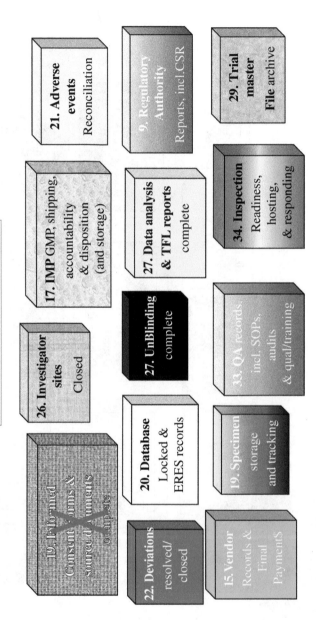

PLATE 17

Legend:

Chapter Reference

14. Study Close-out Activities

21. Adverse events Reconciliation

9. Regulatory Authority Reports, incl.CSR

29. Trial master File archive

17. IMP GMP, shipping, accountability & disposition (and storage)

27. Data analysis & TFL reports complete

34. Inspection Readiness, hosting, & responding

26. Investigator sites Closed

27. UnBlinding complete

33. QA records incl. SOPs, audits & qual/training

19. Informed Consent Forms & source documents complete

20. Database Locked & ERES records

19. Specimen storage and tracking

22. Deviations resolved/ closed

15. Vendor Records & Final Payments

➤ *Study Close = out is similar to Site Close-out, except for signed ICFs and source documents*

Legend:

PLATE 18

29. Example of Structure of Files for Essential Documents

Sponsor Files

At the trial level:
- Investigator's brochure and amendments
- Clinical trial protocol and amendments
- Informed consent form template
- Sample case report form
- Trial management
- Submissions to regulatory authority(ies)
- Safety reporting to regulatory authority(ies) and all investigators
- Investigational product release and shipments
- Statistical analysis plan
- Centralized monitoring procedures
- Other study plans and procedures
… etc.

For each Contract Research Organization
- Qualification
- Financial agreements
- Essential documents for delegated responsibilities as transferred from the CRO
- …etc.

For each central laboratory:
- Qualification
- Financial agreements
- Tracking of laboratory specimen or media
- …etc.

For each Investigator/Institution:
- Investigator's regulatory agreement
- Financial agreements
- Investigator's and staff qualification and training
- IRB/IEC submissions, approvals, and communication
- Subject screening and enrollment logs
- Investigator delegation of study duties
- Investigational product accountability
- Investigator selection, initiation, monitoring and closeout reports
- Protocol and study deviation logs
- Safety reports from the investigator
- … etc.

Contract Research Organization Files

- Qualification
- Contracts
- Essential documents for delegated responsibilities
- Standard operating procedures
- …etc.

Central Laboratory Files

- Qualifications
- Financial agreements
- Tracking of laboratory specimen or media
- Standard operating procedures
- …etc.

Investigator/Institution Files

At the site level:
- Investigator's regulatory agreement
- Financial agreements
- Investigator's and staff qualification and training
- IRB/IEC submissions, approvals, and communication
- Subject identification code list
- Subject screening and enrollment logs
- Investigator delegation of study duties
- Investigational product accountability
- Investigator initiation report
- Protocol and study deviation logs
- Safety reporting to the sponsor
- Other study reporting to the sponsor
- … etc.

For each subject:
- Subject signed informed consent forms
- Source documents for subject eligibility and protocol procedures
- Case report forms
- … etc.

PLATE 19

Typical Document Development Process

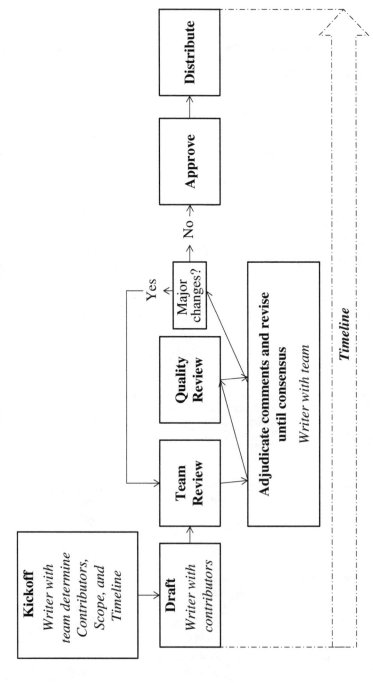

d) No waiver of rights (ICH E6(R2) 4.8.4)
   - No information given to or communication with study subjects may waive or appear to waive the subject's legal rights or release the investigator or sponsor from liability for negligence
e) Sufficient time to consider (ICH E6(R2) 4.8.7)
   - The subject will receive sufficient time to consider the information for the study prior to consenting to participate in the study.
f) Minimum elements of consent
   - A subject must be consented on the minimum required elements of consent (Section 19.2.5.3 (ICH E6(R2) 4.8.10)) and all aspects of the trial prior to study participation. (ICH E6(R2) 4.8.5) Additional local elements may be required.
g) Understandable language (ICH E6(R2) 4.8.6)
   - All the information given to study subjects must be in writing and in a language/manner understandable to the subject (Section 19.2.5.4).
h) Demonstrate understanding (ICH E6(R2) 4.8.7)
   - The subject will have all questions answered to their satisfaction regarding the IRB/IEC-approved information prior to undergoing the study-related procedures.
i) Signed consent (ICH E6(R2) 4.8.8)
   - The subject will personally sign and date consent forms prior to participating in the study
j) Copy of consent (ICH E6(R2) 4.8.11)
   - The subject will receive a copy of their signed and dated consent form prior to participation in the trial
k) New information (ICH E6(R2) 4.8.2) (ICH E6(R2) 4.8.11)
   - A subject must receive, in a timely manner, any new or updated required elements of consent (Section 19.2.5.3) that may affect their willingness to continue participating in the study and this communication must be documented and signed and dated by the study subject.
l) Documented consent process
   - All of the above steps in the process of consenting must be documented (Section 19.2.5.5) in the study records.

There are specific situations when consent is required and also when it may be waived or delayed (Section 19.2.5.2), and additional safeguards are given for vulnerable populations (Section 19.2.5.2.5).

19.2.5.2 Situations for Informed Consent

Signed informed consent is required by or on behalf of all individuals who are volunteering to be clinical trial subjects.

The following presents how consent may be obtained depending on the mental and health capabilities or circumstances of the research subject.

19.2.5.2.1 No Legally Acceptable Representative is Required

No legally acceptable representative (LAR) is required under the following circumstances:

- Adult subjects who are capable of independent and full communication with the individual administering consent may individually and independently undergo the consent process without representation by a legally acceptable individual and personally sign and date the informed consent forms. All study subjects, however, have the right to have family member(s) or other individual(s) present to support them during the consent process.
- Subjects who are volunteering to participate in a nontherapeutic trial (i.e., a trial in which there is no anticipated direct clinical benefit to the subject, e.g., a phase 1 trial for measuring pharmacokinetics) undergo the consent process without representation by a legally acceptable individual and may personally sign and date the informed consent forms. (ICH E6(R2) 4.8.13).
- Subjects who are volunteering to participate in a nontherapeutic trial and an LAR is not required as described in Section 19.2.5.2.2 (ICH E6(R2) 4.8.14).

19.2.5.2.2 The Subject is Represented by a Legally Accepted Representative

The research subject may not be able to personally or wholly undergo the informed consent process; e.g., if they are a minor or a patient with severe dementia. The subject is then represented by a legally accepted representative (ICH E6(R2) 4.8.12). In the case of:

a) Minors:
- The minor will be informed about the trial to the extent compatible with their understanding, and if capable, they will sign "assent." The parent(s) or legal guardian, as required, will also sign and date the consent form.

b) Adults incapable of independent and full communication with the individual administering consent:
- The subject will be informed about the trial to the extent compatible with the subject's understanding. If capable, the subject will sign "assent." The legally accepted representative will also sign and date the consent form.

c) Nontherapeutic trials:
- The legally accepted representative is required to sign and date the consent form if (ICH E6(R2) 4.8.14):
  - The trial must enroll subjects who are unable to personally provide consent.
  - The foreseeable risks to and impact to well-being of the subjects are minimized and low
  - The IRB/IEC review and approval are explicitly specified for such subjects
  - Unless an exception is justified, the trial is conducted on patients having thedisease for the intended indication and the subjects are withdrawn if they appear to be unduly stressed.

19.2.5.2.3 The Subject or their Legally Accepted Representative is Unable to Provide Consent Prior to Trial Participation

If consent from the subject or their legally accepted representative is not possible (e.g., a trial that is evaluating an investigational article in emergency situations) (ICH E6(R2) 4.8.15):

a) The protocol procedures and documentation requirements must be reviewed by the governing IRB/IEC for relevant ethical concerns and compliance with applicable regulatory requirements.
b) The subject many then be enrolled in the study and undergo protocol procedures but a follow-up consent may be required with the subject or their legally accepted representative once possible.

19.2.5.2.4 The Subject or Their Legally Accepted Representative Is Unable to Read

When the subject or their legally accepted representative is unable to read (ICH E6(R2) 4.8.9):

a) An impartial witness (a person, who is independent of the trial, who cannot be unfairly influenced by people involved with the trial) will attend the informed consent process and read the informed consent form and any other written information supplied to the subject. (ICH E6(R2) 3.1.7).
b) The witness will observe the process to ensure that all information was explained to the subject or their LAR was accurate, complete, and without coercion
c) The witness will ensure that the subject or their legally accepted representative demonstrated understanding of the protocol information.
d) The subject or their legally accepted representative will orally provide consent and sign and date, if capable of doing so
e) The witness will then personally sign and date the informed consent form. (ICH E6(R2) 4.8.9)

19.2.5.2.5 Vulnerable Populations

Vulnerable subjects are those individuals whose willingness to volunteer in a clinical trial may be unduly influenced by the expectation, whether justified or not, of benefits associated with participation, or of a retaliatory response from senior members of an hierarchy in case of refusal to participate. Examples are members of a group with a hierarchical structure, such as medical, pharmacy, dental, and nursing students, subordinate hospital and laboratory personnel, employees of the pharmaceutical industry, members of the armed forces, and persons kept in detention. Other vulnerable subjects include patients with incurable diseases, persons in nursing homes, unemployed or impoverished persons, patients in emergency situations, ethnic minority groups, homeless persons, nomads, refugees, minors, and those incapable of giving consent (ICH E6(R2) 1.61). The governing IRB/IEC should pay special attention to trials that may include vulnerable subjects (Chapter 8 IRB/IEC Roles and Responsibilities).

19.2.5.3 Minimum Elements of Consent

ICH E6(R2) 4.8.10 stipulates a list of requirements that must be addressed during the informed consent discussion and in the written informed consent form and any other written information to be provided to subjects. We will refer to these requirements as "minimum elements." Descriptions of the minimum elements for adequate informed consent of human subjects are displayed in Table 19.1.

19.2.5.4 Developing Consent Information and Documents
19.2.5.4.1 General

Qualified individuals should prepare and review information that will be provided to potential research subjects to ensure that the information conforms to GCP requirements. While the IRB/IEC has final approval of the content of subject information, in practice, either the sponsor and/or the investigator will prepare these materials and both will need to review all materials. The sponsor will typically contribute information related to the investigational product and study procedures. A QC checklist containing the following can be very helpful to ensure that study information provided to subjects meet GCP requirements:

- The required elements with checkboxes for the reviewer to indicate if the item is present or not
- Fields for the reviewer to indicate comments or instructions for the consent developer

The key elements to consider when creating consent documents and materials can be summed up as "ELF":

- Minimum required **E**lements of consent (Section 19.2.5.4.2)
- **L**anguage understandable to the subject (Section 19.2.5.4.3)
- **F**ormat that makes information easy to read and comprehend (Section 19.2.5.4.4)

19.2.5.4.2 "E"

Section 19.2.5.3 describes the minimum elements required for consenting documents. The drafted consent materials and form must contain these and any other elements per local requirements.

There should also be signature blocks for the subject and/or LAR, person obtaining consent, and others as required (e.g., assent, witness) to sign.

Once the consent form is drafted, as a quality control measure, we recommended a check of the form to ensure that all the elements were addressed.

Table 19.1 Descriptions of minimum elements for adequate informed consent of human subjects

ICH E6(R2) 4.8.10	Description
a) That the trial involves research.	Participants will need to know that the study is a clinical research study and that it is not approved therapy.
b) The purpose of the trial.	This is to answer the question, Why is this trial being conducted? This reason is typically to study the investigational product in the stated study population and to find out the stated objectives of the trial. The participant is being asked to participate in the trial because they are part of the stated study population.
c) The trial treatment(s) and the probability for random assignment to each treatment.	State the names of the trial treatment(s), including controls and combination products. If there is randomization, the chance of being assigned to any product or group will also be stated.
d) The trial procedures to be followed, including all invasive procedures.	List and describe all of the trial procedures that the participant will undergo and when they will occur. A chart or table showing the visit times and what will be done at each visit is a good supplement for this information.
e) The subject's responsibilities.	The responsibilities of the subject are generally about their rights and how they may ensure that rights are protected. For example: • Their participation in the study is voluntary • They must read and understand the information contained in the consent form • They understand the requirements of the procedures that they will undergo • They understand the timing of the study, when it starts, when it ends, how long it is, and when they need to do the study procedures • They understand the risks and potential benefits associated with the trial and that they have considered those risks and benefits • They will ask questions of the PI and/or study staff about the study and report any problems to the PI immediately

(Continued)

Table 19.1 (Continued)

ICH E6(R2) 4.8.10	Description
	• They will contact the governing IRB/EC if they have any questions or complaints about the conduct of the study or their participation in the study
	• They may discontinue from the study at any time but will contact the PI/study staff if they want to do so
	• Use the study treatment only as directed and for the purposes of the study
	• Maintain a copy of signed consent form for their records
f) Those aspects of the trial that are experimental.	Identify study treatments or procedures that are not approved or that are experimental in the trial. This does not only include the investigational product being studied, but also any assessments (egg, diagnostic procedure, or questionnaire) that is not approved for or is not standard of care for the intended use.
g) The reasonably foreseeable risks or inconveniences to the subject and, when applicable, to an embryo, fetus, or nursing infant.	Describe all foreseeable risks and inconveniences associated with the study treatments and each study procedure for the participant. Also specify potential risks to an embryo, fetus, or nursing infant; i.e., for males or females of child-bearing potential, or nursing females.
	A statement that there unknown risks should also be included.
h) The reasonably expected benefits. When there is no intended clinical benefit to the subject, the subject should be made aware of this.	No claims of benefit from taking the investigational product may be made, either implicitly or explicitly, unless it is has been established (and recognized by the regulatory authorities) that the safety or efficacy may be better than the standard of care or a placebo comparator. In this case, clarify that the participant may benefit only if they receive the investigational product.
	It is acceptable, however, to state that researchers may learn more about the study indication or treatment or that information helps others with the indication in the future.
	Generally, specify that there is no guarantee or proof of benefit, if such is the case for the study.
i) The alternative procedure(s) or course(s) of treatment that may be available to the subject, and their important potential benefits and risks.	Given that the subject is voluntarily consenting to be in the study, they may be informed that they have alternatives to participating in the study. Their choices if they do not take part in the study are; egg,
	• Get alternative available treatments, therapies, or procedures for the indication.
	• Participate in another study
	• Get no treatment
	Describe alternative available treatments, therapies, or procedures (approved or standard of care) and the important potential benefits and risks for these alternatives.

j) The compensation and/or treatment available to the subject in the event of trial-related injury.	As research volunteers, study participants should not be responsible for the cost of treatment in the event of trial-related injury. The sponsor generally will take the financial responsibility, but the compensation may be arranged among the sponsor and/or other parties.
	The consent form needs to only inform the potential research participant that compensation and/or treatment will be available to them in the event of trial-related injury. Specifying what is covered may be helpful. The consent form is not place to describe the details of the arrangements for payments among payers.
k) The anticipated prorated payment, if any, to the subject for participating in the trial.	Research volunteers may be *reasonably* compensated for their time, effort, and expenses for their involvement in the study, depending on the complexities and inconveniences of the study. Financial incentives must not be in amounts or methods that would be coercive, present undue influence, or persuade subjects to stay in the study when they otherwise would have withdrawn. For example, it is reasonable to reimburse or compensate for travel expenses, but a promise to receive (egg, give a voucher or coupon) the study drug once it is approved without cost is coercive.
	Specify how and when payments will be made and when payments may not be made. Compensation should accrue as the study progresses and should generally be on schedule with completion of visit procedures. However, a small proportion of payment may be withheld until study completion, provided that such incentive is not coercive, or such delay is not detrimental.
l) The anticipated expenses, if any, to the subject for participating in the trial.	Specify what expenses, if any, the subject will incur for their involvement in the study. The subject may be responsible for procedures that are part of their standard of care for their condition, i.e., those procedures the patient would undergo regardless of their participation in the study. The subject should not bear any cost for any procedures and study treatments that are solely for the purpose of the study, unless approved by an IRB/EC and/or regulatory authority.
m) That the subject's participation in the trial is voluntary and that the subject may refuse to participate or withdraw from the trial, at any time, without penalty, or loss of benefits to which the subject is otherwise entitled.	It is important that the potential research participant understands that their involvement in the study is completely voluntary, and that they may discontinue from the study at any time and for any reason. They will not be penalized or lose any study-related entitlement as a result of their withdrawal.
	Depending on the safety issues in the study, subjects may be asked as a safety precaution to continue with safety procedures if they want to discontinue study treatment.

(Continued)

Table 19.1 (Continued)

n) That the monitor(s), the auditor(s), the IRB/IEC, and the regulatory authority(ies) will be granted direct access to the subject's original medical records for verification of clinical trial procedures and/or data, without violating the confidentiality of the subject, to the extent permitted by the applicable laws and regulations and that, by signing a written informed consent form, the subject or the subject's legally acceptable representative is authorizing such access.

The subject or their legally accepted representative will, via the informed consent form, agree as to which of their study information, including personal identification information, may be seen by whom. A clinical trial may be audited at any time (scheduled or unscheduled) by the sponsor, IRB/IEC, or the regulatory authority(ies) and sponsors have regulatory responsibility to monitor the trial (see Chapter 33 Quality Assurance Components; Chapter 34 Regulatory Authority Inspections). At the clinical site, all study records, including original medical records that contain subject personal identification information, may be reviewed by representatives of any of these players.

Representatives of the sponsor, for example, also includes CROs that have been contracted to perform clinical site monitoring, auditing, or other tasks that include access to the subject's medical records. Informed consent information must disclose what records may be seen by whom so that volunteer is aware of and agrees to this requirement. Based on this requirement, it follows that no representative may have access to the records unless there is signed consent for them to do so.

o) That records identifying the subject will be kept confidential and, to the extent permitted by the applicable laws and/or regulations, will not be made publicly available. If the results of the trial are published, the subject's identity will remain confidential.

Any information that may identify the individual subject must be protected. Identification of the individual research volunteer may come from a variety of sources, including demographics, national or local identification numbers or pictures, genetic information obtained from biological samples, or medical records. Countries or localities may have different legal requirements regarding what type of information must be kept confidential.

The identity of the subject must be protected so that access is available only to those who are authorized per the subject's consent. This access refers to anywhere or any time during and after the study; egg;

- Review of study records at the clinical site
- Collection and analysis of data and biological specimens
- Sharing of medical records (egg, with other physicians, or health facilities for the management of adverse events)
- Reporting of study information or results (egg, clinical study report, publications)
- Sharing of the study results or study information in the future (egg, sharing biological specimens, study data, genetic information)

The subject will be informed of how the records that contain their identity will be shared, with whom, and until when, and of any rights they have to withdraw information. Likewise, the subject will be informed of any information that may *not* be protected or the *inability* to withdraw information.

ICH E6(R2) 4.8.10	Description
p) That the subject or the subject's legally acceptable representative will be informed in a timely manner if information becomes available that may be relevant to the subject's willingness to continue participation in the trial.	Freely given informed consent should be obtained from every subject prior to clinical trial participation (ICH E6(R2) 2.9). The subject will be given all information about the study that will enable them to make a decision about participating in the study. However, once the study begins, the dissemination of this information to the subject does not end. Any new information that may influence the subject's continued participation in the study will also be provided. New information includes, egg, • Apparent positive or negative information that may arise from the study data (egg, adverse drug reactions or positive side effects; efficacy response, or no response) • Alternative newly approved or standard of care treatments or therapies • Changes to study procedures • Changes to subject responsibilities regarding logistics or costs for participating in the trial We note that it is unethical for a study to continue when the study data reveal that the risks are outweighing the benefits. Likewise, if it is proven that the investigational product is of significant benefit as compared with available treatments or therapies, it is unethical to continue the trial without the treatment from the general population, unless it is possible to provide the general population access to the product.
q) The person(s) to contact for further information regarding the trial and the rights of trial subjects, and whom to contact in the event of trial-related injury.	Subjects may have questions during the trial and should actually be encouraged to ask questions at any time regarding the study procedures, their rights as trial subjects, any trial-related injury, or any question regarding their participation in the study. They should be given the contact name(s) and method(s) for directing such questions at any time. Trial site personnel are usually the most appropriate contact for questions regarding trial procedures and IRB/IEC should be included for questions regarding the rights of trial subjects.

(Continued)

Table 19.1 (Continued)

r) The foreseeable circumstances and/or reasons under which the subject's participation in the trial may be terminated.	Study volunteers have the right to withdraw their consent from participating in the study at any time. At the same time, circumstances may arise that forbid the individual subject for continuing to receive the study treatment, or from continuing in the study, or the continuation of the study as whole. These are typically for risk/benefit reasons but can be for any reason. Examples of foreseeable circumstances and/or reasons under which subject's participation in the trial may be terminated are:
	• The subject incurs a new illness or condition, or progression of preexisting condition that prevents further administration of the study treatment
	• The subject experiences an unacceptable number or severity of adverse events
	• The subject uses or needs to use medications or therapies that are prohibited for the study
	• The subject is not complying with study requirements, either putting the subject at safety risk or affecting the quality of data collected
	• The study itself is terminated for lack of safety (egg, unacceptable number, or severity of adverse events experienced by a number of subjects), lack of efficacy, business (egg, not financially feasible), regulatory compliance issues, or other.
s) The expected duration of the subject's participation in the trial.	The subject will need to know how long they will be expected to participate in the study. This includes from the first of any screening procedures until the last study procedure is performed. It is helpful to break down the approximate duration of each period in the study, egg, screening, treatment, safety follow-up, and survival follow-up.
	If the end of a subject's participation is contingent upon the enrollment of other subjects in the trial (egg, the end of study will be 2 years after the last subject enrolled in the study receives their first study treatment), then a reasonable estimate of how long enrollment of all subjects in the trial should be made. The subject should also be informed if this estimate changes over the course of the study.
t) The approximate number of subjects involved in the trial.	The total number subjects participating in the entire trial, and if available, the anticipated number of subjects participating at the same clinical site as the subject, should be stated in the consent information.

19.2.5.4.3 "L"

The oral or written information to be provided to subjects must (ICH E6(R2) 4.8),

- Be in a language that is understandable to the subject:
  - The subject will be given consent materials and consent forms in a language understandable to them.
  - Written and oral consent materials must be formally translated by qualified translators (and back-translated to verify the translation) to meet this requirement if necessary.
  - The process used for translating consent materials and forms must be documented.
- Be at a language level that is as nontechnical as possible:
  - The education level to read and understand written consent materials and forms must be at the site's regionally required minimum education level. Use simple paragraph and sentence structures. Consider using lists, graphics, or tables to present information.
  - Describe the study and protocol procedures as nontechnical as possible. Use simple and familiar words and phrases and avoid technical jargon and abbreviations.
  - Language regarding legal rights should be simple and relevant. The consent form must not contain any statements that are not relevant to the subject, e.g., agreements between the investigator/institution and sponsor on compensation for injury to the subject.
  - Use the site's IRB/EC standard and preferred language for consent materials and forms, if available.
- Not contain language that is coercive
  - A subject must *voluntarily* participate in the study so they must not be coerced in any way.
  - No promises or claims about the safety or effectiveness of the investigational article may be explicitly or implicitly stated (e.g., "improved," "better than," "superior to," "cures," "relieves," "eliminates," "safe," and "well tolerated") unless such statements have been approved by the applicable regulatory authority.
  - Although an IRB/EC will review the actual materials for consenting, investigator and site staff interacting with prospective study subjects may not make such promises or claims.
  - It is best practice to use language such as "you are being asked to" or "you should" instead of "you must"
  - It is best practice for the sponsor to avoid interactions with the subject to remove any chance for or the perception of possible coercion.
- Not contain language that waives or appear to waives of the subject's legal rights
- Not contain language that releases the investigator, institution, or sponsor from liability for negligence

19.2.5.4.4 "F"

The format of any document or materials should be tailored for the intended user. The general population will most likely read what appears to be:

- easy to read
- interesting
- short
- important

As such, consent documents or materials should be formatted with these goals in mind. Some format and layout recommendations:

- Balance empty and used space
- Sort information by logical order or importance
- Consider using lists, graphics, or tables to present information
- Consider vision impairments and reading problems

19.2.5.5 Documentation of Consent

The following evidence of appropriate consent must be recorded and maintained in the study records:

- Sample consent form (initial and, if applicable, updated) approved by the IRB/IEC
- That the subject had sufficient time to consider study participation prior to signing consent
- That the subject had opportunity to ask and had all their questions answered, and demonstrated understanding of the consent information, prior to signing consent
- Consent form for each subject personally signed and dated by the subject and/or LAR
- If applicable, the consent form is personally signed and dated by a witness
- Consent form for each subject personally signed and dated by the individual who administered consent to the subject
- That the subject and/or LAR received a copy of their signed and dated consent form prior to the subject undergoing study procedures
- That the consent form was signed and dated by the subject and/or LAR prior to the subject undergoing study procedures
- All of the above documentation for any new information provided to the subject that may affect their decision to continue to participate in the study

19.2.6 Confidentiality of Subject Identity

Any information that identifies the subject must be kept confidential. Controls should be in place to limit access and prevent accidental breach. The IRB/IEC-approved and subject-signed consent will specify what identification may be retained by the clinical site, how that information may be used, and who may have access to the information. Because the existence of the subject needs to be authenticated, the clinical research site will maintain some information that fully identifies the subject, such as their full name, date of birth, and a governmental or other institutionally issued identification number. However, an unambiguous subject identification code that allows identification of all the data reported for each subject should be used for research data records that are transmitted externally to the clinical site (ICH E6(R2) 5.5.5). It is also encouraged that only the study identification is used in oral communication within the clinical site to avoid unintended breach of the subject's confidentiality. The documentation that contain all subject authentication identity and the linked study identification number, known as the study identification code list (Chapter 29 Essential Documents), must be maintained with authorized access, and only the approved study identification may be revealed in both oral and written study communication. Extra steps should be taken to omit or redact other unapproved study identification from research records that should not contain such confidential information.

In addition to protecting the identity of the subject, their health information, including medical history and study results, must also be maintained in confidence. Access of subject's health information should be limited to only those individuals who need to review the information to make trial conduct or subject care decisions, or for trial monitoring, auditing, or inspection. All efforts should be made to not discuss or document the health status of research subjects while revealing their identity in unauthorized settings.

19.2.6.1 Protection of Biological Specimens

Biological specimens, such as blood or tissue samples, collected from study subjects are components of the human subject and therefore the same principles for confidentiality and accountability apply. This is to say that specimens should be labeled and used only as approved by the IRB/IEC and as specified in the informed consent and trial protocol. The specimens will have to be tracked to ensure appropriate custody and must be retrievable if the option for withdrawal of the specimen was made available to the subject. Specimens collected and stored for future research, i.e., not for the purposes of the specific study protocol, may also be used only in accordance with the provisions approved by the approved by the IRB/IEC and as specified in the informed consent. As needed, documentation should be maintained to track specimen from collection to all usage and transfers and final destruction (ICH E6(R2) 8.3.25).

19.2.7 Compensation to Subjects

Depending on local regulatory requirement(s), research subjects may be entitled to compensation for trial-related injury as well as for their time, effort, and expenses for their involvement in the study. Records of approval of payments and all payments must be maintained.

19.2.7.1 Trial-Related Injury

If required by the applicable regulatory requirement(s), the sponsor will be responsible for protecting the investigator/institution against *bona fide* claims arising from the trial and or compensating the subject for trial-related injury.

- The sponsor should provide insurance or should indemnify (legal and financial coverage) the investigator/the institution against claims arising from the trial, except for claims that arise from malpractice and/or negligence.(ICH E6(R2) 5.8.1). If required, the sponsor will secure and show evidence of trial insurance prior to initiation of the trial. A sponsor may present coverage for each individual trial protocol or "basket" coverage for multiple trials. That the sponsor will provide insurance coverage indemnifying the investigator/institution against claims arising from the trial, except for claims that arise from malpractice and/or negligence, will be written in an agreement between the sponsor and the investigator/institution. (Chapter 15 Trial Resourcing and Outsourcing).
- Additionally, the sponsor's policies and procedures should address the costs of treatment of trial subjects in the event of trial-related injuries in accordance with the applicable regulatory requirement(s) (ICH E6(R2) 5.8.2). That the subject will be compensated for trial-related injury will be stated in the informed consent documents for trial subjects (Chapter 19 Informed Consent and Other Human Subject Protection).

19.2.7.2 Time, Effort, and Expenses

When trial subjects receive compensation, the method and manner of compensation should comply with applicable regulatory requirement(s). (ICH E6(R2) 5.8.3).

- IRBs/IECs will review the details of the amounts, methods, and timing of compensation to trial subjects.
- The subject will be given the details of the amounts, methods, and timing of compensation in the informed consent forms and will have opportunity to consider the information before agreeing to participate in the study.
- The sponsor will include amounts to be paid to subjects in the trial budget with the investigator and may reimburse the investigator for payments made to subjects. It is not advisable for the sponsor to make payments directly to subjects (unless for compensation for trial-related injury) to avoid the potential for coercion. (Chapter 15 Trial Resourcing and Outsourcing).
- The investigator will make the payments to the subjects.

Compensation may be provided to appropriately compensate subjects for their time, travel, and/or efforts, and may not be used to unduly influence potential human subjects to participate in research activities. Some points to consider when deciding on appropriate compensation:

- Compensation is usually monetary but may be certificates or vouchers of cash value, or the service, such as transportation or accommodation, may be provided. Subjects may also be reimbursed for expenses.
- The amount or type of compensation must not be so large that it could be construed as undue influence. The amount or type of compensation should be comparable to what would be reasonable for the subject population's socioeconomics in the trial site locality.
- If possible, compensation should be prorated based on participation; i.e., the subject will be paid for study procedures and visits that they completed. Compensation should not be withheld or be contingent upon completion of all study procedures.

19.2.8 Medical Care for Subjects

When study subjects are in the trial, they will undergo study treatment(s) or procedures that may result in an adverse event. Additionally, the research subjects may experience other health conditions that are not associated with study treatment while they are in the study. A qualified investigator is responsible for the medical care of the well-being of the trial subject for any health issues that arise during the study. The medical care given to, and medical decisions made on behalf of, subjects should always be the responsibility of a qualified physician or, when appropriate, of a qualified dentist (ICH E6(R2) 2.7). Sponsors will therefore select investigators who have the training, experience, and qualifications to manage the subject's medical care, making clinical decisions regarding management of study-related adverse events, ensuring that treatment is provided for study-related adverse events, determining when study treatment needs to be withdrawn in the interest of the subject, referring the subject for medical care for intercurrent illness(es), and determining when the subject needs to be withdrawn from the study if it is in the subject's best interest. Key points regarding medical care are:

- Protection of the well-being of the trial subjects refers to the provision of medical care for their physical and mental integrity (ICH E6(R2) 1.62).
- All trial-related medical (or dental) decisions should be the responsibility of a qualified physician (or dentist, when appropriate), who is an investigator or a sub-investigator for the trial (ICH E6(R2) 4.3.1).
- For issues related to the subject's participation in the trial (e.g., adverse events that occur either during or following their participation in the trial), the investigator/institution should ensure that adequate medical care is provided to the subject. (ICH E6(R2) 4.3.2).

- If the investigator becomes aware of signs or symptoms of for other health issues that the subject experiences during the study (egg, intercurrent illness(es)), the investigator should immediately inform the subject of the subject's need to seek medical care for the intercurrent illness(es). (ICH E6(R2) 4.3.2).
- It is recommended that the investigator inform the subject's primary physician about the subject's participation in the trial if the subject has a primary physician and if the subject agrees to the primary physician being informed (ICH E6(R2) 4.3.2).
- If the administration of the investigational product is prematurely discontinued for a subject, every effort should be made to encourage the subject to continue to undergo safety follow-up study procedures.

19.2.9   Subject Withdrawal from the Study

Research subjects have the right to freely withdraw from a clinical trial at any time during the trial. If a subject withdraws prematurely from the trial, the investigator should make a reasonable effort to ascertain the reason(s), while fully respecting the subject's right to voluntarily give his/her reason(s) for withdrawing prematurely from the trial. (ICH E6(R2) 4.3.1).

19.2.10   Summary of Study Records Related to Human Subject Protection

Study records that will be maintained as evidence of protection of the rights, safety, and well-being of human subjects are displayed in Table 19.2.

Please see Chapter 29 Essential Documents for additional information regarding the collection and maintenance of essential documents.

19.3   Summary

The protection of human research subjects includes protection of their rights, safety, and well-being. Humans are volunteering to participate in a study in which a product that does not have proven safety and efficacy so they are entitled to certain rights regarding the research:

- Request to participate in a trial with an investigational product that has been designed to minimize risk and is continuously assessed for the benefits of its potential safety versus risk
- Provision and understanding of all known and new information about the investigational product and study procedures that have been reviewed and approved by a qualified ethics committee

Table 19.2 Essential documents pertaining to the protection of the rights, safety, and well-being of human subjects

Responsibility	Essential document(s)
a) Regulatory authority(ies) review of trial information	Regulatory authority(ies) authorization/approval/notification (ICH E6(R2) 8.2.9; 8.3.4)
b) Investigational product manufacturing and handling	• Certificate of analysis of investigational product (ICH E6(R2) 8.2.16; 8.3.9) • Instructions for dispensing investigational product (ICH E6(R2)8.2.14) • Investigational product accountability (ICH E6(R2) 8.3.23; 8.4.1)
c) Qualified individuals involved in development of study information for research subjects and consent process	Signature sheet; i.e., investigator delegation log (ICH E6(R2) 8.3.25)
d) Instructions for revealing the identity of the investigational product in case of emergency	Decoding procedures for blinded trials (ICH E6(R2)8.2.17)
e) Procedures for informed consent	Site selection and/or initiation report (ICH E6(R2) 8.2.19/20; 8.3.10)
f) Safety reporting and monitoring	• Investigator reporting to sponsor of SAEs (ICH E6(R2)8.3.16) • Sponsor/Investigator reporting to regulatory authority(ies) of SUSARs (ICH E6(R2) 8.3.17) • Sponsor notifications of safety information to investigators (ICH E6(R2) 8.3.18)
Ethics review	
Ethics review of study information given to trial subjects	• Qualified IRB/IEC (ICH E6(R2) 8.2.8) • Dated, documented approval/favorable opinion of IRB/IEC of initial review of trial information (ICH E6(R2) 8.2.7) • Dated, documented approval/favorable opinion of IRB/IEC of continuing review of trial information (ICH E6(R2) 8.3.3)
Informed consent	
Informed consent documents and process	• Initial study information given to trial subjects (ICH E6(R2) 8.2.3) • Updated information given to trial subjects (ICH E6(R2) 8.3.3) • Signed consent forms (ICH E6(R2) 8.3.12) • Process of consent (ICH E6(R2) 8.3.13) • Subject screening log; i.e., subjects who underwent study procedures (ICH E6(R2) 8.3.20) • Sponsor verification of process and document of subject consent (ICH E6(R2) 8.3.10)

(Continued)

Table 19.2 (Continued)

Responsibility	Essential document(s)
Confidentiality of subject identity	
Confidentiality of subject study information and protection of their identity	• Subject identification code list (ICH E6(R2) 8.3.21; 8.4.3) • Record of retained biological specimen; i.e., body fluids/tissue samples, if any (ICH E6(R2) 8.3.12)
Compensation to subjects	
Compensation for injury and study participation	• Financial aspects of the trial (payments that the sponsor makes to the investigator for payments to the subjects) (ICH E6(R2) 8.2.4) • Insurance statement for payments to subjects for trial-related injuries (ICH E6(R2) 8.2.5) • Signed agreement between the sponsor and the investigator for the sponsor to indemnify the investigator for claims for *bona fide* trial-related injuries (ICH E6(R2) 8.2.6)
Medical care	
Ensuring medical care for the treatment of non- and study-related adverse events	Source documentation of actions and outcomes to provide medical care (ICH E6(R2) 8.3.13)
Subject withdrawal	
Ability for the subject to withdraw from the study	Documentation of subject withdrawal and their reason for withdrawal from the study (ICH E6(R2) 8.3.13)

- Voluntary consent to participate in the trial before initiation of any of the trial procedures
- Monitoring of all safety events and care for adverse effects that are related to the investigational product
- Protection of their identity and study information
- Payment for injury related to the investigational product and the trial procedures
- As required, reasonable payment (without potential for coercion) for their time, effort, and expense related to their participation in the trial
- Ability to withdraw from the study at any time without repercussions

Knowledge Check Questions
1) What are the general measures for protecting human subjects?
2) What are the minimum elements of informed consent?
3) What are the different situations or groups of individuals for consenting?
4) What is the process for administering consent to a research subject?
5) What are some situations for protecting the confidentiality of research subjects?
6) What are the rights of research subjects?
7) How may research subjects be compensated?

Reference

1 International Council for Harmonisation of Technical Requirements for Pharmaceuticals for Human Use (ICH), Integrated Addendum to ICH E6(R1):Guideline for Good Clinical Practice, E6(R2) (2016). Current Step 4 version dated 9 November 2016. https://www.ich.org/page/efficacy-guidelines

20

Data Collection and Data Management

Karen A. Henry

GCP Key Point
All clinical trial information should be recorded, handled, and stored in a way that allows its accurate reporting, interpretation and verification (Source: ICH E6(R2) 2.10 [1])

20.1 Introduction

How data are collected and managed has a direct effect on data quality for analyses. We can apply the commonly used expression, "garbage in, garbage out" to refer to the fact that input of poor quality data will result in the output of poor quality data.

Plate 8 Individual Study – Data Framework/Information Flow Among Key Trial Documents displays the data framework/information flow between key documents for a clinical trial. The data flow for an individual study starts with the protocol and ends with the clinical study report (CSR). However, these data may also be further integrated with data collected from multiple clinical trials executed during development of the investigational product for analysis in the preparation of an application for approval for marketing of the investigational product.

When a sponsor submits an application for approval for marketing of the investigational product, a reviewing regulatory authority may choose to perform its own data analyses based on the sponsor's submitted datasets and/or may rely solely on the content of the submitted CSR to assess data quality in conjunction with inspections of essential documents and processes at the investigator(s) and sponsor for a trial. The quality of the data will be scrutinized because the data results from a clinical trial will be used to verify and determine the safety and efficacy of an investigational product.

The Fundamentals of Clinical Research: A Universal Guide for Implementing Good Clinical Practice, First Edition. P. Michael Dubinsky and Karen A. Henry.
© 2022 John Wiley & Sons, Inc. Published 2022 by John Wiley & Sons, Inc.
Companion website: www.wiley.com/go/dubinsky/clinicalresearch

In this chapter, we will describe the tool used for data collection (the case report form [CRF]), and the processes and procedures for systems and operations for collecting and accumulating the trial data for analysis, identifying incorrect data and data discrepancies, and for managing changes to the data. The good clinical practice (GCP) responsibilities for data quality are key to assuring that the clinical trial data are credible.

20.2 Objectives

The objectives of this chapter are:

1) Define the general GCP responsibilities for data quality
2) Describe data flow in a clinical trial
3) Describe considerations for source data recording
4) Describe considerations for development and implementation of the CRF
   a) CRF definition
   b) CRF design
   c) CRF content
   d) CRF development process
   e) CRF amendments
5) Describe considerations for database development
6) Describe data management processes
   a) Data entry
   b) Data monitoring and cleaning
   c) Data merging and reconciliation
7) Describe considerations for locking a database
8) Describe the data management plan
9) Describe quality-by-design considerations involving clinical trial data

20.3 GCP Responsibilities for Data Quality

Compliance with the ICH Good Clinical Practice Guideline provides not only public assurance that the rights, safety and well-being of trial subjects are protected, but also that the clinical trial data are credible. The Guideline should be followed when generating clinical trial data that are intended to be submitted to regulatory authorities. (ICH E6(R2) Introduction). All players are responsible for implementing systems with procedures that assure the quality of every aspect of the trial. (ICH E6(R2) 2.13). These quality assurance systems and procedures include all those planned and systematic actions that are established to ensure that the trial is performed and the data are generated, documented (recorded), and reported in compliance with GCP and the applicable regulatory requirement(s).

(ICH E6(R2) 1.46). The different players involved in conducting a clinical trial, namely the sponsor and investigator(s), have different responsibilities for ensuring the credibility of clinical trial data.

20.3.1 Investigator Responsibilities for Data Quality

Data for the clinical trial will generally be created at the investigator site from the trial assessments as described in the clinical trial protocol and recorded on source documents (Section 20.5 Source Data and Source Documents). The investigator will then report the trial data via the CRF (Section 20.8.1 Data Entry) that the sponsor created to collect the data. The investigator has specific responsibilities for the generation and reporting of the trial data as follows:

- The investigator/institution should maintain adequate and accurate source documents and trial records that include all pertinent observations on each of the site's trial subjects. Source data should be attributable, legible, contemporaneous, original, accurate, and complete. Changes to source data should be traceable, should not obscure the original entry, and should be explained if necessary (e.g., via an audit trail). (ICH E6(R2) 4.9.0).
- The investigator should ensure the accuracy, completeness, legibility, and timeliness of the data reported to the sponsor in the study CRFs and in all required reports. (ICH E6(R2) 4.9.1).
- Data reported on the CRFs, that are derived from source documents, should be consistent with the source documents or the discrepancies should be explained. (ICH E6(R2) 4.9.2).
- Any change or correction to a subject's CRF should be dated, initialed, and explained (if necessary) and should not obscure the original entry (i.e., an audit trail should be maintained); this applies to both written and electronic changes or corrections. (ICH E6(R2) 4.9.3). Changes from the sponsor will be verified and maintained.
- If the investigator/institution retains the services of any individual or party to perform trial-related duties and functions, the investigator/institution will implement procedures to ensure the integrity of any data generated (ICH E6(R2) 4.2.6).

20.3.2 Sponsor Responsibilities for Data Quality

The sponsor will be creating systems and procedures for the collection, management, analysis, and reporting of trial data as follows. The sponsor has responsibility for quality assurance of all trial data as follows:

- The sponsor is responsible for implementing a quality management system to identify and mitigate risk to ensure the reliability of trial results. (ICH E6(R2) 5.0).
- The sponsor should utilize appropriately qualified individuals to handle the data and verify the data (ICH E6(R2) 5.5.1).

- The sponsor is responsible for implementing and maintaining quality assurance and quality control systems with written SOPs to ensure that data are generated, documented (recorded), and reported in compliance with the protocol, GCP, and the applicable regulatory requirement(s). (ICH E6(R2) 5.1.1).
- Quality control should be applied to each stage of data handling to ensure that all data are reliable and have been processed correctly. (ICH E6(R2) 5.1.3).
- The sponsor should obtain the investigator's/institution's agreement to comply with procedures for data recording/reporting (ICH E6(R2) 5.6.3).
- Sponsors should provide guidance to investigators and/or the investigators' designated representatives on making such corrections. Sponsors should have written procedures to assure that changes or corrections in CRFs made by sponsor's designated representatives are documented, are necessary, and are endorsed by the investigator. The investigator should retain records of the changes and corrections. (ICH E6(R2) 4.9.3).
- The sponsor has responsibility for monitoring the investigation to verify that the reported trial data are accurate, complete, and verifiable from source documents. (ICH E6(R2) 5.18.1).
- The sponsor is responsible for securing agreement from all involved parties to ensure direct access to all trial-related sites, source data/documents, and reports for the purpose of monitoring and auditing by the sponsor, and inspection by domestic and foreign regulatory authorities. (ICH E6(R2) 5.1.2).
- The sponsor should ensure that the investigator has control of and continuous access to the CRF data reported to the sponsor. The sponsor should not have exclusive control of those data. (ICH E6(R2) 8.1).
- A sponsor may transfer any or all of the sponsor's trial-related duties and functions to a CRO, but the ultimate responsibility for the quality and integrity of the trial data always resides with the sponsor. The CRO should implement quality assurance and quality control. (ICH E6(R2) 5.2.1).
- The sponsor, or other owners of the data, should retain all of the sponsor-specific essential documents pertaining to the trial (see 8. Essential Documents for the Conduct of a Clinical Trial). (ICH E6(R2) 5.5.6).
- Any transfer of ownership of the data should be reported to the appropriate authority(ies), as required by the applicable regulatory requirement(s). (ICH E6(R2) 5.5.10).

20.4 Data Flow in a Clinical Trial

The flow of data for an individual clinical trial begins with the requirements in the trial protocol and culminates as conclusions on trial results in the CSR (Plate 8 Individual Study – Data Framework/Information Flow Among Key Trial Documents). The data for the individual clinical trial may be further integrated with other trial data in an application for approval for marketing the investigational product. As presented in Plate 8 Individual Study - Data Framework/Information Flow Among Key Trial Documents,

- The protocol describes the study objectives, the endpoints that will be used for evaluating the objectives, and the study assessments that will provide the data for the endpoints (Chapter 18 The Clinical Trial Protocol and Amendments);
- The protocol endpoints and study assessments will determine the types of and methods for analysis of the data that will be described in the study's statistical analysis plan (SAP) (Chapter 27 Study Design and Data Analysis);
- Study treatment administration information and the results of the study assessments, in conjunction with GCP requirements, will determine the data that will be generated and recorded in the source documents;
- Data from source documents will be transcribed into the CRFs;
- CRF data will be entered into and/or accumulate in the trial database, and other trial data may be collected in other media for submission to the sponsor;
- Data in the database, and from other media, will be translated into datasets (Chapter 27 Study Design and Data Analysis);
- The datasets will be used for data analysis according to the methods described in the SAP and for the production of data results in the form of tables, figures, and/or listings (Chapter 27 Study Design and Data Analysis);
- Finally, the tables, figures, and/or listings containing trial results will be used for interpretation and presentation in the CSR (Chapter 28 The Clinical Study Report), integrated reports, and publications.

Given this path, considerations will be given for the accuracy and reliability of data at each step in the data flow. In this chapter, we will focus on the flow of data from the source documents, through the CRFs, and into the clinical trial database.

20.5 Source Data and Source Documents

20.5.1 Definitions

Data in a clinical trial are generated from the study protocol assessments. In the ICH Guideline, the source data (study information) are conceptually differentiated from the source documents (records/media that hold the data); that is,

- *Source data* are all *information* in original records and certified copies of original records of clinical findings, observations, or other activities in a clinical trial necessary for the reconstruction and evaluation of the trial. Source data are contained in source documents (original records or certified copies) (ICH E6(R2) 1.51).
- *Source documents* are original documents, data, and records (e.g., hospital records, clinical and office charts, laboratory notes, memoranda, subjects' diaries or

evaluation checklists, pharmacy dispensing records, recorded data from automated instruments, copies or transcriptions certified after verification as being accurate copies, microfiches, photographic negatives, microfilm or magnetic media, X-rays, subject files, and records kept at the pharmacy, at the laboratories and at medico-technical departments involved in the clinical trial) (ICH E6(R2) 1.52).

Original source documents may be in a variety of media as described above.

When a copy is made of the original record (e.g., a print out of laboratory results which are first/originally recorded into an electronic system), the copy has to be "certified" as true, accurate, and complete. Certification for a ***certified copy*** constitutes attestation, via computerized and/or human validation, that the data in the copy are a true, accurate, and complete copy of the data in the original source.

The source documents at the clinical trial site consist of all data as required by the study assessments (e.g., safety and efficacy assessments, as appropriate) described in the study protocol for the individual subject. The study assessments include:

- Documentation of GCP procedures, e.g., informed consent
- Data supporting the subject's medical history and eligibility for the trial
- Randomization information
- Data from the clinical pharmacology, safety, and or efficacy assessments
- Investigational drug administration information
- Other records showing medical care for the treatment and management of adverse events experienced by the subject

20.5.2 Purpose

Source data as recorded in source documents are part of the essential documents for a trial and are evidence of trial conduct necessary for the reconstruction and evaluation of the trial (Chapter 29 Essential Documents).

20.5.3 Creating Source Data and Documents

As source documents will be relied upon for the reconstruction and evaluation of the trial, processes and procedures should be implemented for the recording of source data in source documents. The processes and procedures include:

- Ensuring that all personnel who will create trial data are qualified by training and experience.
- Training all personnel to employ good documentation practices (GDPs) for creating and changing records for the trial to ensure that trial information is accurate and true. (Chapter 29 Essential Documents)
- Ensuring and documenting that electronic data processing system(s) for the recording of source data meet GCP and applicable regulatory requirements for controlled access, audit trials, and system validation.

- Since the order of trial assessments in the clinic may vary from the order in which a sponsor may organize data collection, source document templates may be created at the investigational site to help facilitate the recording and completeness of source data. The templates may reflect the data that need to be collected, but the order for the collection may be tailored to how clinical assessments are completed. The templates will reflect the data as required by the CRFs, and also conform to good documentation principles, requiring the name (and perhaps the signature) and date of the individual recording the data. (Chapter 29 Essential Documents)
- Ensuring that source data are recorded to protect subject identity (Chapter 19 Informed Consent and Other Human Subject Protection)
- Ensuring that source documents are maintained and stored for short-term and long-term use under protective and backup conditions with controlled access, and are organized so that they are readily retrievable and legible (Chapter 29 Essential Documents).
- Ensuring that source documents are made available for trial monitoring, audits, and inspections and are retained as required by GCP and applicable regulatory requirements.

20.6 Development and Implementation of the Case Report Form (CRF)

20.6.1 Definition

A CRF is a printed, optical, or electronic document designed to record all of the protocol-required information to be reported to the sponsor on each trial subject. (ICH E6(R2) 1.11). CRFs are the property of the sponsor and are the sponsor's medium for collecting the data from the investigator.

20.6.2 CRF Design

The sponsor is required to ensure that CRFs are clear, concise, and consistent along with protocols and other operational documents. Additionally, quality management by a sponsor includes the design of efficient tools and procedures for data collection and processing, as well as the collection of information that is essential to decision making (ICH E6(R2) 5.0). To these ends, several factors should be considered when designing the CRF. The factors include, but are not limited to:

- Objectives for the data in a CRF:
  - The data will be analyzed in support of the protocol objectives and based on the protocol objectives and endpoints (Chapter 18 Clinical Trial Protocol and Amendments)

- The data will be reported in a CSR, which has requirements for inclusion of specific study information (Chapter 28 The Clinical Study Report)
- The data should be easily recorded, in a standardized format, clean, concise, informative, conform to good documentation principles, and retrievable (Chapter 29 Essential Documents)
- The data should be verifiable and available as soon as possible for trial monitoring (Chapter 22 Monitoring Overview; Chapter 21 Safety Monitoring and Reporting)
- The data should be unambiguous and need minimalized number of corrections
- The data that are collected and the process for collecting the data must comply with the protocol, clinical study reporting, GCP, and applicable regulatory requirements.

- Trial procedures: The types, number, order, and blinding of trial procedures will determine the length, format, and organization of the CRF.
- CRFs are completed from source documents: Whether data will be transcribed from source documents or entered directly into the CRFs (Note: data that will not be recorded as source but will be entered directly into CRFs must be identified in the clinical trial protocol (ICH E6(R2) 6.4.9).
- Subject identifiers and sorting variables: Which identifiers will be used to ensure uniqueness of each record and to keep data associated with a subject, their study visit, etc.? A code that is linked to a subject or other subject identifiers that are approved by the IRB/IEC and the subjects via their consent form may be used (Chapter 19 Informed Consent and Other Human Subject Protection).
- Database restrictions: Data entered into the CRFs should be easily integrated into a database that will be used to store and process the aggregated data. It is wise to prioritize the practicality for data to be entered into the CRFs by the clinical trial site over database design restrictions to avoid "garbage in-garbage out" consequences and, instead, consider making the database design more robust.
- Must-have versus nice-to-have data: In addition to required GCP information, such as informed consent date and time, the CRF should be designed to collect only the data required to support the analyses of the trial endpoints as stated in the study protocol, which should require data from assessments that are needed to ensure the scientific integrity of the study design. Sponsors should consider the burden on study subjects to obtain study data and the cost and management of each data point (e.g., subject's age as a number that is not calculated) when determining what data are to be collected. If the data are not needed, do not collect it.
- Budget: CRF developers should consider the cost of proposed CRF designs without compromising the objectives for collecting the data, noting that each data point has an associated cost potentially to the research subject (e.g., for the associated assessment), site staff (e.g., for collection and data entry), and to the sponsor (e.g., for storage, cleaning, and analysis).

- Print and/or electronic medium: Data may be collected via print, electronic, and/or other media as available with advancing technology. Whichever medium or combination are used, considerations should be given to the objectives for data quality.
- Confirmation of data: All data in a CRF must be attributable; i.e., it should be clear who created the record or how (e.g., report from an instrument) the record was created, so the record should have an associated signed initials or signature. Additionally, the investigator is responsible for attesting to the accuracy of the data and therefore the entire CRF should be reviewed and signed by the investigator.
- Reconciliation pages: Some clinical trial assessments, by nature, have cause and effect properties, such as:
  - If a research subject took medication during the study, there should be an associated adverse event or health condition that was treated
  - If a research subject experienced an adverse event, there may be associated concomitant medications or procedures to treat the adverse event
  - In practice, if a laboratory or radiographical test, physical examination, or other study assessment results in an abnormality that is considered clinically significant, then the abnormal result is recorded as an adverse event
  - If the research subject reports an adverse event (e.g., back pain) during the course of the study and the start date and time of an adverse event were prior to the start date and time for the first study treatment (i.e., the subject had back pain in the past), the adverse event should be recorded as part of the subject's medical history.

  These data will be reconciled across the CRF so the information needed for the reconciliation (e.g., start and stop dates and times) should be recorded for each type of study information (adverse event, concomitant medication or procedure, medical history) and should have similar formatting.
- Audience: A CRF should be designed for their audience or end-user. The investigator staff and potentially research subjects for self-assessments will be entering trial data. The CRF should be designed to facilitate entry by site staff (e.g., consider location and handling of data entry media) and entry by research subjects (e.g., consider location, dexterity, possible visual impairments, etc.). The sponsor may also enter trial data (e.g., summary scores, data corrections), sponsor monitors will review and verify data against source documents. The format of CRF data will be of concern to the sponsor's statisticians who will be analyzing the final clean data and potentially the regulatory authorities who may receive and analyze trial data as well.
- CRF template organization: Consideration should be given to how the template for the CRF is organized for viewing and data entry:
  - Should data be grouped by study visit or by data type? In practice, generally, the CRF will be organized by the flow of trial assessments; e.g., starting with

documentation of informed consent, demographic data, screening visit data, assessment of eligibility, followed by study treatment visit. The grouping of data will also depend on their timing and how the data will be analyzed; e.g., study assessments that are associated with study visits will generally be grouped by visit; however, adverse events and concomitant medications and procedures data may be grouped together because their start and end dates and time may not coincide with study visit dates and may continue across multiple visits. Further, the cumulative data will be integrated for analysis.

– Consideration should also be given to the need for an individual's access to the full CRF or parts of the CRF; e.g., in a partially blinded trial where only efficacy assessments are blinded, CRF design should ensure that the blinded raters do not have access to the full CRF and their access is limited to only those modules they need for their data entry.

- Data standards and future use: Standards should be applied to how data will be recorded and formatted to facilitate the integration and analysis of individual trial data and data across multiple studies. For example,

  – Will the data be recorded as categorical (i.e., select one or more from pre-listed categories), continuous, or open ended answers (i.e., blank spaces to write sentences? For example, determine if sex is recorded from prescribed categories of Male/Female, M/F, 1/0, 0/1, or as open text. Note that open text data would have to be coded into categories before they can be analyzed. As another example, will age be recorded as a discrete number or will it be calculated from a date of birth? Note that local regulatory requirements may forbid the use of dates of births, which are regarded as personal subject identifiers.

  – What units of measures will be used? It is helpful to provide conversions when data recorders use different units of measures (e.g., inches versus centimeters).

  – What is the reason for missing data? Clarify the reason for missing data with specific options; e.g., Not Done (assessment was not completed), Not Available (information was not available), Not Applicable (the question is not applicable).

  – What is the acceptable range (upper and lower limits) for data (e.g., height, weight, and age)?

  – What lengths and formats will be applied to data fields? For example, data that have a range of 1–99, but may occasionally be 100 or higher, should be assigned three digits instead of two digits. Another example is the format to record dates should be universally unambiguous; i.e., if the study is global a format that uses characters instead of numbers for the month should be used (e.g., dd/MMM/yyyy, MMM/dd/yyyy, Month dd, yyyy, and dd Month yyyy).

20.6.3 CRF Content

The CRF will display general study information and be designed to collect data for the protocol-specific procedures.

- General study information includes:
  - Table of contents/Index of CRF modules
  - CRF completion instructions: instructions for who is completing which parts of the CRF, approval for the CRF, what information should be recorded and not recorded, the formats for data entry (e.g., for dates), and how to make corrections to the data.
  - Study identifiers: the name of the sponsor, study title, study or protocol identification name and/or number, and the CRF version number/date
  - Subject identifiers: the clinical trial site number and an identification number for the subject (as approved by IRB/ICF)
  - Study visit identifiers: the protocol visit number/type (e.g., Visit 1/ Screening Visit)
  - Procedure identifiers: the procedure name (e.g., Vital Signs)
  - Fields to record dates and, if critical, the time, for each study procedure, as appropriate (e.g., dates for Visit 1/Screening, date for Vital Signs procedure if different from the Visit 1/Screening date, and the time the vital signs were taken)
  - Signatures for the data recorder for each set of data and for the whole CRF, and signature of the investigator for approval of the whole CRF
- Study assessments/CRF modules: The typical study protocol-specific fields in a CRF are:
  - Informed consent form version, and date and time of administration
  - Subject demographics (age, sex, race/ethnicity)
  - Eligibility criteria (each inclusion and exclusion criteria), if the subject met all criteria, if the subject was excluded from the study or included in the study and any explanations as necessary
  - Medical and surgical history, general and protocol-specific (e.g., history that pertains to the indication under study), diagnosis or description, and start and end date and time,
  - Physical exam (for each body system)/vital signs (systolic and diastolic blood pressure, body temperature, height, weight)
  - Other safety, pharmacology, and/or efficacy assessments, for example,
    - o Laboratory testing (testing status; i.e., done, not done with reason, and if any clinically significant results, which would be also recorded as adverse events; and/or laboratory data if centralized testing is not done)
    - o Diagnostic procedures, e.g., radiographic scans
    - o Neuropsychological instruments
    - o Quality of life instruments
  - Study drug identification, dose, and time (if a blinded trial, then the study drug identification code is provided)
  - Adverse events diagnosis or description, start and end date and time, event severity, whether, meets definition for serious adverse event (SAE), event

relatedness, event outcome, if associated concomitant medication or procedure, treatment or study action taken (Chapter 21 Safety Monitoring and Reporting)
– Concomitant medications and procedures start and end dates and associated adverse event
– Study treatment/study termination date and reason for end of treatment/end of study
– Subject diaries (if data are to be transcribed from subject diaries)

20.6.4 CRF Development Process and Testing

The CRF is the tool for collecting the data and is the property of the sponsor.

20.6.4.1 Resources for CRF Development

CRF and graphic designers will follow the sponsor's standard operating procedures for CRF development. CRF designers may wait to have the final or mature draft protocol before drafting the CRF. The protocol will describe the required assessments and other activities and their timing that will be recorded in the CRF. The study design will also inform the designers of randomization and blinding requirements. The CRF standard templates, the SAP (if available) and previous CRFs are also helpful resources to the CRF designer.

20.6.4.2 Development Process

In practice, the CRF will typically be developed by CRF and graphics designers with review and input from sponsor's medical monitor, trial manager, data manager, statistician, trial monitor, clinical pharmacologist, as appropriate. The process for developing the CRF is similar to that of developing any document:

- Draft and review unique modules (i.e., a sample of each type of module to appear in the CRF) until there is consensus
- Approval of the unique pages
- Draft and review the full CRF until there is consensus
- Prepare the CRF completion instructions
- Test the final draft CRF with the completion instructions (i.e., enter sample data to test the CRF. It is also helpful for the draft study CRF to be reviewed and "tested" by a staff member who will be responsible for data collection and recording at the investigator site).
- Approval of the final full CRF and completion instructions

Once the CRF and completion instructions are approved, all those involved with data entry and management will be trained on the CRF before its implementation. Samples of the final CRFs and completion instructions will be maintained as Essential Documents.

20.6.4.3 Amending the CRF

Changes to the CRF may occur for different reasons, for example:

- The CRF has errors; e.g., it is missing an assessment at a study visit
- The logistics for CRF completion are problematic; e.g., sections that are to be blinded are not
- The protocol is amended to change study assessments

The development of the amended CRF will be similar to the development of the new CRF as described above. The final amended CRF(s) and a log of the changes and the reasons for the changes to the CRF will be maintained as Essential Documents.

20.7 Database Development

A database is the system used to store the data in a structured format such that the data may be sorted and/or filtered as desired by the user. Clinical trial data from CRFs are usually entered into a database that has been structured to store the data for a clinical trial.

Electronic data entry and database systems for processing clinical trial data must conform to GCP and applicable regulatory requirements to bear certain properties to ensure that integrity of the trial data are maintained (ICH E6(R2) 5.5.3, 5.5.4):

- The systems are validated; i.e., ensure that data are complete, accurate, reliable, and consistent with the intended result
- Standard operating procedures are established for the use of the systems. The SOPs will address:
  - System setup, installation, and use.
  - System validation and functionality testing, data collection and handling, system maintenance, system security measures, change control, data backup, recovery, contingency planning, and decommissioning.
  - The responsibilities of the sponsor, investigator, and other parties with respect to the use of these computerized systems
  - Training for all users of the systems
- The systems will be designed to maintain data, and audit trails (i.e., changes to data will be documented in the system such that the old data are not deleted, the new data are entered and who, when, and why a change was made to the data will be recorded), and edit checks for implausible data.
- The systems and data within the system will be restricted to authorized users only and the system will maintain records of system access
- A list of the individuals who are authorized to make data changes will be maintained
- The data in the systems will be adequately backed up

- The systems will safeguard the blinding, if any (e.g., maintain the blinding during data entry and processing)
- Documentation of metadata (i.e., context, content, and structure of the systems) regarding upgrades to the systems or migration of data from or to the system will be maintained.
- If data are transformed during processing, it should always be possible to compare the original data and observations with the processed data.

20.8   Data Management Processes

The sponsor should utilize appropriately qualified individuals to handle the data and verify the data (ICH E6(R2) 5.5.1). Data for a clinical trial will be entered into the clinical trial database via the study CRF. These data will be verified against source documentation, may be merged with other data, and will be "cleaned," "locked," and transformed into datasets for statistical analysis.

20.8.1   Data Entry

An individual entering data should have authorized access to the system and be trained on how to enter and correct data. Care should be taken to follow data entry instructions for:

- The format of data (e.g., for dates, or the addition of leading zeros in partially completed numeric fields)
- Completing-related data fields
- Entering the appropriate reason for missing data
- Making changes to data
- Signing off on the data

It is helpful if the individual entering data is familiar with the trial protocol so that they can discern anomalies in the source data and correct them before entering in the database.

20.8.2   Data Monitoring and Cleaning

Data entry systems should have quality control checks in place to ensure that the entered data are accurate and complete. These checks include,

- Human observation, where an individual observes the data entry by another
- Human verification of the entered data against the source documents (Chapter 22 Monitoring Overview; Chapter 23 Investigator/Institution Selection; Chapter 24 Investigator/Institution Initiation; Chapter 25 Investigator/Institution Interim Monitoring; Chapter 26 Investigator/Institution Close-Out)

- Edit checks that are programmed in the system to identify discrepant, missing, out-of-range, or incomplete data at the time of data entry
- After data entry, data can be manually and/or electronically reviewed again for discrepant, missing, out-of-range, or incomplete data
- System-programmed edit checks will produce a data query report of the incorrect data and submitted to the clinical trial site for adjudication. The response from the clinical trial site (no change, clarification, or revision) will be reviewed by a sponsor representative and the process will continue until there is an appropriate resolution to the data query. All changes to the data will be recorded as described above.
- Data may be manually reviewed by sponsor staff to identify anomalies that may not be detectable by programmed edits (e.g., the accuracy of verbatim terms to describe adverse events or concomitant medications or procedures). These anomalies may be queried as well and any changes would be recorded as described above.
- Data may be reviewed by type of data (e.g., all adverse events), by subject, by study visit, by site, or other key variable of interest to meet the requirements for monitoring and oversight of trial data (Chapter 14 Trial Management; Start-up, On-Study, and Close-Out).

20.8.3 Data Merging and Reconciliation

Data may also be entered into ancillary databases and transferred to the sponsor to merge with the data in the clinical trial database. For example, the sponsor may choose to use a central laboratory for the testing of clinical tissue samples. The central laboratory will record the testing results into their database and transfer the data to the sponsor at agreed timepoints. Quality control procedures should be established to ensure the integrity of merged data.

Additionally, the sponsor's team for the review, processing, and reporting of SAEs may maintain SAE data in a separate database. These systems may not be merged with the study's larger clinical database, but the adverse events data across the systems should be reconciled to ensure consistency.

20.9   Database Lock

Locking a clinical trial database refers to the process of preventing further edits to the database. This process includes:

- Formatting the data so that they are transferrable or transcribable into datasets while preventing changes to the original data or to the destination datasets
- Setting access permissions so that the data may be read but not changed

The purpose of locking the database is to assure data integrity during data transfers and for statistical analysis for results reporting. Data must be thoroughly verified against source documents (i.e., monitored) and cleaned (i.e., reviewed, queried, and resolved) as described above prior to locking the database. A database will be locked prior to unblinding of trial treatment. Parts of the database may be "frozen" for interim data analyses per the protocol design and/or SAP (Chapter 27 Study Design and Data Analysis). The unlocking of a database should be permitted only if absolutely necessary and the reason for the unlocking and audit trails for the changes to the data must be documented and maintained. Clinical trial data should be retained in accordance with GCP and the applicable regulatory requirements (Chapter 29 Essential Documents).

20.10 The Data Management Plan

The totality of procedures regarding data collection and management may be described in standard operating procedures and/or a Data Management Plan. The Data Management Plan will be prepared to document and assist the data management team with following data collection and management procedures for a specific trial. Examples of information in the Plan include,

- Processes for creation and approval of the CRF and the CRF completion instructions
- Processes for amending the CRF
- Identification and description of the systems to be used for data entry, of access permissions, and of training procedures for these systems
- Identification and description of the systems to be used for data storage and processing, entry of access permissions, and of training procedures for these systems
- Timing and processes for data transfers and merging
- Procedures used for data cleaning; i.e., creating system edit checks, generating data queries, manual review, processes for communicating with the clinical site and resolving data queries, documentation of changes to the trial data
- Timing and processes for database lock and unlocking
- Procedures to maintain data blinding, if applicable.

20.11 Quality-by-Design Considerations Regarding Clinical Trial Data Collection and Management

A number of principles and operational considerations that promote GCP, quality, and compliance may guide how data are collected and managed. Data principles and trial operations considerations to foster quality for trial data include:

- The goal for data collection and management is to collect data:
  - In support of the protocol objectives
  - In a standardized, clean, concise, informative, timely manner

- – That can be easily recorded, read, entered, and verified
- – With minimalized number of corrections
- – For reporting study methods and results in the CSR
- – To demonstrate compliance with GCP and applicable regulatory requirements

- Protocol design: The scientific integrity of the trial and the credibility of the data from the trial depend substantially on the trial design (ICH E6(R2) 6.4).
- Protocol objectives, endpoints, and assessments: Study assessments should be appropriate and feasible to generate the data needed to measure the study endpoints. Only data that are required to support the analysis of protocol endpoints and GCP requirements should be collected to avoid undue burden to research subjects and additional costs to investigators and sponsors.
- Source documents: Source documents should be designed to allow secure, accurate, and complete recording of trial source data that are needed to support the CRF and GCP requirements. Personal identification information of trial subjects should be protected through each stage of data handling.
- CRF design: The CRF should be designed to facilitate data entry by different users, including research subjects, and to ensure accurate and complete data entry required for the study analysis.
- Data entry and database systems: These systems should be compliant with GCP and applicable regulatory requirements to ensure the integrity, validity, and reliability of the data.
- Data quality: Procedures should be implemented to thoroughly verify, review, reconcile, and correct data that are entered into databases.
- Locking the database: The databases should be prepared to prevent further editing when data are transcribed into datasets for transfer and/or analysis.
- Written procedures: A written and trained on standard operating procedures and/or trial-specific Data Management Plan that describe data collection and management processes are helpful for the data management team to ensure compliance with the processes and procedures.
- Qualified staff: All individuals involved in data collection and management should be trained and qualified to perform their study tasks.
- Data integration: All systems designs from the CRF to the locked database should be structured and formatted to facilitate the integration of data from multiple clinical trials for analysis for the ultimate application for approval for marketing the investigational product.

20.12 Summary

How data are collected and managed has a direct effect on data quality for analyses. Many factors are to be considered regarding the processes and procedures that are related to data collection and management. Both the investigator and sponsor have responsibilities to ensure the quality of trial data that are collected from clinical trials and that are used for submission to regulatory authority(ies) as part of applications for approval for marketing an investigational product. Trial data stem from the protocol, CSR, and GCP requirements and flow from source documents, into clinical trial databases via CRFs that the sponsor creates for data collection. Data in CRFs will be verified against source documents, data from other sources may be merged with the database, and all data in the database will be reviewed and cleaned prior to locking the database to prevent further editing of the data.

Through each stage of data handling, personal identification information of trial subjects should be protected, data entry and database systems must meet GCP and applicable regulatory requirements to ensure data integrity, written processes and procedures should be established in standard operating procedures and/or a trial-specific Data Management Plan, and all individuals involved in data collection and management should be appropriately trained to perform their assigned duties.

Knowledge Check Questions

1) What is a CRF?
2) What are the responsibilities of an investigator regarding data collection?
3) What are the responsibilities of a sponsor regarding data collection and management?
4) What are pathways for data in a clinical trial?
5) What are source data and source documents?
6) What are some design considerations for creating:
a) Source documents?
b) CRFs?
c) Electronic data processing systems?
7) What are some quality control checks to ensure data quality?
8) What procedures should be written regarding data collection and management?
9) When may the database be locked and unlocked?
10) What are the key quality-by-design considerations for data collection and management?
11) Overheard:

The data will be recorded in source documents at the site. We will then have the site monitors enter the data in a simple spreadsheet; the data do not have to be entered into the trial database because we store data for only enrolled subjects in the database.

Trial manager when asked how will data for subjects who fail screening be collected in preparation for analysis for the CSR.

Comment and discuss:

d) What are the pros and cons of entering trial data into a spreadsheet? What are some considerations for determining what data should be entered into the clinical trial database?

Reference

1 International Council for Harmonisation of Technical Requirements for Pharmaceuticals for Human Use (ICH), Integrated Addendum to ICH E6(R1):Guideline for Good Clinical Practice, E6(R2), E6(R2), Current Step 4 version dated 9 November 2016. https://www.ich.org/page/efficacy-guidelines

21

Safety Monitoring and Reporting

Karen A. Henry

GCP Key Point

A trial should be initiated and continued only if the anticipated benefits justify the risks. (ICH E6(R2) 2.2)

21.1   Introduction

The goal of a clinical trial/study is to discover or verify the clinical, pharmacological, and/or other pharmacodynamic effects of an investigational product(s), and/or to identify any adverse reactions to an investigational product(s), and/or to study absorption, distribution, metabolism, and excretion of an investigational product(s) with the object of ascertaining its safety and/or efficacy (ICH E6(R2) 1.12 Clinical Trial/Study [1]). As experiments on human subjects were conducted through the ages, regulations, and guidelines were largely reactively established to prevent harm in order to protect the rights, safety, and well-being of trial subjects (Chapter 1 History). The ICH Good Clinical Practice (GCP) is one such current guideline of international ethical and scientific quality standard for designing, conducting, recording, and reporting trials that involve the participation of human subjects. Compliance with this standard provides public assurance that subject rights, safety, and well-being are protected (ICH E6(R2) Introduction).

In the ICH E6(R2) Guideline, the rights, safety, and well-being of the trial subjects are the most important considerations and should prevail over interests of science and society (ICH E6(R2) 2.3). All players involved in clinical trial conduct have responsibilities for the protection of subject's rights, safety, and well-being, which are not only for the duration of the trial, but which continue after trial

The Fundamentals of Clinical Research: A Universal Guide for Implementing Good Clinical Practice, First Edition. P. Michael Dubinsky and Karen A. Henry.
© 2022 John Wiley & Sons, Inc. Published 2022 by John Wiley & Sons, Inc.
Companion website: www.wiley.com/go/dubinsky/clinicalresearch

treatment has ended (Chapter 19 Informed Consent and Other Human Subject Protection). Additionally, all players are responsible for assessment of risks versus the benefits for subjects to participate in a trial to determine if a trial should be initiated and for continuous assessment to determine if subjects should continue to participate in the trial and if the trial should be continued (ICH E6(R2) 2.2). The assessment of risk versus benefit occurs at the subject, investigator site, trial, and investigational product levels; that is, assessments should be made for the individual research volunteer, for all subjects participating in the individual trial, and for all subjects receiving the investigational product across all trials. It is unethical to initiate or continue a clinical trial if it is determined that the risks will or do outweigh the benefits for human subject participation.

In this chapter, we will focus on the responsibilities that are specific to the protection of subject safety for a clinical trial. Safety management refers to processes and procedures implemented to avoid and/or reduce, identify, record, evaluate, report, and if necessary, take action on, adverse events (AEs) associated with the subject's participation in the clinical trial. The Guideline describes general responsibilities for safety management and details are outlined in ICH E2A on Clinical Safety Data Management [2] (ICH E6(R2) Introduction).

21.2 Objectives

The objectives of this chapter are:

1) Describe general responsibilities for safety management
2) Describe key concepts for safety management before the trial commences
3) Describe key concepts for safety management during the trial
4) Describe key concepts for safety management after trial participation
5) Define safety reporting terms
6) Describe procedures for safety reporting
   a) Investigator responsibilities
   b) Sponsor responsibilities
   c) IRB responsibilities
   d) Records to be maintained for safety reporting
7) Describe the Safety Management Plan (SMP)
8) Describe Quality by Design Considerations for safety monitoring and reporting

21.2.1 General Responsibilities for Safety Management

Safety management refers to processes and procedures implemented to avoid and/or reduce, identify, record, evaluate, report, and if necessary, take action on,

AEs associated with the subject's participation in the clinical trial. *All* players involved in the conduct of a clinical trial are responsible for:

1) Assessment of risks versus the benefits for subjects to participate in a trial to determine if a trial should be initiated and for continuous assessment to determine if subjects should continue to participate in the trial and if the trial should be continued (ICH E6(R2) 2.2).
2) Assessment of risks versus the benefits at the subject, investigator site, trial, and investigational product levels; that is, assessments should be made for the individual research volunteer, for all subjects participating in the individual trial, and for all subjects receiving the investigational product across all trials.

For their assessment of risks versus the benefits for subjects to enroll and continue to participate in a trial:

1) The IRB/IEC and regulatory authority(ies) will review study information (e.g., protocol and investigator's brochure) prior to implementation of the trial protocol and review reported AEs and changes to the protocol and IB during the trial.
2) The sponsor will establish and implement procedures and processes before the trial starts and make changes during the trial to avoid/and or reduce the occurrence of AEs.
3) The investigator and sponsor will establish and implement processes for safety management for identifying, recording, evaluating, reporting, and if necessary, take action on, AEs associated with the subject's participation in the clinical trial during, and after trial treatment is administered.

21.2.2 Key Concepts for Safety Management Before the Trial Commences

Three main concepts apply for safety management to allow assessment of risk versus benefit to the human research subject before the trial commences:

1) The available nonclinical and clinical information on an investigational product should be adequate to support the proposed clinical trial (ICH E6(R2) 2.4, ICH E6(R2) 5.12.1). *The sponsor will consider and provide the following information needed for review by the regulatory authority(ies) and IRBs/IECs so that they may make an informed assessment of benefit-risk for the implementation of the trial:*
   a) The clinical trial protocol will describe the rationale for conducting the trial and the selection of and dosing regimen for treatments.
   b) The investigator's brochure (IB) will contain product properties and pharmacology and toxicology data from preclinical and safety and efficacy data from

previous human experience that justify the proposed protocol objectives and procedures. The IB will provide the investigators and others involved in the trial with the information to facilitate their understanding of the rationale for, and their compliance with, many key features of the protocol, such as the dose, dose frequency/interval, methods of administration, and safety monitoring procedures. Nonclinical and clinical experience (ICH E6(R2) 7.1).

c) Other information, (e.g., the chemistry, manufacturing, and control of the investigational product) as required.

2) The study will be designed to avoid and/or reduce AEs:

a) The sponsor should decide which risks to reduce and/or which risks to accept. The approach used to reduce risk to an acceptable level should be proportionate to the significance of the risk. Risk reduction activities may be incorporated in protocol design and implementation, monitoring plans, agreements between parties defining roles and responsibilities, systematic safeguards to ensure adherence to standard operating procedures, and training in processes and procedures. Predefined quality tolerance limits should be established, taking into consideration the medical and statistical characteristics of the variables as well as the statistical design of the trial, to identify systematic issues that can impact subject safety or reliability of trial results. Detection of deviations from the predefined quality tolerance limits should trigger an evaluation to determine if action is needed (ICH E6(R2) 5.0.4 Risk Control).

Note: The goal to avoid and/or reduce adverse events does not imply that adverse events associated with the investigational product should be under-reported. The goal is to consider product and study design before use of the investigational product to reduce subject risk.

b) The protocol will contain (Chapter 18 The Clinical Trial Protocol and Amendments):

i) Eligibility criteria for subject participation to avoid and/or reduce anticipated AEs as a result of the subject's exposure to the investigational product(s), including any marketed product that is used as a control. The inclusion criteria will allow only those participants who are part of the study population and for whom the study treatment is intended. At the same time, the exclusion criteria will contain criteria to ensure that enrolled subjects do not have any health conditions or contraindications to the investigational product that will increase their risk for adverse effects with treatment or their general participation in the trial

ii) Only those assessments that are necessary to adequately measure and evaluate the protocol endpoints

3) Systems and processes will be created for the reporting and assessment of AEs:

a) The protocol will contain (Chapter 18 The Clinical Trial Protocol and Amendments):

i) Specifications of safety parameters; i.e., definitions for AEs and what the investigator should report to the sponsor (ICH E6(R2) 6.8.1); e.g., the sponsor may predefine that events associated with disease progression will not be classified and reported as AEs, or how events that are associated with a concomitant treatment, device, or procedure should be reported. For example, if the study drug cannot be administered without the use of a device, will the investigator attempt to parse events associated with the drug versus the device and report accordingly? And likewise for combination investigational and approved product therapies.

ii) Specifications for how serious adverse drug reactions in a blinded trial will be handled between the investigator and sponsor.

iii) Specifications for coding the characteristics of AEs:
   1) Start and end date and time of the event
   2) Severity grading (e.g., mild, moderate, and severe)
   3) Relationship to the study treatment (e.g., not related, possibly or probably related, and definitely related)
   4) Seriousness (e.g., serious or not serious per the definitions)
   5) Action (e.g., modified or stopped treatment, provided medication, and medical procedure)
   6) Outcome (e.g., resolved, unresolved, and resolved with sequela(e))

iv) Instructions for reporting AEs that the subject experiences with non-study drug administration procedures or assessments (e.g., a reaction at the site of blood draw), as required by IRB/IEC or regulatory authority (ies). The ethical concern is that the subject would not experience the event had they not been in the trial and safety issues may occur with these procedures for individual subjects or may be systematic to a site or the trial and should be evaluated and addressed.

v) Definitions for other types of events of special interest that must be reported to the sponsor; for example, pregnancies by the trial participant or their partner, investigational product overdosing, high risk events associated with the product or class of products that the sponsor may want to closely monitor.

vi) The timing and methods for reporting assessing, recording, and analyzing safety events (ICH E6(R2) 6.8.2). The timing for the reporting of safety events will be based on ICH E2A and applicable regulatory requirements (see Section 21.2.6.2).

vii) Procedures for eliciting reports of and for recording and reporting AE and intercurrent illnesses (ICH E6(R2) 6.8.3).

viii) The type and duration of the follow-up of subjects after AEs (ICH E6(R2) 6.8.4).

ix) Procedures for centralized assessment of AEs by an independent data monitoring committee (IDMC) or other committee for assessment specific types of events of special interest. The sponsor may consider establishing an IDMC to assess the progress of a clinical trial, including the safety data and the critical efficacy endpoints at intervals, and to recommend to the sponsor whether to continue, modify, or stop a trial. The IDMC should have written operating procedures and maintain written records of all its meetings. (ICH E6(R2) 1.2, 5.5.2).

x) Actions to be taken for medical care for subjects who experience AEs associated with treatment and/or trial participation.

b) In practice, the sponsor may develop and implement an SMP that outlines procedures and processes for safety management; i.e., what will be reported when and by whom and how AEs will be reviewed in aggregate (Chapter 14 Trial Management; Start-up, On-Study, and Close-Out; Section 21.2.7). All investigator and sponsor representatives involved in the identification, assessment, review, and evaluation of safety events will be trained on procedures for these activities.

4) Subjects will be informed of anticipated risks and benefits before participating in the trial as part of the informed consent process (Chapter 19 Informed Consent and Other Human Subject Protection). Subjects may also be asked to record their health conditions in a diary between study visits (Chapter 20 Data Collection and Data Management). When the diary solicits the subject's rating for named types of events (e.g., headache, fever, etc.) these events are known as solicited AEs.

21.2.3 Key Concepts for Safety Management During the Trial

The various players have specified responsibilities for safety management during the trial. The goal is that safety events are reviewed and evaluated during the course of the trial so that all parties may continuously evaluate risk versus benefit for research subjects. Parties will be looking at new events, and changes in the number and severity of previously reported events. During the trial:

1) An IRB/IEC will require the investigator to provide changes to the investigation (e.g., protocol amendments), and will specify the types of and the timing for the reporting of protocol deviations and AEs for the IRB/IEC's continuous review of the study to ensure that the benefits outweigh the risks for participating subjects.

2) The investigator will identify, evaluate, and report AEs to the sponsor and the IRB/IEC per the protocol, IRB/IEC, standard operating procedures, GCP, and regulatory requirements.

3) The sponsor is responsible for the ongoing safety evaluation of the investigational product(s) (ICH E6(R2) 5.16.1). The sponsor will review and evaluate

individual and aggregated site events reported by individual investigator for reporting to other investigators participating in the trial as well to those who are using the investigational product for other trials, and IRBs/IECs and regulatory authority(ies) per the protocol, SMP (if created), standard operating procedures, GCP, and applicable regulatory requirements. The sponsor will also review and evaluate events reported by all clinical trial sites and report as appropriate to investigators, ethics committees, and regulatory authorities.

4) If the sponsor should not have direct access to safety data (e.g., in a blinded trial), the sponsor will engage an IDMC to review blinded data or for another purpose of independent review. The sponsor and any engaged IDMC(s) will follow written procedures (e.g., in a Charter) to evaluate safety data.

5) The sponsor and investigator will consider the advantages and disadvantages for breaking the code of treatment (i.e., unblinding the treatment) for a subject who experiences a serious event while participating in the study. The investigator will inform the sponsor and the IRB/IEC of any unblinding of subject treatment, whether the unblinding was accidental or purposeful for protecting the safety of the subject. The sponsor may consult the regulatory authority(ies) regarding those decisions.

21.2.4 Key Concepts for Safety Management After Trial Completion

Because the long-term effects of the study treatment(s) may be unknown, the goal of safety management after a subject discontinues from trial treatment or after they complete the trial and after the trial ends is to ensure that there are systems in place for the continued reporting and evaluation of AEs that are determined to be associated with the study treatment(s) (see Section 21.2.5).

1) If a subject discontinues receiving study treatment while he/she is participating in the trial, then it is best practice for the subject to be encouraged to remain in the trial to complete at least safety assessments. The sponsor may then integrate and analyze the safety, and possibly efficacy data based on the timing of the last treatment for the subject.

2) If the subject completes the trial, the protocol may require the continued reporting and assessment of AEs for a specified period, depending on the half-life and other properties of the investigational product. Pregnancies may also be reported for a period of time once the subject no longer is administered the study drug.

3) The outcomes of pregnancies are also collected to learn more about the safety of the investigational product with respect to the fetus and expectant mother.

21.2.5 Safety Reporting Definitions

In order for clinical researchers to know what to assess and report, the ICH Guidelines provide terms and their definitions and requirements for when to report events as defined. This is an attempt to standardize what is reported by the different players and to facilitate comparison of the frequency of events for the test and control products in a trial. The ethics committees and regulatory authorities are interested in specific types of events and the impact they have on the research subject. Since the goal is to determine the safety of the investigational product, the focus is primarily on events associated with the use of the investigational product. However, procedures should be implemented, as appropriate, to also assess and evaluate any adverse reaction that the subject experiences with study procedures or assessments (e.g., a reaction at the site of blood draw), for the subject would not experience the event had they not been in the trial.

We are interested in the relatedness to the investigational product, seriousness, and expectedness of an event; i.e., whether they are new to, exacerbations of, or increased in frequency to what has already been reported in connection with use of the investigational product. Specific definitions are therefore provided for an "adverse event" based on its "seriousness," "relatedness," and "expectedness."

21.2.5.1 Adverse Event

AE is any untoward medical occurrence in a patient or clinical investigation subject administered a pharmaceutical product and which does not necessarily have a causal relationship with this treatment. An AE can therefore be any unfavorable and unintended sign (including an abnormal laboratory finding), symptom, or disease temporally associated with the use of a medicinal (investigational) product, whether or not related to the medicinal (investigational) product (ICH E6(R2) 1.2).

Simply stated, an AE is an event that has occurred during the trial, whether or not it is related to the investigational product.

21.2.5.2 Adverse Drug Reaction (ADR)

In the preapproval clinical experience with a new medicinal product or its new usages, particularly as the therapeutic dose(s) may not be established, all noxious and unintended responses to a medicinal product related to any dose should be considered adverse drug reactions. The phrase responses to a medicinal product means that a causal relationship between a medicinal product and an AE is at least a reasonable possibility, i.e., the relationship cannot be ruled out. If the investigational product is marketed, a response which is noxious and unintended and which occurs at doses normally used in man for prophylaxis, diagnosis, or therapy of diseases or for modification of physiological function is also an ADR (ICH E6(R2) 1.1).

Simply stated, an ADR is an event that has a causal relationship with the investigational product; i.e., the event occurred with or after the administration of the investigational product, and has a scientific causal relationship with the investigational product.

21.2.5.3 Serious Adverse Event (SAE) or Serious Adverse Drug Reaction (Serious ADR)

Any untoward medical occurrence that at any dose (ICH E6(R2) 1.50):

a) Results in death,
b) Is life-threatening,
c) Requires inpatient hospitalization or prolongation of existing hospitalization,
d) Results in persistent or significant disability/incapacity, OR
e) Is a congenital anomaly/birth defect

Simply stated, a serious adverse event (SAE) or SADR is an event that had serious health consequences for the subject and "serious" is defined as above.

21.2.5.4 Unexpected Adverse Drug Reaction

An adverse reaction, the nature or severity of which is not consistent with the applicable product information (e.g., Investigator's Brochure for an unapproved investigational product or package insert/summary of product characteristics for an approved product) (ICH E6(R2) 1.60).

Simply stated, if an event is documented in the investigator's brochure, the event is considered expected. If the event has not been previously observed or documented in the investigator's brochure with the same severity and frequency as stated in the brochure, the event is considered unexpected. For a marketed product, the information in the approved product label will serve as the basis for determining expectedness.

21.2.5.5 Events Associated with a Placebo

Events known to be associated with placebo treatment will usually not satisfy the criteria for an ADR and, therefore, for expedited reporting; however, refer to the protocol, IRB/EC, and applicable regulatory requirements.

21.2.5.6 Timeframes for Reporting Safety Events

AEs have different requirements for timing for reporting depending on the type of event. Certain types of events will require expedited reporting by the investigator and the sponsor (ICH E2A), while others may be reported in periodic reports to the regulatory authority(ies) or finally in the clinical study report.

a) Expedited Reporting
    i) The types of cases that require expedited reporting are:
        • Single cases of serious, and unexpected ADRs; that is, the event is an adverse drug reaction and is related to the study drug, meets the definition for serious, and is not stated at the severity and frequency in the IB or approved product label.

- Other observations, e.g.,
  - Expected serious ADR that is of greater severity or frequency than is documented in the IB or approved product label
  - A significant hazard to the patient population, such as lack of efficacy with a medicinal product used in treating life-threatening disease
  - A major safety finding from a newly completed animal study (such as carcinogenicity)
  ii) The timing for expedited reporting
  The clock starts for expedited reporting once the sponsor has knowledge of the case and the case meets the minimum criteria for expedited reporting. The sponsor will report these cases to the regulatory authority(ies) and other concerned investigators, who will in turn report to their governing IRB/IEC. Cases for expedited reporting are as follows:
  - Within 7 calendar days:
    - Serious fatal or life-threatening unexpected ADRs
  - Within 15 calendar days:
    - All serious, unexpected ADRs, other than fatal, or life-threatening
b) Other cases not requiring expedited reporting will be reported to the regulatory authority(ies) as follows:
  i) Cases that will be reported with annual or periodic safety reports
  - All SAEs
  ii) In the clinical study report
  - All AEs

21.2.6 Procedures for Safety Reporting

Both the investigator and sponsor both have requirements for safety reporting.

21.2.6.1 Investigator Requirements for Safety Reporting

The investigator will report:

a) AEs and/or laboratory abnormalities identified in the protocol as critical to safety evaluations, to the sponsor according to the reporting requirements and within the time periods specified by the sponsor in the protocol (ICH E6(R2) 4.11.2). The investigator or qualified designee will question the subject regarding their wellbeing and obtain details of any health conditions reported by the subject to determine AEs needed to be reported. The investigator or qualified designee will also review any information recorded in the subject's diary, if used in the study, and discuss as necessary with the subject. All information pertinent to AEs reporting will be documented in the subject's case histories and reported in the case report forms as required.

b) All SAEs immediately to the sponsor except for those SAEs that the protocol or other document (e.g., Investigator's Brochure) identifies as not needing immediate reporting. The immediate reports should be followed promptly by detailed, written reports. The immediate and follow-up reports should identify subjects by unique code numbers assigned to the trial subjects rather than by the subjects' names, personal identification numbers, and/or addresses. The timing for investigator reporting of SAEs will be specified in the protocol or other written instructions (e.g., standard operating procedures, SMP) (see Section 21.2.6.2).

c) To the regulatory authority(ies) and the IRB/IEC per the applicable regulatory requirement(s) related to the reporting of unexpected serious adverse drug reactions. (ICH E6(R2) 4.11.1).

d) Supply the sponsor and the IRB/IEC with any additional requested information (e.g., autopsy reports and terminal medical reports) for reported deaths (ICH E6(R2) 4.11.3).

21.2.6.2   Sponsor Requirements for Safety Reporting

The sponsor will report (from individual subject reports or aggregate data analyses):

a) Events and findings that could adversely affect the safety of subjects, impact the conduct of the trial, or alter the IRB/IEC's approval/favorable opinion to continue the trial to all concerned investigator(s)/institution(s) and the regulatory authority(ies) (ICH E6(R2) 5.16.2).

b) To all concerned investigator(s)/institutions(s), to the IRB(s)/IEC(s), where required, and to the regulatory authority(ies) all adverse drug reactions (ADRs) that are both serious and unexpected (ICH E6(R2) 5.17.1). Such expedited reports should comply with the applicable regulatory requirement(s) (ICH E6(R2) 5.17.2).

c) All safety updates and periodic reports to the regulatory authority(ies), as required by applicable regulatory requirement(s) (ICH E6(R2) 5.17.3).

d) As necessary, events associated with an approved active comparator to the manufacturer or appropriate regulatory authority(ies).

21.2.6.3   IRB/IEC Requirements for Safety Reporting

The IRB/IEC will:

a) Safeguard the rights, safety, and well-being of all trial subjects. Special attention should be paid to trials that may include vulnerable subjects. (ICH E6(R2) 3.1.1)

b) Inform the investigator of the investigator's requirement to promptly report to the IRB/IEC (ICH E6(R2) 3.3.8)

   (a) Deviations from, or changes of, the protocol to eliminate immediate hazards to the trial subjects

 (b) Changes increasing the risk to subjects and/or affecting significantly the conduct of the trial

 (c) All adverse drug reactions (ADRs) that are both serious and unexpected.

 (d) New information that may affect adversely the safety of the subjects or the conduct of the trial.

21.2.6.4 Records of Safety Reporting

Several records regarding safety reporting will be maintained by the investigator and the sponsor (Chapter 29 Essential Documents).

 The investigator will maintain the following:

- All AEs and their characteristics for each trial subject in their case histories
- Reports of safety events submitted to the sponsor, either via the case report form and/or expedited reporting forms
- Reports of safety events to the IRB/IEC and to regulatory authority(ies) as required
- Records of unblinding of subject treatment for safety reasons
- Reasons of safety for subject discontinuation from study treatment
- Reasons of safety for subject discontinuation from the study

The sponsor will maintain the following:

- Documentation of procedures for safety events collection, analyses, and reporting
- Reports of safety events received from the investigator, market surveillance, literature surveillance, or other sources
- Charters and minutes of meetings for IDMC receipt and review of safety events, and recommendations on findings for the trial
- Notifications of expedited reports of safety events to the investigator(s)
- Notifications of expedited reports of safety events to the regulatory authority(ies)
- Records of integrated analyses of safety events
- Annual or periodic reports to the regulatory authority(ies)
- Clinical study report

21.2.7 The Safety Management Plan

The SMP will outline all requirements for the collection, monitoring, analysis, and review of safety data for a trial. The SMP will also outline who is responsible for what and when, and the plans and procedures for training and updating procedures as necessary. The SMP may include the following and additional information as necessary for a specific trial:

1) A description of potential risks and benefits for study subjects
2) A description of how AEs will be solicited and collected from study subjects
3) A description of conditions and procedures for decoding/unblinding study treatment for a study subject

4) Procedures for safety data review: the timing of review, a list of variables to be reviewed, and the methods for review (includes references to procedures for an IDMC)
5) Procedures for discussion of findings for safety data review and actions to be taken for important safety signals
6) Procedures for expedited reporting of safety events. This may include a process flow chart showing timing and who is responsible, consulted, or informed of what during the process.
7) Procedures for reporting to the regulatory authority(ies), investigators, other manufacturers, and others as needed
8) Stopping rules for safety findings

The SMP should be updated as necessary and previous versions maintained.

21.2.8 Quality by Design Considerations for the Monitoring and Reporting of Safety Events

A number of principles and operational considerations that promote GCP, quality, and compliance may guide procedures monitoring and reporting safety events for a trial. Data principles and trial operations considerations to foster quality for safety management include:

- Considerations for avoiding and/or reducing safety events through thoughtful study and product design
- Specifying safety parameters and definitions for safety events, and training all involved in safety reporting and analysis on those definitions and procedures
- Ensuring that procedures for soliciting AEs and supporting information from subjects are clear
- Ensuring that the path for expedited reporting of safety events is clear and the procedures for expedited safety reporting explicitly identify who will be responsible for what and when, and that the timing and processes are realistic and feasible
- Outlining procedures for continuous assessment of safety events and processes for identifying new and reportable events
- Ensuring that trial subjects are aware of all the risks and benefits regarding study participation and that they are updated with information that may affect their decision to remain in the study
- Ensuring that procedures are in place for the continuous review and evaluation of reported safety events to assess the benefit-risk balance for subjects participating the study and that the process includes guidance on appropriate actions to take if the risks outweigh the benefits
- Ensuring procedures are in place for the maintenance of required records of safety data collection, assessment, and reporting

21.3 Summary

Clinical safety data monitoring and reporting is the primary concern of all involved in the planning and conduct of a clinical research study.

The ICH E6(R2) and ICH E2A Guidances contain definitions and responsibilities for safety monitoring and reporting by the investigator, sponsor, and the IRB/IEC. Safety management concepts apply to processes and procedures before the trial begins, during the trial, and posttrial treatment or after the trial ends.

The primary goal of safety reporting is to collect and review AEs associated with the subject's participation in the trial and receipt of study drug(s) (active or placebo, or investigational or approved) to continuously assess the risk-benefit ratio to justify exposing the volunteering subject to the investigational product and other study drugs. As such, some events are considered more serious than others and therefore require expedited reporting and analysis by the investigator, sponsor, IRB/IEC, and regulatory authority(ies). The sponsor may engage an IDMC to assist with the review of safety and other events of significant interest if the trial is blinded or if an independent review is otherwise warranted.

Quality by design principles also apply to safety monitoring and reporting. The protocol should be designed to limit or avoid AEs and systems and procedures should be implemented to ensure the timely and appropriate collection, review, analysis, and reporting of safety events for the trial. Procedures should also be implemented to ensure that required documentation of safety events and the processing and review of events are maintained. An SMP may be created, followed, and updated as necessary to ensure compliance with protocol, GCP, and applicable regulatory requirements.

Knowledge Check Questions

1) What is the general purpose of safety monitoring and reporting?
2) What are some concepts of protocol design that are relevant to safety management?
3) What are the investigator's responsibilities for safety management?
4) What are the sponsor's responsibilities for safety management?
5) What are the IRB/IEC's responsibilities regarding reporting of safety data?
6) What events require expedited reporting and when?
7) When and how are non-expedited events reported?
8) What are the key quality-by-design considerations for safety management?
9) Overheard:
   We do not agree with the investigator's assessment of possibly related for this event so we will down-grade the event to not related.

Sponsor's Chief Medical Officer, citing theoretical mechanism of action models for the investigational product.

Comment and discuss:

a) Whose grading of the event should be used for regulatory reporting purposes?
b) What are advantages and disadvantages for using theoretical models to ascertain safety conclusions for an investigational product?
c) What implications may relatedness for a safety event has on the overall safety outcomes for research subjects in the short run, and for the general public in the long run?

References

1 International Council for Harmonisation of Technical Requirements for Pharmaceuticals for Human Use (ICH), Integrated Addendum to ICH E6(R1):Guideline for Good Clinical Practice, E6(R2), Current Step 4 version dated 9 November 2016. https://www.ich.org/page/efficacy-guidelines
2 International Conference on Harmonisation of Technical Requirements For Registration of Pharmaceuticals For Human Use Ichharmonised Tripartite Guidelineclinical Safety Data Management: Definitions and Standards for Expedited Reporting, E2A, Current Step 4 version dated 27 October 1994 https://www.ich.org/page/efficacy-guidelines

22

Monitoring Overview

Karen A. Henry

GCP Key Point

Monitoring is a Quality Control (operational technique) activity to ensure that a protocol is followed.

22.1   Introduction

Clinical site "Monitoring" is a quality control (QC) activity that is inherent to the definition of good clinical practice (GCP):

> A standard for the design, conduct, performance, monitoring, auditing, recording, analyses, and reporting of clinical trials that provides assurance that the data and reported results are credible and accurate, and that the rights, integrity, and confidentiality of trial subjects are protected (ICH E6(R2) 1.24) [].

This means that the scope of monitoring includes all clinical site activities, from setup to archiving, which are, in whole and in part, checked in real time and controlled for their compliance with the protocol, standard operating procedures (SOPs), GCP, and applicable regulatory requirements. This QC activity complements the ICH E6(R2) principle for systems with procedures that assure the quality of every aspect of the trial should be implemented (ICH E6(R2) 2.13).

In fact, upon review of the Principles of ICH GCP (ICH E6(R2); Chapter 6 GCP Definition and Principles), all of the other 12 principles apply to monitoring, given that monitoring is of all study activities and the principles apply to all of those activities. These principles, therefore, inform us of what will be monitored.

The Fundamentals of Clinical Research: A Universal Guide for Implementing Good Clinical Practice, First Edition. P. Michael Dubinsky and Karen A. Henry.
© 2022 John Wiley & Sons, Inc. Published 2022 by John Wiley & Sons, Inc.
Companion website: www.wiley.com/go/dubinsky/clinicalresearch

The ICH has assigned the responsibility for monitoring to the sponsor (ICH E6(R2) 5.18). For practical reasons, regulatory agencies do not have the bandwidth to perform ongoing monitoring of all registered investigations (the number of investigators active at any one time is numerous and onerous!) so their responsibility is limited to inspections at a quality assurance level. The sponsor and the institutional review board (IRB)/independent ethics committee (IEC) may also perform audits as part of quality assurance responsibilities. The investigations are therefore examined at the QC and quality assurance level.

22.2 Objectives

The objectives of this chapter are to:

1) Define monitoring
2) Describe
   a) Why: The purpose of monitoring
   b) Who: Qualification and role of a monitor
   c) What: A monitor's checklist
   d) Scope: The extent and nature of monitoring
   e) Strategy: On-site and centralized monitoring
      i) Individual on-site review
      ii) Centralized monitoring
      iii) Individual off-site review
   f) When: The timing of monitoring
3) Describe the Monitoring Plan
4) Describe reporting of Monitoring Activities

22.2.1 Definition of Monitoring

Monitoring is the act of overseeing the progress of a clinical trial, and of ensuring that it is conducted, recorded, and reported in accordance with the protocol, SOPs, GCP, and the applicable regulatory requirement(s) (ICH E6(R2) 1.38).

In GCP, qualified individuals are expected to supervise, manage, and control all study processes and data, to ensure complete, clear, and accurate documentation that reflect how the trial is conducted, and to ensure that the trial status and activities are communicated in accordance with the protocol, SOPs, GCP, and applicable regulatory requirement(s).

22.2.2 Why: The Purpose of Monitoring

As it is for all GCP activities, the primary concern of monitoring is three-fold (ICH E6(R2) 5.18.1):

1) Protect the rights and well-being of human subjects.
2) Maintain data integrity.
3) Ensure compliance with the currently approved protocol, GCP, and applicable regulatory requirement(s).

The purpose of monitoring, therefore, is to *verify* that:

1) The rights and well-being of human subjects are protected.
2) The reported trial data are accurate, complete, and verifiable from source documents.
3) The conduct of the trial is in compliance with the currently approved protocol, GCP and applicable regulatory requirement(s).

This is to say that, from setting up the trial through archiving its documentation, all trial activities will be guided by these intentions and, conversely, the intentions will guide how the trial activities are conducted (Chapter 31 Quality Responsibilities).

Additionally, as we review the principles of GCP, we note how all 13 principles apply to monitoring (see Chapter 6 GCP Definition and Principles). To summarize, trial monitoring will review study processes and data to check ICH E6 principles as follows in Table 22.1.

22.2.3 Who: Qualification and Role of a Monitor

22.2.3.1 Monitor Selection

The Monitor is appointed by the sponsor (ICH E6(R2) 5.18.2(a)). The sponsor may engage a qualified employee, an independent contractor, or a member of a Contract Research Organization (CRO) as a Monitor. The responsibility for monitoring may be wholly assigned to a CRO, the sponsor may choose to retain responsibility for centralized monitoring and assign only site monitoring to the CRO, or the sponsor may choose to divide the responsibility in another manner that meets the business objectives of the organization. Regardless of how monitoring responsibilities are divided, if a CRO is retained, the CRO will assume the regulatory responsibility(ies) assigned and the sponsor maintains responsibility for all oversight of the CRO and overall study conduct.

22.2.3.2 Monitor Training

The Monitor must be appropriately trained and will have the scientific and/or clinical knowledge needed to monitor the trial adequately (ICH E6(R2) 5.18.2(b)).

Table 22.1 GCP principle and associated trial monitoring application.

ICH E6(R2) GCP Principle	Trial Monitoring Application
#2.1 Clinical trials should be conducted in accordance with the ethical principles that have their origin in the Declaration of Helsinki, and that are consistent with GCP and the applicable regulatory requirement(s).	The investigator's decisions for medical care and study conduct are foremost in the best interest of the subject's rights and well-being.
#2.2 . . . A trial should be initiated and continued only if the anticipated benefits justify the risks.	Risks and benefits are continuously reviewed and weighed. Information for assessing risk versus benefit is derived from not only the specified trial, but all clinical trials using the investigational product, and nonclinical and manufacturing information about the investigational product that may relate to and adversely affect human subjects.
#2.3 The rights, safety, and well-being of the trial subjects are the most important considerations and should prevail over interests of science and society.	The rights, safety, and well-being of trial subjects are never compromised, regardless of available resources or scientific or business objectives.
#2.4 The available clinical and nonclinical information on an investigational product should be adequate to support the proposed clinical trial.	The initial and any proposed changes to the protocol must be supported by available clinical and nonclinical information.
#2.5 Clinical trials should be scientifically sound, and described in a clear, detailed protocol.	The protocol will be revised as necessary if monitoring identifies deviations that reflect deficiencies in how information is presented.
#2.6 A trial should be conducted in compliance with the protocol that has received prior IRB/IEC approval/favorable opinion.	Only procedures that have been approved by an IRB/IEC may be conducted, and any conducted procedure that is not exactly in accordance with the approved protocol is considered a deviation from the protocol. In real life, this means, for example, that if a procedure is completed on 23 June and the IRB/IEC stamp of approval is 24 June, then the completed procedure is a deviation from the approved protocol. Likewise, if a procedure is completed at 08 : 11 and the approved protocol prescribes it to be done 08 : 00 with a window of $\pm$10 minutes, then that procedure is a deviation from the protocol.

Table 22.1 (Continued)

ICH E6(R2) GCP Principle	Trial Monitoring Application
#2.7 The medical care given to, and medical decisions made on behalf of, subjects should always be the responsibility of a qualified physician or, when appropriate, of a qualified dentist.	The investigator and all delegated personnel who will make medical decisions or generate study data regarding medical care of a subject must have complete and current documentation of appropriate qualification required by the institution and local regulatory requirements to perform such procedures.
#2.8 Each individual involved in conducting a trial should be qualified by education, training, and experience to perform his or her respective tasks(s).	All persons, whether conducting sponsor or investigator responsibilities, must have evidence of qualification to perform their assigned delegated task.
#2.9 Freely given informed consent should be obtained from every subject prior to clinical trial participation.	Documentation must be present for all subjects participating in a clinical trial showing all required aspects of administration of informed consent prior to undergoing any trial procedure. If the procedure and consent are performed on the same day, then the relative timing must also be documented.
#2.10 All clinical trial information should be recorded, handled, and stored in a way that allows its accurate reporting, interpretation, and verification.	The goal is that a reviewer of trial conduct (e.g., monitor, auditor, inspector, or other authorized individual) should be able to analyze or reconstruct, at any time as required by the protocol, GCP, or applicable regulations, exactly how the trial was executed based on the records.
#2.11 The confidentiality of records that could identify subjects should be protected, respecting privacy and confidentiality rules in accordance with the applicable regulatory requirement(s).	The identity and confidentiality of subject information must be maintained at all time during and after the study. Institutional and local regulatory requirements will guide on which subject identifiers may be used in clinical trials, and the subject will further determine which of their identifiers may be used on study records and who may see those records via their signed informed consent form. Technically, a Monitor may not review any of a subject's study records unless a duly executed informed consent is in place for the subject.

(Continued)

Table 22.1 (Continued)

ICH E6(R2) GCP Principle	Trial Monitoring Application
#2.12 Investigational products should be manufactured, handled, and stored in accordance with applicable good manufacturing practice (GMP). They should be used in accordance with the approved protocol.	The "chain of custody" for the investigational product starts with its release from the manufacturing facility to its disposal at a location approved by the sponsor. The sponsor is responsible for all activities related to the investigational product outside of the clinical site and the investigator is responsible for all such activities that occur at the site, with sponsor oversight of investigator-related activities. The sponsor is therefore responsible for monitoring the entire chain from manufacturing to disposal. At the clinical site, the sponsor will verify receipt, storage, handling, and administration of the investigational products in accordance with the approved protocol.
#2.13 Systems with procedures that assure the quality of every aspect of the trial should be implemented.	Quality systems include both quality control (e.g., monitoring) and quality assurance (e.g., SOPs, training, audits) measures that ensure adherence to the protocol, SOPs, GCP, and applicable regulatory requirements.

They should be familiar with the therapeutic area being studied; i.e., the clinical study population and medical conditions and typical treatments associated with the disease under study. This scientific/clinical knowledge enables them to identify issues or discrepancies with study assessments, the management of medical care for the subject, as well as safety reporting.

22.2.3.3 Monitor Familiarity with the Study Information
The Monitor will be thoroughly familiar with the sponsor's SOPs, GCP, and applicable regulatory requirement(s) (ICH E6(R2) 5.18.2(c)), both for the study at large and those specific to the individual clinical site, to ensure the site's compliance and to be able to identify any noncompliance at the clinical site and for the general study. Understanding who has regulatory responsibility for what clinical trial activity and the required SOP procedures help the Monitor to make decisions and resolve issues. For example, when negotiating the content of subject information and informed consent forms, it is important to be aware that the regulatory decision on the final content lies with the IRB/IEC, and not with the sponsor or

investigator. Additionally, the knowledge and application of GCP principles can be helpful in applying and prioritizing resources; i.e., whether the underlying risk is to subject safety, data integrity, or compliance.

The Monitor will also be thoroughly familiar with the investigational product(s), the protocol, written informed consent form and any other written information to be provided to subjects (ICH E6(R2) 5.18.2(c)). Knowledge of the properties of the investigational product or its class of products helps the Monitor to understand and monitor the shipping, handling, and storage requirements. Additionally, the monitor will ensure that only procedures as outlined in the informed consent form are those that are performed for a subject who has a fully executed consent.

The qualification and training of each and all monitors must be documented (ICH E6(R2) 5.18.2(b)).

22.2.3.4 Monitor's Role

The Monitor acts as the main line of communication between the sponsor and the investigator (ICH E6(R2) 5.18.4(a)). The Monitor, therefore, must be able to visit the clinical site, have access to and be able to read and understand study records, and communicate with the investigator and site staff and the sponsor. The Monitor, therefore, must be fluent in the written and spoken language of the investigator and site staff. Information that is communicated between the sponsor and the investigator includes:

- Regulatory information
  - Investigator and site qualifications and resources (Chapter 23 Investigator/Institution Selection)
  - Investigator agreements (Chapter 23 Investigator/Institution Selection)
  - Trial insurance (Chapter 23 Investigator/Institution Selection)
  - Study and site status notifications, applications, submissions, and reporting to the sponsor and IRB/IEC (Chapter 8 IRB/IEC Roles and Responsibilities; Chapter 25 Investigator/Institution Interim Monitoring)
  - Auditing and inspections (Chapter 34 Regulatory Authority Inspections)
  - Essential documents (Chapter 29 Essential Documents)

- Protocol procedures
  - Receipt of all trial information to conduct the trial (Chapter 23 Investigator/Institution Selection)
  - Investigator and staff knowledge of the trial (Chapter 23 Investigator/Institution Selection)
  - Investigational product supplies and usage (Chapter 17 The Investigational Product (Clinical Supplies))
  - Compliance with the protocol and protocol deviations (Chapter 18 The Clinical Trial Protocol and Amendments)

- Subject recruitment, consent, and eligibility (Chapter 19 Informed Consent and Other Human Subject Protection)
- Facilities and equipment for protocol procedures (Chapter 25 Investigator/ Institution Interim Monitoring)
- Safety reporting (Chapter 21 Safety Monitoring and Reporting)
- Source documentation (Chapter 20 Data Collection and Data Management)
- Case report form (CRF) completion and data corrections (Chapter 20 Data Collection and Data Management)
- Laboratory testing, supplies, and samples
- Administrative
  - Contracting (Chapter 15 Trial Resourcing and Outsourcing)
  - Budget and payments (Chapter 15 Trial Resourcing and Outsourcing)
  - Trial personnel contact and communication (Chapter 14 Trial Management; Start-up, On-Study, and Close-Out)

The Monitor verifies that study conduct is compliant with the protocol, GCP, and applicable regulatory requirements. (See Section 22.2.4.) As the liaison between the sponsor and the investigator, the Monitor not only verifies, but also takes measures to ensure that the trial is conducted to meet all stated objectives. The Monitor, within the confines of SOPs, GCP, and applicable regulations, will follow-up and facilitate measures to resolve identified deficiencies and deviations with the investigator and staff.

22.2.4 What: The Individual Site Monitoring Checklist

The monitoring checklist will include all study activities that need to be evaluated for compliance with the protocol, SOPs, GCP, and applicable regulatory requirements (Plate 15 Monitoring Overview Checklist). Those activities are driven by both sponsor and investigator responsibilities (see Chapter 9 Investigator and Sponsor Roles and Responsibilities). In addition to acting as the main line of communication between the sponsor and investigator, ICH E6(R2) 5.18.4 outlines the Monitor's responsibilities as follows:

- Appropriate investigator and site selection and continued participation:
  - *(b)* Verifying that the investigator has adequate qualifications and resources that remain adequate throughout the trial period; that facilities, including laboratories, equipment, and staff, are adequate to safely and properly conduct the trial and remain adequate throughout the trial period.
- Investigator compliance with investigational product requirements:
  - *(c)* Verifying, for the investigational product(s):

    o That storage times and conditions are acceptable, and that supplies are sufficient throughout the trial.

    o That the investigational product(s) are supplied only to subjects who are eligible to receive it and at the protocol specified dose(s).

    o That subjects are provided with necessary instruction on properly using, handling, storing, and returning the investigational product(s).

    o That the receipt, use, and return of the investigational product(s) at the trial sites are controlled and documented adequately.

    o That the disposition of unused investigational product(s) at the trial sites complies with applicable regulatory requirement(s) and is in accordance with the sponsor procedures.

- Investigator compliance with the approved protocol:
  - *(d)* Verifying that the investigator follows the approved protocol and all approved amendment(s), if any.
- Subject informed consent:
  - *(e)* Verifying that written informed consent was obtained before each subject's participation in the trial.
- Investigator receives all trial information:
  - *(f)* Ensuring that the investigator receives the current Investigator's Brochure, all documents, and all trial supplies needed to conduct the trial properly and to comply with the applicable regulatory requirement(s).
- Investigator and staff knowledge of the trial:
  - *(g)* Ensuring that the investigator and the investigator's trial staff are adequately informed about the trial.
- Investigator and staff qualifications:
  - *(h)* Verifying that the investigator and the investigator's trial staff are performing the specified trial functions, in accordance with the protocol and any other written agreement between the sponsor and the investigator/institution, and have not delegated these functions to unauthorized individuals.
- Subject eligibility:
  - *(i)* Verifying that the investigator is enrolling only eligible subjects.
- Subject recruitment:
  - *(j)* Reporting the subject recruitment rate.
- Source documentation:
  - *(k)* Verifying that source documents and other trial records are accurate, complete, up-to-date, and maintained.
- Study reporting:
  - *(l)* Verifying that the investigator provides all the required reports, notifications, applications, and submissions, and that these documents are accurate, complete, timely, legible, dated, and identify the trial.

- CRF completion:
  - *(m)* Checking the accuracy and completeness of the CRF entries, source documents and other trial-related records against each other. The Monitor specifically should verify that:
    - o The data required by the protocol are reported accurately on the CRFs and are consistent with the source documents.
    - o Any dose and/or therapy modifications are well documented for each of the trial subjects.
    - o Adverse events, concomitant medications and intercurrent illnesses are reported in accordance with the protocol on the CRFs.
    - o Visits that the subjects fail to make, tests that are not conducted, and examinations that are not performed are clearly reported as such on the CRFs.
    - o All withdrawals and dropouts of enrolled subjects from the trial are reported and explained on the CRFs.
- CRF corrections:
  - *(n)* Informing the investigator of any CRF entry error, omission, or illegibility. The Monitor should ensure that appropriate corrections, additions, or deletions are made, dated, explained (if necessary), and approved by the investigator or by a member of the investigator's trial staff who is authorized to approve CRF changes for the investigator. This authorization should be documented.
- Adverse events reporting:
  - *(o)* Determining whether all adverse events (AEs) are appropriately reported within the time periods required by GCP, the protocol, the IRB/IEC, the sponsor, and the applicable regulatory requirement(s).
- Essential documents:
  - *(p)* Determining whether the essential documents are complete, up-to-date, and maintained (Chapter 29 Essential Documents).
- Deviations reporting and corrective and preventive actions (CAPAs):
  - *(q)* Communicating deviations from the protocol, SOPs, GCP, and the applicable regulatory requirements to the investigator and taking appropriate action designed to correct and prevent recurrence of the detected deviations.

22.2.5 Scope: The Extent and Nature of Monitoring

As stated before, monitoring is the act of overseeing the progress of a clinical trial, and of ensuring that it is conducted, recorded, and reported in accordance with the protocol, SOPs, GCP, and the applicable regulatory requirement(s) and the sponsor has regulatory responsibility for this task.

The quality goal of clinical research is to conduct a clinical trial that is in full compliance with perfectly accurate and complete data. In order to reach this goal and given human and resource limitations, ICH E6(R2) allows for sponsors to determine the appropriate extent and nature of monitoring to ensure that trials are adequately monitored (ICH E6(R2) 5.18.3) via a risk-based approach to quality management (ICH E6(R2) 5.0.1). That is to say, a sponsor will identify critical processes and data to assure human subject protection and the reliability of study results by prioritizing what it monitors (the checklist), how much it monitors (the scope), and how it monitors (the strategy) the investigation.

The extent and nature of monitoring will depend on the characteristics of the trial and the sponsor should develop a systematic, prioritized, risk-based approach to monitoring based on these characteristics, such as those (per ICH E6(R2) 5.18.3) displayed in Figure 22.1.

22.2.6 Strategy: On-site and Centralized Monitoring

Study conduct at the investigator site involves a variety of processes and the collection of a variety of data. Some processes and data may be adequately reviewed remotely (e.g., documentation of investigator qualification) while the Monitor must have on-site and tangible contact with others (e.g., investigational product accountability) for adequate verification. At the same time, some processes and data are so critical to the quality outcome of the trial that it is best for them to be evaluated on-site regardless of whether there is flexibility to review them remotely or on-site.

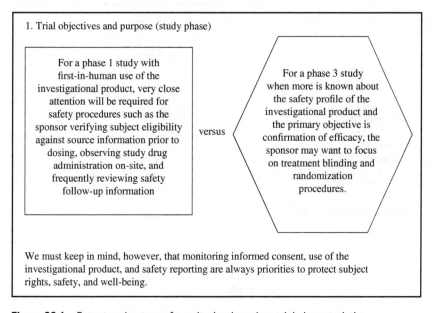

Figure 22.1 Extent and nature of monitoring based on trial characteristics.

2. Protocol design

An open-label single-arm trial with a single visit for administration of an oral medication to 20 healthy volunteers who return a week later for a blood draw that provides information about efficacy

Will have less demand on monitoring resources than…

A two-arm, double-blinded study of a monthly 2-hour intravenous infusion in patients 65 years or older with advanced motor-neuron disease and efficacy is measured by monthly imaging and data from patient diaries.

3. Protocol complexity

A study in which patients may self-administer oral medication.

Will have less demand on monitoring resources than…

A study where live cells have to be counted under a sterile hood before surgically implanted into the brain.

4. Protocol endpoints

Exploratory endpoints

Will have less demand on monitoring than

Primary endpoints

5. Blinding

An open-label study

Will have less demand on monitoring resources than…

A blinded study

6. Size of the trial

A trial of 20 healthy volunteers at a single site

Will have less demand on monitoring resources than…

A global trial of 3000 subjects at 300 sites located in 6 countries

7. Other considerations include:

a. Enrollment rate

Slow enrollment; e.g., one subject per month.

Will have less demand on monitoring resources than…

Rapid enrollment; e.g., 20 subjects per month.

Figure 22.1 (Continued)

b. Site compliance

| A site that has an average of less than two protocol deviations for each subject visit. | Will have less demand on monitoring resources than... | A site that has an average of 10 or more protocol deviations per subject visit |

c. Safety issues associated with the investigational product or study procedures

| A trial with an investigational product that has less than two expected common adverse events per subject or a trial in 18 – 25-year-old healthy volunteers. | Will have less demand on monitoring resources than... | A trial with an investigational product that has more than 10 expected adverse events per subject or a trial in stage IV cancer patients. |

d. Staff turnover

| A site that has tenured investigator and staff with extensive GCP experience | Will have less demand on monitoring resources than... | A site that has naive staff with temporary employment |

e. Sponsor's experience with the investigator and site

| An investigator and site staff who have previously conducted a trial by the sponsor and are familiar with the investigational product. | Will have less demand on monitoring resources than... | An investigator and site staff who have never conducted a trial with the sponsor and have no familiarity with the class of investigational product. |

f. Investigator and site experience with the study population, class of investigational product, disease under study

| An investigator and/or site staff who have conducted no trials in study population, class of investigational product, and/or disease under study. | Will have less demand on monitoring resources than... | An investigator and/or site staff who have conducted no trials in study population, class of investigational product, and/or disease under study. |

Figure 22.1 (Continued)

Given that the sponsor must adequately monitor the trial, the risk-based approach to monitoring gives the sponsor the opportunity to prioritize processes and data that are critical to assure human subject protection and the reliability of study results (ICH E6(R2) 5.0.1; Chapter 13 Risk Assessment and Quality Management). The sponsor will then determine if the critical process or data will be monitored on-site or in a centralized manner:

- *On*-site monitoring refers to the review and assessment of study activities at the site where the clinical trial is being conducted (ICH E6(R2) 5.18.3).
- In centralized monitoring, the sponsor can remotely evaluate ongoing and/or cumulative data collected from trial sites (ICH E6(R2) 5.18.3).

For the monitoring of individual clinical site activities, the sponsor may also determine if a specific activity may be monitored *off*-site; that is, via remote review of the study activity, considering the constraint to maintain confidentiality of subject identity (Chapter 19 Informed Consent and Other Human Subject Protection) and study information, and remote access to source documentation.

SOPs that will be followed for a trial may provide high-level guidance for monitoring all trials (e.g., templates for monitoring reports, procedures for reporting suspected fraud or misconduct). However, any strategy the sponsor decides to use for a specific study and the rationale for the choice should be documented; e.g., in a study-specific Monitoring Plan (see Section 22.2.8).

22.2.6.1 On-site Review

The Monitoring Plan (Section 22.2.8) will outline what critical processes and data will be monitored at the clinical site when remote access to source documentation is not available. On-site review is required for "critical" source data verification, such as:

- Informed consent prior to any study-specific procedure:
  Review informed consent records to verify that the full process for consent was completed and signed and that informed consent was obtained from the subject prior to the subject undergoing any study-specific protocol procedure
- Adherence to eligibility criteria:
  Review source documentation to verify that the subject met all eligibility criteria (or appropriate waivers were obtained and documented) prior to the administration of the investigational product(s) or randomization, if applicable.
- Primary endpoint data:
  Review testing, test results and other source records to verify the collection of data for the primary endpoint(s) and that the data are correctly entered in the CRF.
- Safety events that lead to the discontinuation of study treatment or subject withdrawal:

Review source records to verify information for adverse events (e.g., verbatim term, date of onset, severity, seriousness) that led to the discontinuation of study treatment or the subject's participation in the study and ensure they are correctly and timely reported.

- Processes that support subject safety and ethical treatment, such as medical consultation and unscheduled visits:
  Verify that a subject received or was referred for appropriate medical care for adverse events resulting from their participation in the trial. As necessary, the subject should undergo appropriate clinical procedures at unscheduled site visits (that is, not on the protocol schedule) for evaluation of such events.
- Randomization and blinding procedures:
  Review all relevant study documentation and procedures and interview study personnel to ensure that randomization and blinding procedures were followed and that the blinding per the protocol has been maintained. If incorrect randomization or accidental or intentional unblinding occurred, the deviation should have been reported timely to the sponsor and IRB/IEC as required. Investigative and corrective and preventive actions should always be performed and documented for incorrect randomization or accidental unblinding.
- Investigational product administration and accountability:
  Review site records of investigational product accountability and verify against sponsor shipping records; investigational product dispensed, administered, destroyed; and unused supplies; thereby accounting for all investigational product(s) received at the site.

22.2.6.2 Centralized Monitoring Checklist

Clinical sites should transmit study CRFs and other data to the sponsor in a timely manner as the data are collected during the course of the study. The sponsor will therefore have ongoing access to study data and can review data for individual subject(s), individual site, all sites, or any subset as needed. Data review can be completed from e.g., data entry reports, listings of individual subject data, or summaries of data in aggregate, to name a few. Centralized monitoring consists of:

- Routine review of ongoing and/or cumulative submitted data to assess individual site characteristics and performance metrics to determine need for targeted on-site monitoring.
- Routine review of ongoing and/or cumulative submitted data to assess study performance metrics to determine needs for protocol or CRF amendments, changes in risk management or monitoring specifications, or changes in other study or operating procedures.

Submitted data may be reviewed for:

- Missing or incomplete data; i.e., identify data that have no explanations for their absence. Data should be noted as not applicable, not available, or other notation to assure that a response was not overlooked.
- Range checks; e.g., comparing the subject's data (such as age) with the minimum and maximum parameters per the eligibility criteria
- Inconsistent or discrepant data; e.g., "pregnant males"
- Data outliers
- Data trends such as the range and consistency of data within and across sites
- CRF completion accuracy, volume, and timing
- Procedures "out of window"; i.e., to identify procedures that were not completed within the window (e.g., ±1 day) in the protocol
- Number and type of protocol or GCP deviations
- Rate and type of subjects who fail screening
- Delays in data reporting
- Data plausibility or unexpected lack of variability

Note: Data analyses to evaluate study endpoints, such as safety or efficacy, should only be performed according to the protocol and statistical analysis plan. Consideration should be given to study blinding when conducting centralized monitoring.

22.2.6.3 Off-site Review

A sponsor, having the responsibility for monitoring, may consider remotely monitoring study activities that do not require a visit to the clinical site. The decision for this type of remote monitoring will be based on risk and an available infrastructure to facilitate this strategy. Clinical sites will have to provide the sponsor with documentation of data and processes while ensuring that subject and study confidentiality are maintained. Examples of documented study processes and data that may be remotely reviewed are:

- Verification of source data when remote access to source documentation is available
- Verification of the investigator's delegation of responsibilities against investigator and site staff qualification
- Reconciliation of site files and sponsor files for content and versions of documents
- Confirmation of IRB/IEC submissions, review, and approvals
- Reconciliation of screening and enrollment records against randomization and investigational product administration records

Note: Records with subject personal identification (e.g., subject identification code list, signed informed consent forms) must NOT be transmitted outside of the clinical site. Subject personal identification must be redacted from any documentation that must be transmitted outside of the clinical site. The subject's signed consent will guide on which of their personal identification may be transmitted on study documentation.

22.2.7 When: The Timing of Monitoring

Since the aim of monitoring is to ensure the protection of human subjects, integrity of the data, and overall compliance, monitoring activities will generally occur (Plate 7 Monitoring):

1) Before the study; i.e., selecting investigators and initiating the investigation (see Chapter 23 Investigator/Institution Selection; Chapter 24 Investigator/ Institution Initiations). The purpose of
   a) Site selection and pre-study visits are to assess (review records, procedures, systems, and knowledge) for *suitability* to conduct the specified study
   b) Investigator initiation is to assess (review records, procedures, systems, and knowledge) for *qualification and preparedness* to conduct the specified study.
2) During the study; i.e., once the first subject is consented and through the last study contact with the last subject on study (see Chapter 25 Investigator/ Institution Interim Monitoring). Interim monitoring assesses (review records, procedures, systems, and knowledge) for *ongoing compliance* with the specified study requirements.
3) After the study; i.e., after the last contact with the last subject on study, or the last data point for the study is collected and through archiving the records and destruction of the records (see Chapter 26 Investigator/Institution Close-out). The purpose of study and site close-out is to assess (review records) for *completed compliance* with the specified study requirements and prepare records for archiving.

The applicable SOPs and/or Monitoring Plan will outline the specifications for the timing and frequency of monitoring for the trial.

22.2.8 The Monitoring Plan

In addition to the requirements specified in SOPs that apply to monitoring all clinical trials for an organization, the Monitoring Plan is created for a specific protocol. The Monitoring Plan is defined as "a description of the methods, responsibilities, and requirements for monitoring the trial" (ICH E6(R2) 1.38.1).

Given that the sponsor may use a risk-based approach to monitoring, the sponsor may decide on what study processes and data will be monitored and how they will be monitored for a specific study. This monitoring strategy and the rationale for the chosen monitoring strategy will be documented in the Monitoring Plan (ICH E6(R2) 5.18.7).

The Monitoring Plan will contain the following:

- Rationale for the monitoring strategy:
  Consideration should be given to the characteristics of the trial (Section 22.2.4; ICH E6(R2) 5.18.3) to determine the rationale for the chosen monitoring strategy.
- The monitoring strategy:
  - Describe what processes and data will be reviewed on-site
  - Describe what processes and data will reviewed by centralized monitoring

- Monitoring responsibilities of all the parties involved:
  Describe in detail who will monitor which aspects of study conduct; for example, if a CRO and the sponsor employees will share on-site versus centralized responsibilities for monitoring or if the sponsor employees will perform on-site selection visits and the CRO will perform all other visits.
- Various monitoring methods to be used and the criteria for use, for example, describe:
  - Criteria for on-site visits, e.g. timing and frequency visits, waived visits, on-site/off-site
  - Procedures for the monitor to follow for each type of visit
  - Percent of CRF data that will be verified against the source for which process or data
  - Criteria and process for managing non-compliance (protocol and study deviations and issue escalation)
  - How monitoring results will be reported for each on-site versus centralized monitoring, or other trial-related communication
  - Criteria for acting on centralized monitoring outcomes; e.g., what rate of CRF completion is acceptable? how many protocol deviations warrant a visit to the site?
  - Monitor and site training procedures

- References to applicable policies and procedures that will be followed for monitoring
  - Maintain a list of policies and procedures, including their versions and effective dates, that were effective during the course of the study. This enables a reviewer (i.e., monitor, auditor, or inspector) to identify how a procedure was to be performed at a specific time during the study.
- Maintain a record of change history for revisions or amendments to the Monitoring Plan.

22.2.9 Reporting Monitoring Activities

The Monitor will follow the Monitoring Plan, SOPs, GCP, and applicable regulatory requirements to communicate monitoring results to the sponsor.

The Monitoring Plan or SOPs may provide a report template that should be used for each type of monitoring result (e.g., site selection visit, interim monitoring, remote contact, centralized monitoring) and prescribe a time frame for submitting documentation of monitoring communication to the sponsor.

Some sponsors may also require that the investigator receives a copy of the documented monitoring results, depending on the reason for the monitoring.

Communication of monitoring results comprises the following (ICH E6(R2) 5.18.6):

- A written report to the sponsor after each site visit or trial-related communication to include:
  - The date, site, name of the Monitor, and name of investigator or other(s) contacted.
  - A summary of what the Monitor reviewed.
  - Sufficient detail to allow verification of compliance with the Monitoring Plan.
  - Statements concerning the significant findings/facts, deviations and deficiencies, conclusions, actions taken or to be taken, and/or actions recommended to secure compliance.
- The report is to be reviewed by a qualified sponsor representative.
- Follow up on observations and actions to be taken.
- All documentation of monitoring results is retained in the sponsor's files (ICH E6(R2) 8.3.10).

22.3 Summary

Definition and Why:
- Clinical trial monitoring is the oversight and QC of clinical site activities from site selection to site closeout to ensure:
  - Protection of research subjects
  - Trial is conducted according to protocol, SOPs, GCP, and applicable regulations
  - Complete and accurate documentation of the evidence of trial conduct, e.g.:
    - o Informed consent
    - o Trial procedures
    - o CRFs
    - o Investigator staff and facility
    - o Use of investigational product

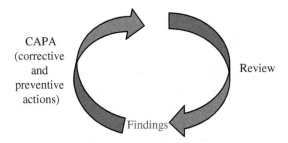

Figure 22.2 GCP principle and associated trial monitoring application.

- Monitoring is a continuous process during which processes and data are reviewed from start-up to the archiving of a clinical trial in Figure 22.2. Deficiencies and deviations that are identified during the review are promptly addressed to correct and prevent their reoccurrence of the deficiencies or deviations.

Who:
- The sponsor, who is the responsible party, may outsource some or all of monitoring activities to individual, independent monitors, or CROs. Any monitoring activity that is not written in agreements with a contractor is assumed to be the responsibility of the sponsor.
- Monitors must have knowledge of the protocol, investigational product as outlined in the investigator's brochure, informed consent and other study documents, and GCP, and applicable SOPs and regulatory requirements. They act as liaisons between the investigator and sponsor and provide reports of all monitoring communications to the sponsor.

What:
- The monitoring checklist will include all study activities that need to be evaluated for compliance with the protocol, SOPs, GCP, and applicable regulatory requirements. Those activities are driven by both sponsor and investigator responsibilities

Scope:
- Monitors will review clinical trial processes or data as specified in written procedures such as SOPs and/ or a study-specific Monitoring Plan.
- The sponsor may determine the extent and nature of monitoring (what and how much) by prioritizing critical trial processes and data to be monitored based on risk of various characteristics of the trial. Critical trial processes and data to be monitored, and the rationale for their choosing them, will be described in the study-specific Monitoring Plan.

Strategy:

- The sponsor may review trial processes and data on-site, off-site, or in a centralized manner. It is highly recommended that critical trial processes and data are reviewed on site or with direct remote access to source documentation.
- Centralized monitoring provide the sponsor with the ability to evaluate study processes and data on an on-going basis, generating data characteristics of data at the individual subject, site, and/or overall study level. Assessing the outcomes of centralized monitoring enable the sponsor to determine where adjustments (increase or reduction) may be made to oversight of individual investigator(s) study conduct, or where adjustments to the protocol or study processes may be necessary.

The Monitoring Plan

- A written procedure that outlines the methods, responsibilities, and requirements for monitoring the trial. This document may be updated as needed with tracking of all revisions and amendments.

Reporting Monitoring Activities

- Organizations may have templates that a Monitor may use to report different types of monitoring results. All results of monitoring activities must be documented and communicated to a qualified sponsor representative for evaluation of site and study performance.
- Outcomes of monitoring that reflect deficiencies or deviations in study conduct must be documented, addressed, and prevented according to procedures SOPs (e.g., Corrective and Preventive Action System [CAPA]), GCP, and applicable regulatory requirements).

Knowledge Check Questions

1) Who is responsible for monitoring?
2) What is the scope of monitoring?
3) What are the qualifications of a monitor?
4) When must monitoring occur?
5) What are the considerations for determining the scope and nature of monitoring?
6) What methods can be used for monitoring?
7) What clinical trial activity or materials may NOT be monitored off-site?
8) What clinical trial activity or materials may be monitored off-site?
9) What is of utmost concern for all participants in the conduct of a clinical trial?
10) How are the procedures for monitoring documented?
11) How are monitoring activities reported?
12) What are some consequences of inadequate monitoring?

Reference

1 International Council for Harmonisation of Technical Requirements for Pharmaceuticals for Human Use (ICH), Integrated Addendum to ICH E6(R1):Guideline for Good Clinical Practice, E6(R2) 2016. Current Step 4 version dated 9 November. https://www.ich.org/page/efficacy-guidelines

23

Investigator/Institution Selection

Karen A. Henry

GCP Key Point
*Investigator/Institution Selection is a monitoring activity to assess (review records and knowledge) for **suitability** to conduct the specified study.*

23.1   Introduction

In order for the sponsor to test the investigational product on humans, the sponsor will need to locate physicians or dentists who have access to the study population and who are suitable to administer the investigational product. Selecting the investigator/institution is like the selection of any personal physician or dentist: we want to ensure that the physician or dentist and staff have the qualifications and knowledge to attend to our medical need and have adequate equipment and facilities. The general considerations for investigation and site selection are:

1) What are the criteria for the selection?
   a) Regulatory; e.g., resources, licensing of the physician, or dentist and staff
   b) Medical; e.g., clinical specialty of the physician or dentist and staff
   c) Administrative; e.g., cost, location
2) How we will perform the search?
3) What are the consequences if we make a poor selection?

In contrast to a personal search for a physician or dentist, searching for a clinical investigator and clinical site must also consider that an investigational product cannot be administered as part of usual clinical care but only under strict good clinical practice (GCP) conditions. The considerations, the criteria for selection, how the search is performed, and the consequences of poor investigator selection

The Fundamentals of Clinical Research: A Universal Guide for Implementing Good Clinical Practice, First Edition. P. Michael Dubinsky and Karen A. Henry.
© 2022 John Wiley & Sons, Inc. Published 2022 by John Wiley & Sons, Inc.
Companion website: www.wiley.com/go/dubinsky/clinicalresearch

for a clinical trial are specialized. In GCP, the principal ethical concerns for investigator selection are:

- Clinical trials should be conducted in accordance with the ethical principles that have their origin in the Declaration of Helsinki, and that are consistent with GCP and the applicable regulatory requirement(s) (ICH E6(R2) 2.1 [1]).
- The medical care given to, and medical decisions made on behalf of, subjects should always be the responsibility of a qualified physician, or when, appropriate, of a qualified dentist (ICH E6(R2) 2.7).
- Each individual involved in conducting a trial should be qualified by education, training, and experience to perform his or her respective task(s) (ICH E6(R2) 2.8).

Investigator selection is a monitoring activity that serves to confirm that the investigator and site are suitable to conduct the trial; it is the first monitoring phase of the trial (Chapter 22 Monitoring Overview; Plate 7 Monitoring). In this chapter, we will review and discuss the procedures for selecting investigator(s)/institution(s) for conducting clinical research.

23.2 Objectives

The objectives of this chapter are to describe:

1) Who are involved in investigator selection?
2) What are the criteria for investigator selection?
   a) Regulatory
   b) Protocol
   c) Administrative
3) How are investigator(s)/institution(s) identified?
4) The investigator/institution selection visit
5) What are the consequences of poor selection investigator(s)/institution(s) selection?

23.2.1 Who are Involved in Investigator Selection

The key players in investigator selection are the sponsor and the investigator. The sponsor, an individual, company, institution, or organization which takes responsibility for the initiation, management, and/or financing of a clinical trial (ICH E6(R2) 1.53) is responsible for selecting the investigator(s)/institution(s) (ICH E6(R2) 5.6.1). The physician or dentist who will have access to the study population to receive the investigational product usually has supporting staff and facilities that constitute or are part of the institution. As defined in ICH E6(R2),

- The investigator is a person responsible for the conduct of the clinical trial at a trial site. If a trial is conducted by a team of individuals at a trial site, the investigator is the responsible leader of the team and may be called the principal investigator (ICH E6(R2) 1.34).
- The institution is any public or private entity or agency or medical or dental facility where clinical trials are conducted (ICH E6(R2) 1.30).
- The trial site is the specific location(s) where trial-related activities are actually conducted (ICH E6(R2) 1.59).

The goal of investigator selection is therefore to confirm that the investigator(s), staff, and facilities are *suitable* to conduct the clinical study to meet the scientific and ethical objectives of the trial:

1) Protect the rights and well-being of human subjects.
2) Maintain data integrity.
3) Compliance with the currently approved protocol, GCP, and applicable regulatory requirement(s).

The sponsor will ensure that each investigator should be qualified by training and experience and should have adequate resources to properly conduct the trial for which the investigator is selected. If a coordinating committee and/or coordinating investigator(s) are to be utilized in multicenter trials, their organization and/ or selection are also the sponsor's responsibility (ICH E6(R2) 5.6.1).

23.2.2 What: Criteria for Qualifications and Fit

Clinical trials are governed by regulatory and ethical requirements, protocol requirements, and business objectives. The general criteria for the qualifications and fit of the ideal candidate(s) can therefore be grouped into the following:

a) Regulatory and ethical – the applicable regulations and GCP
b) Protocol – the trial-specific procedures
c) Administrative – the constraints of timelines, personnel resources, and finances

Qualifications refer to the evidence that show that the investigator and site meet the regulatory requirements for participating in the conduct of the trial; such as licensing and accreditation of the principal investigator, staff, and facilities. Characteristics of "fit" are; e.g., whether the investigator has adequate resources, motivation, and interest to conduct the trial.

23.2.2.1 The Investigator/Institution Selection Checklist

The checklist for investigator and site selection includes all study activities that need to be evaluated for the investigator and site suitability to comply with the protocol, SOPs, GCP, and applicable regulatory requirements. Those activities are largely driven by the investigator responsibilities (see Chapter 9 Investigator and Sponsor Roles and Responsibilities) and responsibilities of the Monitor (see Chapter 22 Monitoring Overview) (Figure 23.1):

A checklist ensures that there is systematic evaluation of the qualifications and fit of the investigator and site. The Monitor's responsibilities for investigator selection are shown in Table 23.1.

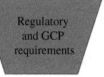

Regulatory and GCP requirements

1) Regulatory and GCP requirements – i.e., requirements for investigator qualifications and responsibilities that are laid out by GCP and local regulations:

- ICH E6(R2) 4: The investigator is responsible for:

    o Investigator qualification and agreements

        • Provide evidence of education, training, and experience to assume the responsibility for the proper conduct of the trial and to meet applicable regulatory requirement(s)

        • Complying with GCP and applicable regulatory requirements

        • Permit monitoring, auditing, and inspection

    o The investigational product

    o Maintaining adequate resources:

        • Demonstrate ability to recruit the subject population;

        • Have sufficient time to conduct the trial;

Figure 23.1 Investigator/institution responsibilities to review for selection.

- Have adequate staff and facilities, including specialized expertise, equipment, facilities, or laboratories;

- Informing all persons assisting with the trial of the protocol, IP, and their trial duties

o The medical care of trial subjects

o Communication with institutional review board (IRB)/independent ethics committee (IEC)

o Compliance with the protocol

o Complying with randomization and unblinding procedures

o Informed consent of trial subjects

o Maintaining records and reports of the investigation

o Submitting progress reports as required

o Reporting safety events

o Complying with procedures in the event of premature termination or suspension of a trial

o Submitting final reports to the IRB/IEC and sponsor

Figure 23.1 (Continued)

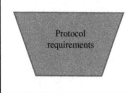

2) Protocol requirements – i.e., clinical and
operational procedures that are required by
the specific protocol

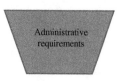

3) Administrative requirements – i.e., business or
non-regulatory:

- Timelines

- Personnel resources

- Data collection media and processes

- Financial

  ○ Sponsor's budget

  ○ Investigator's budget

Figure 23.1 (Continued)

Table 23.1 Investigator/institution selection checklist.

Site characteristic or activity	Monitor's responsibility to assess and confirm (review records, procedures, systems, and knowledge) *suitability* to conduct the specified study per *ICH E6(R2) 5.18.4*

Appropriate investigator and site selection and continued participation:	*b)* Verifying that the investigator has adequate qualifications and resources that can remain adequate throughout the trial period; that facilities, including laboratories, equipment, and staff, are adequate to safely and properly conduct the trial and can remain adequate throughout the trial period:
	• Qualification and experience of the investigator, subinvestigators, and all staff who will be delegated study tasks:
	  – Evidence (e.g., a current curriculum vitae) of education, training, and experience with knowledge of the therapeutic area under study
	  – Evidence of applicable regulatory qualification; e.g., licensing

Table 23.1 (Continued)

Site characteristic or activity	Monitor's responsibility to assess and confirm (review records, procedures, systems, and knowledge) *suitability* to conduct the specified study per *ICH E6(R2) 5.18.4*
	– GCP knowledge (Experience conducting clinical investigations is always preferred.)
	– Ability to communicate with the sponsor and sponsor's representatives; i.e., there are no language or physical barriers that hinder communication
	• The investigator is personally willing and able to conduct the trial or supervise qualified staff who are delegated trial duties
	• The investigator and trial staff are motivated and have sufficient time to conduct the trial
	• Study duties will be delegated to only qualified individuals.
	• A list of trial staff and their assigned duties will be maintained.
	• All facilities and equipment are adequate and operational (e.g., capacity, temperature monitors, backups) and calibration records where applicable are maintained.
	• Laboratory facilities are adequate and operational and certification records are current and staff members are qualified.
	• Foreseen and unplanned personnel and facilities or equipment changes can be managed appropriately to maintain their adequacy during the course of the trial.
Investigator compliance with investigational product requirements:	c) Verifying, for the investigational product(s):
	• Investigator(s) and relevant staff are familiar with the investigational product(s) properties and class of the investigational product(s).
	• Qualified individuals can receive, prepare, and administer the investigational product.
	• Investigational product can be stored for times and conditions as required.
	• The investigator can retain sufficient supplies of investigational product.
	• Administration of the investigational product(s) can be only to eligible subjects and at the protocol specified dose(s).
	• Subjects can be provided with necessary instructions on proper use, handling, storage, and return the investigational product(s).
	• The receipt, use, and return of the investigational product(s) at the trial sites can be controlled and documented adequately.
	• The disposition of unused investigational product(s) at the trial sites can comply with applicable regulatory requirement(s) and is in accordance with the sponsor procedures.

(Continued)

Table 23.1 (Continued)

Site characteristic or activity	Monitor's responsibility to assess and confirm (review records, procedures, systems, and knowledge) *suitability* to conduct the specified study per *ICH E6(R2) 5.18.4*
Investigator compliance with the approved protocol:	*d)* Verifying that the investigator is able to follow the approved protocol and all approved amendment(s), if any: • The investigator and staff will implement only a protocol or its amendments that have received the approval or favorable opinion of the IRB/IEC. • The investigator and staff are able to follow the approved protocol and all approved amendment(s), if any.
Subject informed consent:	*e)* Verifying that written informed consent can be obtained before each subject's participation in the trial. The investigator and staff are familiar with and are able to comply with the requirements for: • A study participant to be consented only with an informed consent form that has been reviewed and approved by the IRB/IEC • Specific information (required elements) to be contained in the informed consent form • Subject information and the administration of consent to be in a language understandable to the subject • Administration of and the signed and dated consent of a subject prior to their participation in the trial • The person administering consent to sign and date the consent form • Providing the subject with a copy of their signed and dated consent • The process for administering consent • Documentation of the process of consent for each study participant • Updating the informed consent form with new information that may influence the subject's decision to continue participation in the trial • Specific consenting procedures for minors, patients with cognitive impairment, vulnerable populations, emergency situations, and other trial circumstances, as applicable to the trial or clinical site location • Complying with local and other regulatory requirements
Investigator receives all trial information:	*f)* Ensuring that the investigator receives the current Investigator's Brochure, all documents, and all trial supplies needed to conduct the trial properly and to comply with the applicable regulatory requirement(s). The investigator has received: • The current Investigator's Brochure • The current protocol

Table 23.1 (Continued)

Site characteristic or activity	Monitor's responsibility to assess and confirm (review records, procedures, systems, and knowledge) *suitability* to conduct the specified study per *ICH E6(R2) 5.18.4*
	• The current informed consent form and all information to be provided to subjects • CRFs and instructions for completion of CRFs and for making corrections to CRFs • Instructions for reporting of adverse events • Instructions for randomization and maintaining study blinding and conditions and instructions for unblinding • Instructions for reporting the study status to the sponsor • Instructions for reporting protocol and trial deviations to the sponsor • Laboratory procedures and instructions for the receipt of laboratory supplies, as applicable • Instructions for the receipt of investigational product supplies and instructions for storage, handling, administration and return or destruction of the IP • Other trial instructions, supplies, and equipment, as needed
Investigator and staff knowledge of the trial:	*g)* Ensuring that the investigator and the investigator's trial staff are adequately informed about the trial. • The investigator and staff are familiar with and have knowledge of all trial information that were received.
Investigator and staff compliance:	*h)* Verifying that the investigator and the investigator's trial staff can perform the specified trial functions, in accordance with the protocol and any other written agreement between the sponsor and the investigator/institution, and will not delegate these functions to unauthorized individuals. • Investigator(s) and staff can perform the specified trial functions according to the protocol and any other written agreement between the sponsor and the investigator/institution • Investigator(s) and staff can perform only duties for which they are qualified • Subinvestigator(s) and other site staff can perform only duties that will be delegated by the investigator
Subject eligibility:	*i)* Verifying that the investigator can enroll only eligible subjects: • The investigator is aware of and understands the enrollment eligibility criteria for the trial • The investigator and staff are able to provide evidence to support the eligibility (i.e., meeting all inclusion criteria and eligibility) of each subject enrolled in the trial (i.e., randomized, if applicable, or received investigational product).

(Continued)

Table 23.1 (Continued)

Site characteristic or activity	Monitor's responsibility to assess and confirm (review records, procedures, systems, and knowledge) *suitability* to conduct the specified study per *ICH E6(R2) 5.18.4*
Subject recruitment:	*j)* Reporting the subject recruitment rate: • The investigator can recruit subjects for the trial per the enrollment rate • The investigator can comply with the recruitment reporting requirements (e.g., medium and frequency) to the sponsor.
Source documentation and other study records:	*k)* Verifying that source documents and other trial records can be accurate, complete, kept up-to-date and maintained: • Investigator and staff are familiar with and have the capacity to comply with the requirements for accurate, complete, and up-to-date source documentation and the maintenance of source documents. • The investigator or qualified delegated staff members are familiar with ALCOAC principles for good documentation practices. • The investigator can make all source documents and other study records available for monitoring, audits, and inspections by authorized personnel.
Study reporting:	*l)* Verifying that the investigator can provide all the required reports, notifications, applications, and submissions, and that these documents can be accurate, complete, timely, legible, dated, and identify the trial. That is, the investigator can provide all the required reports, notifications, applications, and submissions to the sponsor and IRB/IEC, as applicable. For example, • Submissions to the IRB/IEC for review and approval/favorable opinion of the initial and any amendments to the protocol • Submissions to the IRB/IEC for review and approval/favorable opinion of the initial and updates to the Investigator's Brochure • Submissions to the IRB/IEC for review and approval/favorable opinion of the initial and updates to the informed consent and any information, including advertising materials, to be provided to subjects • Submissions, at least annually, to the IRB/IEC for continuing review and renewal of approval/favorable opinion of trial information • Submissions of reports of study status to the sponsor • Submissions of safety reports to the IRB/IEC and the sponsor • Submissions of protocol and trial deviations to the IRB/IEC and the sponsor • Notification to the IRB/IEC and sponsor, as required, of the premature termination or suspension of a trial • Submissions of final reports of study status to the IRB/IEC and the sponsor

Table 23.1 (Continued)

Site characteristic or activity	Monitor's responsibility to assess and confirm (review records, procedures, systems, and knowledge) *suitability* to conduct the specified study per *ICH E6(R2) 5.18.4*
Case Report Form completion:	*m)* The accuracy and completeness of the CRF entries, source documents and other trial-related records can be checked for: • The investigator or qualified delegated staff members are completing the CRFs as instructed and submit CRFs in a timely manner. • The Monitor is able to verify the accuracy and completeness of the CRF entries against source documents and other trial-related records. • The data required by the protocol are reported accurately on the CRFs and are consistent with the source documents. • Any dose and/or therapy modifications are well documented for each of the trial subjects. • Adverse events, concomitant medications, and intercurrent illnesses are reported in accordance with the protocol on the CRFs. • Visits that the subjects fail to make, tests that are not conducted, and examinations that are not performed are clearly reported as such on the CRFs. • All withdrawals and dropouts of enrolled subjects from the trial are reported and explained on the CRFs.
CRF corrections:	*n)* The Monitor or other sponsor representative will inform the investigator of any CRF entry error, omission, or illegibility, and ensure that appropriate corrections, additions, or deletions can be made, dated, explained (if necessary), and approved by the investigator or by a member of the investigator's trial staff who is authorized to approve CRF changes for the investigator. This authorization can be documented. • The investigator or delegated qualified staff member(s) are familiar with the methods for receiving and assessing CRF errors and for making corrections to the CRFs. • The authorization of delegated staff member(s) to make changes to CRFs can be documented.
Adverse events reporting:	*o)* Determining whether all adverse events (AEs) can be appropriately reported within the time periods required by GCP, the protocol, the IRB/IEC, the sponsor, and the applicable regulatory requirement(s). The investigator and relevant staff must be aware of and will follow the protocol, regulatory, GCP, and other applicable requirements for: • Assessing and identifying adverse events and serious adverse as defined in the study protocol • The collection and follow up period for adverse events

(Continued)

Table 23.1 (Continued)

Site characteristic or activity	Monitor's responsibility to assess and confirm (review records, procedures, systems, and knowledge) *suitability* to conduct the specified study per *ICH E6(R2) 5.18.4*
	• Recording adverse events • Determining expectedness of adverse events • Expedited reporting of adverse events and providing updates on the status, treatment, and outcomes of adverse events • Providing a subject with or referring them for appropriate medical care for adverse events resulting from their participation in the trial. As necessary, the subject should undergo appropriate clinical procedures at unscheduled site visits (that is, not on the protocol schedule) for evaluation of such events.
Essential documents:	*p)* Determining whether the investigator can maintain the required essential documents (Chapter 29 Essential Documents): • All evidence of trial conduct (records and reports) must be maintained as essential documents the clinical site • All essential documents must be complete, legible, and available upon request to the sponsor, IRB/IEC, regulatory or health authority(ies), or their representatives for monitoring, auditing, or inspections, as applicable • All applicable essential documents can be reconciled between the sponsor's and the investigator's files • All essential documents will be maintained for a minimum period as stated in the protocol and applicable regulatory requirements • Retain essential documents that should be in the investigator/institution files until notified for destruction
Deviations reporting and corrective and preventive actions (CAPAs):	*q)* Informing the investigator and staff that the Monitor and/or sponsor representative(s) will communicate identified deviations from the protocol, SOPs, GCP, and the applicable regulatory requirements to the investigator and take appropriate action designed to correct and prevent recurrence of the detected deviations. Ensuring that the investigator and staff are aware of and understand the requirements for: • Identifying, recording, and reporting deviations from the protocol, SOPs, GCP, and the applicable regulatory requirements • Investigating, identifying the root cause, and implementing corrective and preventive actions for identified deviations.

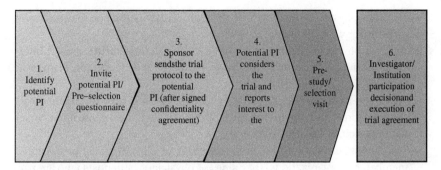

Figure 23.2 Process for investigator selection.

23.2.3 How: Process for Investigator(S)/Institution(s) Selection

Before entering an agreement with an investigator/institution to conduct a trial, the sponsor should provide the investigator(s)/institution(s) with the protocol and an up-to-date Investigator's Brochure, and should provide sufficient time for the investigator/institution to review the protocol and the information provided (ICH E6(R2) 5.6.2).

In practice, the process for selecting a qualified investigator and clinical site is generally similar to that of a personal selection of primary care physician or dentist, or for that matter, to contract any service (Figure 23.2). Once the general criteria for the qualifications and fit of the ideal candidate are determined, we would:

1) Identify potential candidates
2) Ask a few questions of the potential candidates to broadly determine if they can meet critical needs (e.g., location) without disclosing too much of the details of all needs (for privacy or proprietary reasons) and narrow the pool of candidates.
3) Recontact the shorter list of candidates to and provide additional details of the needed service.
4) The shorter list of candidates assess their own interest and fit for the service. This feedback may reduce the pool of candidates.
5) Invite the now narrow pool of candidates for in-person interaction.
6) Decide on the selection and execute a contract, as applicable.

With respect to clinical research, the process for selecting a clinical investigator(s) and clinical site(s) is a similar process that in practice typically includes:

1) The sponsor identifies potential investigator(s)/institution(s); e.g.,
   - Look for physicians/dentists who are located within the target trial geographic region. This location depends on the region where testing will occur to meet the regulatory and business objectives and where subjects with the indication being studied are located.

- Consider physicians/dentists who have previously participated as a clinical investigator with the sponsor.
- Seek out physicians/dentists who are trained in the therapeutic area of interest, considering those who are known experts or key opinion leaders in the field.
- Solicit referrals, perhaps from other clinical investigators, the members of the sales force, investigator recruiting firms, or others who come into contact with physicians/dentists in the field.
- Search public databases (such as registries of clinical trials, professional membership organizations) for names of physicians or dentists who are participating in similar research
- Consider using umbrella organizations that recruit and/or contract with clinical investigators
- Evaluate available information on regulatory or health authority inspection findings of the potential PI or the clinical site
- Ensure the non-selection of physicians or dentists who are debarred or have impeding practicing restrictions

2) The sponsor invites potential investigator(s)/institution(s); i.e.,

- Contact the potential investigator(s)/institution(s). This introduction may be by sponsor staff such as the medical monitor or trial manager/monitor, or a contracted recruiter.
- At this point, minimum general trial information (e.g., indication, study phase) is provided to maintain propriety confidentiality. A questionnaire may be useful to obtain standard information. The questionnaire may contain queries for:
  - The number of subjects with indication/minimum enrollment criteria
  - The number of competing trials
  - A summary of the investigator's and other key site staff (e.g., subinvestigator and the coordinator of the trial) clinical trial experience (e.g., number of years and types of trials)
  - The contact information for the investigator and key site staff (e.g., subinvestigator and the coordinator of the trial)

3) The sponsor sends detailed trial information to potential investigator(s)/institution(s):

- It is advisable to execute an agreement between the parties to keep all exchanged information confidential prior to sending detailed protocol and investigational product information. The agreement is between the institution/investigator on behalf of all subinvestigators and trial staff and the sponsor on behalf of sponsor personnel or CROs. The agreement is that neither the investigator/institution nor the sponsor representatives will disclose confidential information about the other.

- At this point, a protocol synopsis may be used if a fully developed protocol is not yet available and all known information about the investigational product should be provided.
  NOTE: The full protocol and an Investigator's Brochure must be provided prior to executing an agreement for trial conduct between the investigator/institution and the sponsor.
- The sponsor should track all distributions and record the experience of this process with the potential site. This experience may be a preview of the investigator and site performance during study participation. Likewise, the investigator/institution should track their experience with the sponsor as this experience may be a preview of the sponsor's demands and expectations, responsiveness, and management of the trial.
4) The potential investigator(s)/institution(s) consider the trial (ICH E6(R2) 5.6.2) and report their interest to the sponsor:
- The potential investigator, perhaps in collaboration with their potential trial team, may consider the following with respect to trial:
  - Scientific interest
  - Technical expertise
  - Available and demands on resources
  - Previous experience with the sponsor
  - Financial feasibility
- The potential investigator reports whether they are interested in participating in the trial to the sponsor and have any questions answered.
5) If the potential investigator is interested in pursuing participation in the trial and the sponsor remains interested in pursuing them, then a prestudy/selection visit to the clinical site may be arranged:
- This is the time for the sponsor AND investigator to assess the site's qualification and ability to conduct the trial.
- Before entering an agreement with an investigator/institution to conduct a trial, the sponsor should provide the investigator(s)/institution(s) with the protocol and an up-to-date Investigator's Brochure, and should provide sufficient time for the investigator/institution to review the protocol and the information provided (ICH E6(R2) 5.6.2).
6) The potential investigator and the sponsor decide whether the potential investigator/institution is suitable to conduct the study and process a clinical trial agreement between the investigator/institution and the sponsor.
7) After a decision is made between the sponsor and the investigator regarding the investigator's suitability and interest to participate in trial conduct, a written agreement between the investigator/institution and the sponsor will be executed (ICH E6(R2) 5.6.3). This agreement may also include the financial arrangements (Chapter 15 Trial Resourcing and Outsourcing).

23.2.4 The Site Selection Visit

23.2.4.1 The Selection Checklist

The checklist above may be modified if certain characteristics or activities are not required by the specific protocol. The evaluation of characteristics and activities may occur on- or off-site, but all relevant items must be confirmed to ensure appropriate selection of the investigator and site prior to initiation of the trial at the site. The sponsor's representative(s) will follow standard operating procedures and the study-specific Monitoring Plan for guidance on when and how the visit may be conducted and reported site (Chapter 22 Monitoring Overview).

23.2.4.2 Preparing for the Visit

The sponsor and the investigator will decide on a time that is convenient for both parties for the site selection visit. The Monitor and other sponsor representatives (such as the study Medical Monitor) who have the knowledge and expertise to perform the assessment of the investigator/institution, and the investigator, the study coordinator, and other key site personnel who have the information necessary to provide to the sponsor may attend the visit.

23.2.4.3 The Visit

The evaluation should be treated like an interview: the sponsor is interviewing the investigator to assess if the investigator/institution is suitable for conducting the study and the investigator is interviewing the sponsor to determine if the investigator/institution is capable of and interested in conducting the study. This should be an active rather than a passive assessment; i.e., interactive questioning and discussions, rather than one-way presentations. The evaluation will include tours of the facilities and review of available written procedures or maintenance records.

23.2.4.4 The Selection Report

Once all the criteria have been evaluated, the Monitor will complete a report that describes the items reviewed and any findings and follow-up that are necessary (Chapter 22 Monitoring Overview). The report will be reviewed by a qualified sponsor representative who is responsible for selecting investigators. This pretrial monitoring report will be maintained in the sponsor's files (ICH E6(R2) 8.2.19) and a summary may be communicated to the investigator/institution informing them of the selection or non-selection.

23.2.4.5 Follow-up

If the investigator/institution is selected to participate in trial conduct, the Monitor will follow-up on any outstanding items to ensure complete qualification of the investigator/institution. The investigator/institution should be informed of the next steps for trial initiation.

23.2.5 Consequences of Poor Investigator(s)/ Institution(s) Selection

Similar to a personal experience of choosing a physician/dentist, making a decision without careful and thorough evaluation of the potential physician/dentist may have significant undesirable consequences. It may not be possible to screen to avoid all possible negative consequences as some are unforeseeable or uncontrollable; e.g., natural disasters, unanticipated changes. We can, however, perform due diligence in the moment and continuously monitor and implement change control methods to prevent unfavorable outcomes.

In clinical research, we aim to prevent the site's failure to comply with the protocol, GCP, and regulatory requirements. Additionally, we want to avoid opposing effects on the business objectives. The goal then is to carefully review all requirements, ensure that the clinical investigator and staff have a thorough understanding of those requirements, anticipate any potential for noncompliance, and determine methods for training on and implementation of measures to prevent potential noncompliance.

The following are some typical consequences of poor investigator/intuition selection:

Subject:
- Violation of rights; e.g.,
  - Failure to administer or inadequately administer consent to a subject
  - Breach of subject confidentiality
  - Misrepresentation of the investigational product as safe and/or effective
- Violation of safety; e.g.,
  - Improper administration of the investigational product
  - Failure to identify and treat adverse events
  - Administration of damaged or contaminated investigational product

Regulatory:
- Violation of protocol procedures; e.g.,
  - Failure to perform protocol procedures as described and at the time they are required
  - Failure to maintain blinding or following randomization procedures
  - Failure to address protocol deviations
- Violation of IRB/IEC procedures; e.g.,
  - Failure to submit to the IRB/IEC for initial and/or continuing review
  - Inadequate communication of study status with the IRB/IEC
- Violation of regulatory requirements; e.g.,
  - Implementing the protocol and/or consent forms that are not approved by the IRB/IEC
  - Failure to maintain adequate case histories and other source documents

- – Documenting what did not happen
- – Investigator's failure to oversee the investigation
- – Unqualified personnel performing study duties
- – Failure to report safety events as required
- Misuse/handling of investigational product; e.g.,
  - – Inadequate accountability for the investigational product
  - – Improper storage of the investigational product

Business:
- No or delayed start-up of the clinical investigational site
- No or slow enrollment at the clinical investigational site
- Increased costs of operations at the site
- Costs related to addressing issues due to negligence

Everything perfect?!
- If the investigator site produces perfect data, and there are no protocol deviations, and no adverse events reported, this may be a sign of a "too good to be true" situation. While this situation is certainly possible, it is highly improbable, given the nature of clinical trials; i.e., they involve human beings as research participants and as conductors of the trials. It is prudent for the Monitor(s) to carefully review such circumstances, and if there are no findings, Bravo!

23.3 Summary

The sponsor is required to select qualified investigators who have adequate resources (i.e., staff, time, and facilities) to conduct the trial. The process of selection investigator/institutions is similar to the process we would use for personal selection of a physician/ dentist, with the addition of meeting requirements that are peculiar to a clinical trial. The sponsor's Monitor, who will be qualified by training and experience, will review all characteristics of the investigator/institution that are necessary for the appropriate and compliant implementation of the study protocol. This review is to ensure the *suitability* of the investigator/institution to comply with all protocol, GCP, and applicable regulatory requirements to avoid the possible dire and costly consequences to poor site selection.

Knowledge Check Questions
1) When does investigator/institution selection occur?
2) Whose responsibility is it for investigator/institution selection?
3) What are considerations for determining the criteria for investigator/institution selection?
4) What are the minimum criteria for investigator/institution selection?
5) What are the consequences of poor investigator/institution selection?

Reference

1 International Council for Harmonisation of Technical Requirements for Pharmaceuticals for Human Use (ICH), Integrated Addendum to ICH E6(R1):Guideline for Good Clinical Practice, E6(R2) (2016). Current Step 4 version dated 9 November 2016. https://www.ich.org/page/efficacy-guidelines

24

Investigator/Institution Initiation

Karen A. Henry

GCP Key Point

*Investigator/Institution Initiation is a monitoring activity to assess (review records, procedures, systems, and knowledge) for **qualification and preparedness** to conduct the specified study.*

24.1 Introduction

Investigator/Institution initiation ensures that the investigator/institution is qualified and prepared to conduct the specified study. It is the second monitoring phase of the trial (Chapter 22 Monitoring Overview): trial initiation is the point at which subjects may be consented for entry into the trial (Chapter 14 Trial Management; Start-up, On-Study, and Close-Out; Plate 7 Monitoring). After the investigator/institution selection is confirmed (Chapter 23 Investigator/Institution Selection), the process for preparing the investigator/institution for trial initiation commences. This process includes the

- Sponsor's review and collection of all documentation of qualification of the investigator, staff, and facilities
- Training of the investigator and staff on the study procedures
- Confirmation of executed written agreements
- Investigator submission to and approval/favorable opinion from the institutional review board (IRB)/independent ethics committee (IEC)
- Sponsor's submission to and authorization/approval/notification by the applicable regulatory authority(ies) prior to initiation (Chapter 14 Trial Management; Start-up, On-Study, and Close-Out).

The Fundamentals of Clinical Research: A Universal Guide for Implementing Good Clinical Practice, First Edition. P. Michael Dubinsky and Karen A. Henry.
© 2022 John Wiley & Sons, Inc. Published 2022 by John Wiley & Sons, Inc.
Companion website: www.wiley.com/go/dubinsky/clinicalresearch

24.2 Objectives

The objectives of this chapter are to describe:

1) Who are involved in investigator/institution initiation?
2) What are reviewed for investigator/institution initiation?
   a) Regulatory
   b) Protocol
   c) Administrative
3) The process for initiation of the investigator/institution
4) The investigator/institution initiation visit

24.2.1 Who are Involved in Investigator/Institution Initiation

The key players in investigator/institution initiation are the sponsor, the investigator, and all sponsor and investigator representatives who are delegated key study duties. The sponsor, an individual, company, institution, or organization which takes responsibility for the initiation, management, and/or financing of a clinical trial (ICH E6(R2) 1.53 [1]), will ensure that trial procedures were reviewed with the investigator and the investigator's trial staff prior to initiating the trial at the investigator(s)/institution(s) (ICH E6(R2) 8.2.20).

The goal of investigator/institution initiation is therefore to confirm that the investigator(s), staff, and facilities are *qualified and prepared* to conduct the clinical study to meet the scientific and ethical objectives of the trial:

1) Protect the rights and well-being of human subjects.
2) Maintain data integrity.
3) Compliance with the currently approved protocol, Good Clinical Practice (GCP), and applicable regulatory requirement(s).

24.2.2 What: Items that are Reviewed for Investigator/Institution Initiation

Clinical trials are governed by regulatory and ethical requirements, protocol requirements, and business objectives. The general items that are reviewed to ensure that the investigator/institution is qualified and prepared for conducting the trial can therefore be grouped into the following:

a) Regulatory and ethical – the applicable regulations and GCP
b) Protocol – the trial-specific procedures
c) Administrative – the constraints of timelines, personnel resources, and finances

Qualifications refer to the evidence that show that the investigator and site meet the regulatory requirements for participating in the conduct of the trial; such as licensing and accreditation of the principal investigator, staff, and facilities. Characteristics of preparedness are whether all personnel, equipment, and facilities are operationally ready to conduct the trial.

24.2.2.1 The Investigator/Institution Initiation Checklist

The checklist for investigator and site initiation includes confirmation of all study characteristics and activities that need to be evaluated for the investigator and site readiness to comply with the protocol, SOPs, GCP, and applicable regulatory requirements. Those activities are largely driven by the investigator responsibilities (see Chapter 9 Investigator and Sponsor Roles and Responsibilities) and responsibilities of the Monitor (see Chapter 22 Monitoring Overview) (Figure 24.1):

A checklist ensures that there is systematic evaluation of the qualifications and fit of the investigator and site. The Monitor's responsibilities for investigator initiation are shown in Table 24.1

1) Regulatory and GCP requirements – i.e., requirements for investigator qualifications and responsibilities that are laid out by GCP and local regulations:

Regulatory and GCP requirements

- ICH E6(R2) 4: The investigator is responsible for:

o Investigator qualification and agreements

- Provide evidence of education, training, and experience to assume the responsibility for the proper conduct of the trial and to meet applicable regulatory requirement(s)
- Complying with GCP and applicable regulatory requirements
- Permit monitoring, auditing, and inspection

o The investigational product

o Maintaining adequate resources:

- Demonstrate ability to recruit the subject population;

Figure 24.1 Investigator/institution responsibilities to review for initiation.

- Have sufficient time to conduct the trial;
- Have adequate staff and facilities, including specialized expertise, equipment, facilities, or laboratories;
- Informing all persons assisting with the trial of the protocol, IP, and their trial duties

o The medical care of trial subjects

o Communication with IRB/IEC

o Compliance with the protocol

o Complying with randomization and unblinding procedures

o Informed consent of trial subjects

o Maintaining records and reports of the investigation

o Submitting progress reports as required

o Reporting safety events

o Complying with procedures in the event of premature termination or suspension of a trial

o Submitting final reports to the IRB/IEC and sponsor

Protocol requirements

2) Protocol requirements –i.e., clinical and operational procedures that are required by the specific protocol

Administrative requirements

3) Administrative requirements – i.e., business or non-regulatory:

- Timelines
- Personnel resources
- Data collection media and processes
- Financial
    o Sponsor's budget
    o Investigator's budget
    o Contract issues

Figure 24.1 (Continued)

Table 24.1 Investigator/institution iniiation checklist.

Site characteristic or activity:	Monitor's responsibility to assess and confirm (review records, procedures, systems, and knowledge) *qualification and preparedness* to conduct the specified study per *ICH E6(R2) 5.18.4*:
Appropriate investigator and site selection and continued participation:	*b)* Verifying that the investigator has adequate qualifications and resources that will remain adequate throughout the trial period; that facilities, including laboratories, equipment, and staff, are adequate to safely and properly conduct the trial and will remain adequate throughout the trial period:

- Qualification and experience of the investigator, subinvestigators, and all staff who will be delegated study tasks:
  - Evidence (e.g., a current curriculum vitae) of education, training, and experience with knowledge of the therapeutic area under study
  - Evidence of applicable regulatory qualification; e.g., current license
  - GCP knowledge (Experience conducting clinical investigations is always preferred.)
  - Ability to communicate with the sponsor and sponsor's representatives; i.e., there are no language or physical barriers that hinder communication
- The investigator is personally willing and able to conduct the trial or supervise qualified staff who are delegated trial duties
- The investigator and trial staff are motivated and have sufficient time to conduct the trial
- Study duties will be delegated to only qualified individuals.
- A list of trial staff and their assigned duties will be maintained.
- All facilities and equipment are adequate and operational (e.g., capacity, temperature monitors, backups) and calibration records where applicable are maintained.
- Laboratory facilities are adequate and operational and certification records are current and staff members are qualified.
- Foreseen and unplanned personnel and facilities or equipment changes will be managed appropriately to maintain their adequacy during the course of the trial.

(Continued)

Table 24.1   (Continued)

Site characteristic or activity:	Monitor's responsibility to assess and confirm (review records, procedures, systems, and knowledge) *qualification and preparedness* to conduct the specified study per *ICH E6(R2) 5.18.4*:
Investigator compliance with investigational product requirements:	*c)* Verifying, for the investigational product(s): • Investigator(s) and relevant staff are familiar with the investigational product(s) properties and class of the investigational product(s). • Qualified individuals will receive, prepare, and administer the investigational product. • Investigational product will be stored for times and conditions as required. • The investigator will retain sufficient supplies of investigational product • Administration of the investigational product(s) will be only to eligible subjects and at the protocol specified dose(s). • Subjects will be provided with necessary instructions on proper use, handling, storage, and return the investigational product(s). • The receipt, use, and return of the investigational product(s) at the trial sites will be controlled and documented adequately. • The disposition of unused investigational product(s) at the trial sites will comply with applicable regulatory requirement(s) and is in accordance with the sponsor procedures.
Investigator compliance with the approved protocol:	*d)* Verifying that the investigator is prepared to follow the approved protocol and all approved amendment(s), if any. • The investigator and staff will implement only a protocol or its amendments that have received the approval or favorable opinion of the IRB/IEC. • The investigator and staff are able to follow the approved protocol and all approved amendment(s), if any.
Subject informed consent:	*e)* Verifying that written informed consent will be obtained before each subject's participation in the trial. The investigator and staff are familiar with and are able to comply with the requirements for: • A study participant to be consented only with an informed consent form that has been reviewed and approved by the IRB/IEC • Specific information (required elements) to be contained in the informed consent form • Subject information and the administration of consent to be in a language understandable to the subject

Table 24.1 (Continued)

Site characteristic or activity:	Monitor's responsibility to assess and confirm (review records, procedures, systems, and knowledge) *qualification and preparedness* to conduct the specified study per *ICH E6(R2) 5.18.4*:
	• Administration of and the signed and dated consent of a subject prior to their participation in the trial
	• The person administering consent to sign and date the consent form
	• Providing the subject with a copy of their signed and dated consent
	• The process for administering consent
	• Documentation of the process of consent for each study participant
	• Updating the informed consent form with new information that may influence the subject's decision to continue participation in the trial
	• Specific consenting procedures for minors, patients with cognitive impairment, vulnerable populations, emergency situations, and other trial circumstances, as applicable to the trial or clinical site location
	• Complying with local and other regulatory requirements
Investigator receives all trial information:	*f)* Ensuring that the investigator received the current Investigator's Brochure, all documents, and all trial supplies needed to conduct the trial properly and to comply with the applicable regulatory requirement(s). The investigator has received:
	• The current Investigator's Brochure
	• The current protocol
	• The current informed consent form and all information to be provided to subjects
	• CRFs and instructions for completion of CRFs and for making corrections to CRFs
	• Instructions for reporting of adverse events
	• Instructions for randomization and maintaining study blinding and conditions and instructions for unblinding
	• Instructions for reporting the study status to the sponsor
	• Instructions for reporting protocol and trial deviations to the sponsor
	• Laboratory procedures and instructions for the receipt of laboratory supplies, as applicable
	• Instructions for the receipt of investigational product supplies and instructions for storage, handling, administration and return or destruction of the IP
	• Other trial instructions, supplies, and equipment, as needed

(Continued)

Table 24.1 (Continued)

Site characteristic or activity:	Monitor's responsibility to assess and confirm (review records, procedures, systems, and knowledge) *qualification and preparedness* to conduct the specified study per *ICH E6(R2) 5.18.4*:
Investigator and staff knowledge of the trial:	*g)* Ensuring that the investigator and the investigator's trial staff are adequately informed about the trial and of the trial supplies. • The investigator and staff are familiar with and have knowledge of all trial information and trial supplies that were received.
Investigator and staff compliance:	*h)* Verifying that the investigator and the investigator's trial staff will perform the specified trial functions, in accordance with the protocol and any other written agreement between the sponsor and the investigator/institution, and will not delegate these functions to unauthorized individuals. • Investigator(s) and staff will perform the specified trial functions according to the protocol and any other written agreement between the sponsor and the investigator/institution • Investigator(s) and staff will perform only duties for which they are qualified • Subinvestigator(s) and other site staff will perform only duties that will be delegated by the investigator
Subject eligibility:	*i)* Verifying that the investigator will enroll only eligible subjects: • The investigator is aware of and understands the enrollment eligibility criteria for the trial • The investigator and staff will provide evidence to support the eligibility (i.e., meeting all inclusion criteria and eligibility) of each subject enrolled in the trial (i.e., randomized, if applicable, or received investigational product).
Subject recruitment:	*j)* Reporting the subject recruitment rate: • The investigator will recruit subjects for the trial per the enrollment rate • The investigator will comply with the recruitment reporting requirements (e.g., medium and frequency) to the sponsor.
Source documentation and other study records:	*k)* Verifying that source documents and other trial records will be accurate, complete, kept up-to-date and maintained: • Investigator and staff are familiar with and will comply with the requirements for accurate, complete, and up-to-date source documentation and the maintenance of source documents.

Table 24.1   (Continued)

Site characteristic or activity:	Monitor's responsibility to assess and confirm (review records, procedures, systems, and knowledge) *qualification and preparedness* to conduct the specified study per *ICH E6(R2) 5.18.4*:
	• The investigator or qualified delegated staff members are familiar with ALCOAC principles for good documentation practices. • The investigator will make all source documents and other study records available for monitoring, audits, and inspections by authorized personnel.
Study reporting:	*l)* Verifying that the investigator will provide all the required reports, notifications, applications, and submissions, and that these documents can be accurate, complete, timely, legible, dated, and identify the trial. That is, the investigator will provide all the required reports, notifications, applications, and submissions to the sponsor and IRB/IEC, as applicable. For example, • Submissions to the IRB/IEC for review and approval/favorable opinion of the initial and any amendments to the protocol • Submissions to the IRB/IEC for review and approval/favorable opinion of the initial and updates to the Investigator's Brochure • Submissions to the IRB/IEC for review and approval/favorable opinion of the initial and updates to the informed consent and any information, including advertising materials, to be provided to subjects • Submissions, at least annually, to the IRB/IEC for continuing review and renewal of approval/favorable opinion of trial information • Submissions of reports of study status to the sponsor • Submissions of safety reports to the IRB/IEC and the sponsor • Submissions of protocol and trial deviations to the IRB/IEC and the sponsor • Notification to the IRB/IEC and sponsor, as required, of the premature termination or suspension of a trial • Submissions of final reports of study status to the IRB/IEC and the sponsor
Case report form completion:	*m)* The accuracy and completeness of the CRF entries, source documents and other trial-related records will be checked for: • The investigator or qualified delegated staff are completing the CRFs as instructed and submit CRFs in a timely manner. • The Monitor is able to verify the accuracy and completeness of the CRF entries against source documents and other trial-related records.

Table 24.1 (Continued)

Site characteristic or activity:	Monitor's responsibility to assess and confirm (review records, procedures, systems, and knowledge) *qualification and preparedness* to conduct the specified study per *ICH E6(R2) 5.18.4*:
	• The data required by the protocol are reported accurately on the CRFs and are consistent with the source documents.
	• Any dose and/or therapy modifications are well documented for each of the trial subjects.
	• Adverse events, concomitant medications, and intercurrent illnesses are reported in accordance with the protocol on the CRFs.
	• Visits that the subjects fail to make, tests that are not conducted, and examinations that are not performed are clearly reported as such on the CRFs.
	• All withdrawals and dropouts of enrolled subjects from the trial are reported and explained on the CRFs.
CRF corrections:	*n)* The Monitor or other sponsor representative will inform the investigator of any CRF entry error, omission, or illegibility, and ensure that appropriate corrections, additions, or deletions will be made, dated, explained (if necessary), and approved by the investigator or by a member of the investigator's trial staff who is authorized to approve CRF changes for the investigator. This authorization will be documented.
	• The investigator or delegated qualified staff member(s) are familiar with the methods for receiving and assessing CRF errors and for making corrections to the CRFs.
	• The authorization of delegated staff member(s) to make changes to CRFs will be documented.
Adverse events reporting:	*o)* Determining whether all adverse events (AEs) will be appropriately reported within the time periods required by GCP, the protocol, the IRB/IEC, the sponsor, and the applicable regulatory requirement(s). The investigator and relevant staff must be aware of and will follow the protocol, regulatory, GCP, and other applicable requirements for:
	• Assessing and identifying adverse events and serious adverse as defined in the study protocol
	• The collection and follow-up period for adverse events
	• Recording adverse events
	• Determining expectedness of adverse events
	• Expedited reporting of adverse events and providing updates on the status, treatment, and outcomes of adverse events

Table 24.1 (Continued)

Site characteristic or activity:	Monitor's responsibility to assess and confirm (review records, procedures, systems, and knowledge) *qualification and preparedness* to conduct the specified study per *ICH E6(R2) 5.18.4*:
	• Providing a subject with or referring them for appropriate medical care for adverse events resulting from their participation in the trial. As necessary, the subject should undergo appropriate clinical procedures at unscheduled site visits (that is, not on the protocol schedule) for evaluation of such events.
Essential documents:	*p)* Determining whether the investigator will maintain the required essential documents (Chapter 29 Essential Documents):
	• All evidence of trial conduct (records and reports) must be maintained as essential documents of the clinical site
	• All essential documents must be complete, legible, and available upon request to the sponsor, IRB/IEC, regulatory or health authority(ies), or their representatives for monitoring, auditing, or inspections, as applicable
	• All applicable essential documents can be reconciled between the sponsor's and the investigator's files
	• All essential documents will be maintained for a minimum period as stated in the protocol and applicable regulatory requirements
	• Retain essential documents that should be in the investigator/institution files until notified for destruction
Deviations reporting and corrective and preventive actions (CAPAs):	*q)* Informing the investigator and staff that the Monitor and/or sponsor representative(s) will communicate identified deviations from the protocol, SOPs, GCP, and the applicable regulatory requirements to the investigator and take appropriate action designed to correct and prevent recurrence of the detected deviations. Ensuring that the investigator and staff are aware of and understand the requirements for:
	• Identifying, recording, and reporting deviations from the protocol, SOPs, GCP, and the applicable regulatory requirements
	• Investigating, identifying the root cause, and implementing corrective and preventive actions for identified deviations.

24.2.3 How: Process for Investigator(S)/Institution(s) Initiation

In general, the sponsor will ensure that the investigator/institution is qualified and prepared to conduct the trial prior to initiating the trial at the clinical site. The sponsor may accomplish this goal via:

1) Central investigators' training and meetings (ICH E6(R2) 5.18.3).
2) Training and initiation of the investigator/institution individually
3) Combination of the above

The sponsor must consider that, whatever method is employed, it assures appropriate conduct of the trial in accordance with GCP.

24.2.3.1 Central Investigators' Training and Meetings

Central investigators' training and meetings involve the gathering of key trial personnel (sponsor and investigator) in one location to discuss and train on study procedures prior to trial initiation. Attendees may include sponsor personnel and representatives (CROs) and investigator/institution personnel and their subcontractors:

- Investigator/institution representatives
  - Principal investigator and subinvestigators
  - Coordinator
  - Specialists
  - Subcontractors
- Sponsor and CRO representatives
  - Medical monitor and other safety management
  - Trial manager
  - Data management
  - Statistics
  - Site monitors
  - Central laboratory representatives
  - Clinical supplies representatives.

The goals of central investigators' training and meetings are:

- Train personnel involved in trial conduct:
  - Investigator
  - Sponsor (trial management, data management, statistics, monitoring, and safety monitoring)
- Present information about the trial at the same time so that all hear the same information
- Answer questions, sharing information, and identify current and potential trial issues as a group
- Motivate for trial participation

Whether central investigators' training and meetings are used for trial initiation will depend on several factors, including:

- Trial phase/size: Single versus multicenter; i.e., the number of sites to be trained
- Trial timelines: Is there sufficient time to arrange and conduct the meeting prior to the business deadline for trial initiation?
- Logistics: Site locations, number of attendees
- Budget: Assessment of the cost individual on-site investigator/institution initiation at versus the cost of travel, accommodations, and meals for attendees and for meeting rooms and supplies for a central investigators' meeting.

The agenda for such meetings would include all those training and initiation preparedness items that can be addressed off-site, such as:

- Trial management and status: Review of the organization and infrastructure for trial management and conduct (e.g., trial monitoring, data management, and laboratories) and contacts for sponsor and investigator representatives timelines.
- Trial protocol: Study background and procedures
- Investigational product information: Review of product properties, safety and efficacy profile, and procedures for shipping and handling, preparation and administration, return and/or destruction, and accountability.
- GCP and regulatory compliance: Review of GCP and applicable regulatory requirements for trial conduct, responsibilities of the investigator, and instructions for monitoring, auditing, and inspections.
- Source documentation and essential documents: Review of procedures for recording and maintaining study data and records, requirements for controlled access to study data and records, audit trials, original and changed study data, the application of ALCOAC principles for good documentation practices.
- Safety reporting: Review of definitions of safety events, guidelines for identifying safety events, procedures for recording and reporting safety events, including expedited reporting, and procedures for reporting to the sponsor, IRB/IEC, as applicable.
- Reporting to sponsor: Procedures for reporting study status to the sponsor, submitting regulatory and administrative documents to the sponsor, and communicating study protocol, regulatory, and administrative issues.
- Special study procedures/testing/central laboratories (hands-on training): Procedures for collecting, processing, shipping, and tracking biological samples and other clinical testing results media. Requirements and procedures for the review and reporting of testing results.
- Case report form (CRF) completion, submission, and queries (hands-on training): Review of procedures for CRF completion, review, approval, submission, addressing queries, and making changes to the CRFs.

If central investigators' training and meetings are employed, the documentation of such training and initiation must be clear and complete and include:

- Confirmation of attendees (signed attendance) for each session
- Confirmation of agenda and content; i.e., details of what was presented and reviewed
- Confirmation of the qualification of the trainers (who conducted the training for each session and what were their credentials)
- Minutes of the meeting; i.e., decisions that affect study design and conduct

24.2.3.2 Individual Investigator/Institution Initiation

The sponsor may choose to initiate each investigator/institution individually, without or with the complements of a centralized meeting. To name a few, this individualized approach has the advantages of:

- Ensuring attendance by required institution staff
- A smaller more familiar setting for the investigator and staff to openly discuss anticipated site-specific and protocol issues
- The sponsor's ability to review staff and study procedures in the actual site setting

On-site investigator/institution initiation should occur:

- To confirm items that can be reviewed only on-site; e.g., the existence and readiness of facilities and equipment
- If the central investigators' training was so long past that a refresher of protocol and study procedures is necessary
- If the key investigator/institution personnel (e.g., principal investigator and study coordinator) did not attend the central meeting

Investigator/Institution initiation reports of the central meeting and/or the individual on-site investigator/institution initiation will be filed in the sponsor's and investigator's files (ICH E6(R2) 8.2.20). Initiation reports for investigators who attend both types of meetings will include copies of the information and materials presented at the centralized meeting, the meeting minutes, and attendance record, and the initiation report for the on-site visit.

24.2.4 The Investigator/Institution Initiation Visit

24.2.4.1 The Initiation Checklist

The checklist above may be modified if certain characteristics or activities are not required by the specific protocol. The evaluation of characteristics and activities may occur on- or off-site, but all relevant items must be confirmed to ensure the investigator and site staff understand their responsibilities, including protocol procedures, study processes, and applicable regulatory requirements. The sponsor's representative(s) will follow standard operating procedures and the study-specific

Monitoring Plan for guidance on when and how the visit may be conducted and reported site (Chapter 22 Monitoring Overview).

24.2.4.2 Preparing for the Visit

The Monitor will confirm the site's readiness for the initiation visit. All "regulatory documents" (i.e., those records that are required to be in place prior to initiation) must have been collected and confirmed complete, such as:

- Investigator and staff qualification (i.e., CVs and licenses)
- Laboratory qualifications (certificates and normal ranges)
- Final executed agreements (between investigator and regulatory authority(ies), between investigator and sponsor, etc.)
- Evidence of trial insurance
- Approval/favorable opinion of the IRB/IEC for protocol, ICF, and other study documents
- Regulatory authority(ies) authorization/approval/notification of protocol

A complete list of required documentation that must be in place prior to initiation of the trial are described in Chapter 29 Essential Documents.

The sponsor and the investigator will decide on a time that is convenient for both parties for the initiation visit. The Monitor and other sponsor representatives (such as the study Medical Monitor) who have the knowledge and expertise to perform the training and assessment of preparedness of the investigator/institution, and the investigator, the study coordinator, and other key site personnel who will be participating in the study conduct may attend the visit. The Monitor will note documents (and their versions) already collected by the sponsor and provided to the investigator, the status of clinical and other study supplies to be provided to or already shipped to the site, and the status of written agreements that are needed prior to site initiation.

24.2.4.3 The Visit

The training and evaluation should be an active rather than a passive assessment; i.e., interactive questioning and discussions, rather than one-way presentations. The evaluation will include confirmation of the sponsor's collection of required qualification records of investigator, staff, and facilities, reconciliation of those records and other study documentation, tours to inspect the facilities and confirmation of available written procedures or processes for maintaining records of equipment.

In practice, sponsors may withhold arrival of investigational product at the site until the day of the initiation visit or thereafter to ensure that subjects do not receive investigational product until the site is confirmed qualified and prepared to conduct the trial. If investigational product was already shipped to the site, the Monitor will perform accountability of opened and unopened product. Likewise, the Monitor will review other study and laboratory supplies that were already shipped to the site.

24.2.4.4   The Initiation Report

Once all the criteria have been evaluated, the Monitor will complete a report that describes the items reviewed and any findings and follow-up that are necessary (Chapter 22 Monitoring Overview). The report will be reviewed by a qualified sponsor representative who is responsible for investigator oversight. This trial initiation report will be maintained in the sponsor's files (ICH E6(R2) 8.2.20) and a copy of the report or a summary of the visit will be communicated to the investigator/institution informing them of their preparedness to initiate the study at their site. The investigator will maintain the copy of the report or the summary of the visit in the investigator's files (ICH E6(R2) 8.2.20).

24.2.4.5   Follow-up

The Monitor will follow-up on any outstanding items to ensure complete qualifications and preparedness of a site to conduct the trial. A site must not consent subjects until all required documentation of site qualification and approval/authorization from the IRB/IEC/regulatory authority(ies) are in place. Subjects may not be administered investigational product until all procedures and supplies relevant to the randomization, blinding, and preparation and administration of investigational product are in place.

24.2.5   Consequences of Inadequate Investigator(s)/Institution(s) Initiation

Investigator/Institution initiation is a process to confirm that the investigator/institution is qualified and prepared to initiate the trial; i.e., commence consenting and screening of research subjects for enrollment in the trial. If,

- the investigator and trial staff are not adequately trained on and have knowledge of the protocol procedures, GCP, and applicable regulatory requirements
- the investigator/institution does not have adequate and qualified facilities, equipment, and clinical supplies
- the investigator and staff are not trained on the nature of and the handling and use of the investigational product
- the investigator and staff are not trained on the collection of data
- ALL evidence of investigator/institution qualification and trial approval documentation are not in place prior to the site consenting the first trial participant

then the sponsor, sponsor's monitor, and/or the investigator are not complying with GCP and applicable regulatory requirements. There is also a risk to subject's rights, safety, and well-being, the quality and integrity of the data, and to the business goals of the trial.

In clinical research, we aim to prevent the site's failure to comply with the protocol, GCP, and regulatory requirements. Additionally, we want to avoid opposing effects on the business objectives. The goal of investigator/institution initiation then is to carefully review all requirements, ensure that the clinical investigator and staff have a thorough understanding of those requirements, ensure that the investigator has all resources and study information and supplies, all required study documentation are in place, and anticipate any potential for noncompliance and train on and implement measures to prevent potential noncompliance.

The typical consequences of inadequate investigator/intuition initiation are similar to those of poor selection:

Subject:

- Violation of rights; e.g.,
  - Failure to administer or inadequately administer consent to a subject
  - Breach of subject confidentiality
  - Misrepresentation of the investigational product as safe and/or effective
- Violation of safety; e.g.,
  - Improper administration of the investigational product
  - Failure to identify and treat adverse events

Regulatory:

- Violation of protocol procedures; e.g.,
  - Failure to perform protocol procedures as described and at the time they are required
  - Failure to maintain blinding or following randomization procedures
  - Failure to address protocol deviations
- Violation of IRB procedures; e.g.,
  - Failure to submit to the IRB/IEC for initial and/or continuing review
  - Inadequate communication of study status with the IRB
- Violation of regulatory requirements; e.g.,
  - Implementing the protocol and/or consent forms that are not approved by the IRB/IEC
  - Failure to maintain adequate case histories and other source documents
  - Documenting what did not happen
  - Investigator's failure to oversee the investigation
  - Unqualified personnel performing study duties
  - Failure to report safety events as required
- Misuse/mishandling of investigational product; e.g.,
  - Inadequate accountability for the investigational product
  - Improper storage of the investigational product

Business:

- No or delayed start-up of the clinical investigational site
- No or slow enrollment at the clinical investigational site
- Increased costs of operations at the site
- Costs related to addressing issues due to negligence

Everything perfect?!

- If the investigator site produces perfect data, and there are no protocol deviations, and no adverse events reported, this may be a sign of a "too good to be true" situation. While this situation is certainly possible, it is highly improbable, given the nature of clinical trials; i.e., they involve human beings as research participants and as conductors of the trials. It is prudent for the Monitor(s) to carefully review such circumstances, and if there are no findings, Bravo!

24.3 Summary

The sponsor is required to ensure that the investigator/institution are prepared to conduct the trial. The process of initiation involves training the investigators and trial staff and evaluating preparedness. Investigator/institution initiation may be conducted via centralized meetings and/or on-site review. Whether initiation is performed via centralized and/or individual on-site evaluation, the documentation of all training and evaluation must show detailed review and provision of instructions for protocol, GCP, and applicable regulatory procedures. The sponsor's Monitor, who will be qualified by training and experience, will review all characteristics of the investigator/institution that are necessary for the appropriate and compliant implementation of the study protocol. This review is to ensure the *qualification and preparedness* of the investigator/institution to comply with all protocol, GCP, and applicable regulatory requirements to avoid the possible dire and costly consequences to inadequate site initiation.

Knowledge Check Questions

---

1) What is the purpose of investigator/institution initiation occur?
2) How may investigator/institution initiation occur?
3) When does investigator/institution initiation occur?
4) Who are involved in investigator/institution initiation occurrence?
5) What items are reviewed during investigator/institution initiation occur?
6) What minimum documentation must be in place for investigator/institution initiation to occur?
7) What are some consequences of inadequate investigator/institution initiation?

Reference

1 International Council for Harmonisation of Technical Requirements for Pharmaceuticals for Human Use (ICH), Integrated Addendum to ICH E6(R1):Guideline for Good Clinical Practice, E6(R2) (2016). Current Step 4 version dated 9 November 2016. https://www.ich.org/page/efficacy-guidelines

25

Investigator/Institution Interim Monitoring

Karen A. Henry

GCP Key Point

*Interim monitoring is a quality control activity to assess (review records, procedures, systems, and knowledge) for **ongoing compliance** with the specified study requirements.*

25.1 Introduction

Interim monitoring is a quality control activity to ensure that the investigator/institution is complying with the protocol, Good Clinical Practice (GCP), and applicable regulatory requirements of the specified study. It is the third monitoring phase of the trial (Chapter 22 Monitoring Overview; Plate 7 Monitoring): interim monitoring takes place during the course of the study; i.e., once the first subject is consented and through the last study contact with the last subject on study (Chapter 14 Trial Management; Start-up, On-Study, and Close-Out). After the investigator/institution initiates the study (i.e., consents the first subject) (Chapter 19 Informed Consent and Other Human Subject Protection), the process for monitoring of all study conduct commences, with the aim to ensure compliance; i.e., confirm compliance or secure compliance for deviation(s) from the protocol, GCP, and applicable regulatory requirements of the specified study. This process includes the

- Sponsor's review of investigator/institution records of study conduct
- Sponsor's review of study data for safety and compliance monitoring
- Sponsor's review of the investigator's implementation of amendments to the study protocol or other study documents

The Fundamentals of Clinical Research: A Universal Guide for Implementing Good Clinical Practice, First Edition. P. Michael Dubinsky and Karen A. Henry.
Companion website: www.wiley.com/go/dubinsky/clinicalresearch

- Sponsor's corrective and preventive actions in response to systemic overall study noncompliance; e.g., amend the study protocol and/or update study instructions
- Sponsor's corrective and preventive actions in response to individual investigator/institution noncompliance; e.g., retraining of investigator and/or staff, facilitate revision of investigator processes or provision of study facilities, termination of investigator
- Sponsor's review and collection of all new documentation of qualification of existing and new investigator, staff, and facilities
- Training of the investigator and staff on new procedures, training new investigator and staff on the study procedures, or retraining investigator and staff on established processes as necessary

25.2 Objectives

The objectives of this chapter are to describe:

1) Who are involved in investigator/institution interim monitoring?
2) What are reviewed during investigator/institution interim monitoring?
   a) Regulatory
   b) Protocol
   c) Administrative
3) The process for interim monitoring:
   a) Centralized monitoring
   b) Monitoring the individual investigator/institution
4) The investigator/institution interim monitoring visit

25.2.1 Who are Involved in Investigator/Institution Interim Monitoring

The key players in investigator/institution initiation are the sponsor, the investigator, and all sponsor and investigator representatives who are delegated key study duties. This is because the sponsor, an individual, company, institution, or organization which takes responsibility for the initiation, management, and/or financing of a clinical trial (ICH E6(R2) 1.53) [1], will monitor the investigation via a risk-based approach that involves on-site monitoring by a qualified monitor and centralized monitoring supported by appropriately qualified and trained persons (e.g., data managers, biostatisticians) (ICH E6(R2) 5.18.3). Additionally, the sponsor's monitor will review trial records and processes at the clinical site in conjunction with the investigator and trial staff, as appropriate and necessary.

The goal of interim monitoring of the investigator/institution is therefore to confirm and ensure the investigator(s), staff, and facilities *comply* with the protocol, GCP, and applicable regulatory requirements in accordance with the study-specific monitoring plan to meet the scientific and ethical objectives of the trial:

1) Protect the rights and well-being of human subjects.
2) Maintain data integrity.
3) Compliance with the currently approved protocol, GCP and applicable regulatory requirement(s).

25.2.2 What: Items that are Reviewed for Investigator/Institution Interim Monitoring

Clinical trials are governed by regulatory and ethical requirements, protocol requirements, and business objectives. The general items that are reviewed to ensure that the investigator/institution is complying with the requirements for study conduct can therefore be grouped into the following:

a) Regulatory and ethical – the applicable regulatory requirements and GCP
b) Protocol – the trial-specific procedures
c) Administrative – the constraints of timelines, personnel resources, and finances

25.2.2.1 The Investigator/Institution Interim Monitoring Checklist

The checklist for investigator and site interim monitoring includes verification of all study characteristics and activities to demonstrate that the investigator and site are complying with the protocol, SOPs, GCP, and applicable regulatory requirements. Those characteristics and activities are largely driven by the investigator responsibilities (See Chapter 9 Investigator and Sponsor Roles and Responsibilities) and responsibilities of the Monitor (see Chapter 22 Monitoring Overview) (Figure 25.1):

A checklist ensures that there is systematic evaluation of the conduct of the study by investigator/institution. The Monitor's responsibilities for investigator selection are shown in Table 25.1.

1) Regulatory and GCPrequirements – ie, requirements for investigator qualifications and responsibilities that are laid out by GCP and local regulations:

Regulatory and GCP requirements

- ICH E6(R2) 4: The investigator is responsible for:

   ○ Investigator qualification and agreements

     • Provide evidence of education, training, and experience to assume the responsibility for the proper conduct of the trial and to meet applicable regulatory requirement(s)

     • Complying with GCP and applicable regulatory requirements

     • Permit monitoring, auditing, and inspection

   ○ The investigational product

   ○ Maintaining adequate resources:

     • Demonstrate ability to recruit the subject population;

     • Have sufficient time to conduct the trial;

     • Have adequate staff and facilities, including specialized expertise, equipment, facilities, or laboratories;

     • Informing all persons assisting with the trial of the protocol, IP, and their trial duties

   ○ The medical care of trial subjects

   ○ Communication with institutional review board (IRB)/independent ethics committee (IEC)

   ○ Compliance with the protocol

   ○ Complying with randomization and unblinding procedures

   ○ Informed consent of trial subjects

   ○ Maintaining records and reports of the investigation

   ○ Submitting progress reports as required

   ○ Reporting safety events

   ○ Complying with procedures in the event of premature termination or suspension of a trial

   ○ Submitting final reports to the IRB/IEC and sponsor

Figure 25.1 Investigator/institution responsibilities to review for interim monitoring.

Figure 25.1 (Continued)

Table 25.1 Investigator/institution interim monitoring checklist.

Site characteristic or activity:	Monitor's responsibility to assess and confirm (review records, procedures, systems, and knowledge) *compliance* with the requirements of the specified study per *ICH E6(R2) 5.18.4*:

Appropriate investigator and site selection and continued participation:	*b)* Verifying that the investigator continues to have adequate qualifications, resources, facilities, including laboratories, equipment, and staff to safely and properly conduct the trial:
	• Qualification and experience of the investigator, subinvestigators, and all staff who will be delegated study tasks:
	  – Evidence (e.g., a current curriculum vitae) of education, training, and experience with knowledge of the therapeutic area under study
	  – Evidence of applicable regulatory qualification; e.g., current license
	  – GCP knowledge (Experience in conducting clinical investigations is always preferred.)
	  – Ability to communicate with the sponsor and sponsor's representatives; i.e., there are no language or physical barriers that hinder communication

(Continued)

Table 25.1 (Continued)

Site characteristic or activity:	Monitor's responsibility to assess and confirm (review records, procedures, systems, and knowledge) *compliance* with the requirements of the specified study per *ICH E6(R2) 5.18.4*:
	• The investigator is personally conducting the trial or supervising qualified staff members who are delegated trial duties
	• The investigator and trial staff are motivated and have sufficient time to conduct the trial
	• Study duties are delegated to only qualified individuals.
	• A list of trial staff and their assigned duties is maintained.
	• All facilities and equipment are adequate and operational (e.g., capacity, temperature monitors, backups) and calibration records where applicable are maintained.
	• Laboratory facilities are adequate and operational and certification records are current and staff members are qualified.
	• Foreseen and unplanned personnel and facilities or equipment changes are managed appropriately to maintain their adequacy during the course of the trial.
Investigator compliance with investigational product requirements:	*c)* Verifying, for the investigational product(s): • Investigator(s) and relevant staff are familiar with the investigational product(s) properties and class of the investigational product(s). • Qualified individuals are receiving, preparing, and administering the investigational product. • Investigational product is stored for times and conditions as required. • The investigator is retaining sufficient supplies of investigational product • Administration of the investigational product(s) is only to eligible subjects and at the protocol-specified dose(s). • Subjects are provided with necessary instructions on proper use, handling, storage, and return the investigational product(s). • The receipt, use, and return of the investigational product(s) at the trial sites are controlled and documented adequately. • The disposition of unused investigational product(s) at the trial sites complies with applicable regulatory requirement(s) and is in accordance with the sponsor procedures.

Table 25.1 (Continued)

Site characteristic or activity:	Monitor's responsibility to assess and confirm (review records, procedures, systems, and knowledge) *compliance* with the requirements of the specified study per *ICH E6(R2) 5.18.4*:
Investigator compliance with the approved protocol:	*d)* Verifying that the investigator is following the approved protocol and all approved amendment(s), if any. • The investigator and staff are implementing only a protocol or its amendments that have received the approval or favorable opinion of the IRB/IEC. • The investigator and staff are following the approved protocol and all approved amendment(s), if any.
Subject informed consent:	*e)* Verifying that written informed consent was obtained before each subject's participation in the trial. The investigator and staff are familiar with and are complying with the requirements for: • A study participant to be consented only with an informed consent form that has been reviewed and approved by the IRB/IEC • Specific information (required elements) to be contained in the informed consent form • Subject information and the administration of consent to be in a language understandable to the subject • Administration of and the signed and dated consent of a subject prior to their participation in the trial • The person administering consent to sign and date the consent form • Providing the subject with a copy of their signed and dated consent • The process for administering consent • Documentation of the process of consent for each study participant • Updating the informed consent form with new information that may influence the subject's decision to continue participation in the trial • Specific consenting procedures for minors, patients with cognitive impairment, vulnerable populations, emergency situations, and other trial circumstances, as applicable to the trial or clinical site location • Complying with local and other regulatory requirements
Investigator receives all trial information:	*f)* Ensuring that the investigator received the current Investigator's Brochure, all documents, and all trial supplies needed to conduct the trial properly and to comply with the applicable regulatory requirement(s). The investigator has received: • The current Investigator's Brochure • The current protocol

(Continued)

Table 25.1 (Continued)

Site characteristic or activity:	Monitor's responsibility to assess and confirm (review records, procedures, systems, and knowledge) *compliance* with the requirements of the specified study per *ICH E6(R2) 5.18.4*:
	• The current informed consent form and all information to be provided to subjects • CRFs and instructions for completion of CRFs and for making corrections to CRFs • Instructions for reporting of adverse events • Instructions for randomization and maintaining study blinding and conditions and instructions for unblinding • Instructions for reporting the study status to the sponsor • Instructions for reporting protocol and trial deviations to the sponsor • Laboratory procedures and instructions for the receipt of laboratory supplies, as applicable • Instructions for the receipt of investigational product supplies and instructions for storage, handling, administration and return or destruction of the IP • Other trial instructions, supplies, and equipment, as needed
Investigator and staff knowledge of the trial:	*g)* Ensuring that the investigator and the members of the investigator's trial staff are adequately informed about the trial and of the trial supplies. • The investigator and staff are familiar with and have knowledge of all trial information and trial supplies that were received.
Investigator and staff compliance:	*h)* Verifying that the investigator and the members of the investigator's trial staff are performing the specified trial functions, in accordance with the protocol and any other written agreement between the sponsor and the investigator/institution, and these functions are delegated to only unauthorized individuals. • Investigator(s) and staff are performing the specified trial functions according to the protocol and any other written agreement between the sponsor and the investigator/institution • Investigator(s) and staff are performing only duties for which they are qualified • Subinvestigator(s) and other site staff are performing only duties that are delegated by the investigator

Table 25.1 (Continued)

Site characteristic or activity:	Monitor's responsibility to assess and confirm (review records, procedures, systems, and knowledge) *compliance* with the requirements of the specified study per *ICH E6(R2) 5.18.4*:
Subject eligibility:	*i)* Verifying that the investigator is enrolling only eligible subjects: • The investigator is aware of and understands the enrollment eligibility criteria for the trial • The investigator and staff have the evidence to support the eligibility (i.e., meeting all inclusion criteria and eligibility) of each subject enrolled in the trial (i.e., randomized, if applicable, or received investigational product).
Subject recruitment:	*j)* Reporting the subject recruitment rate: • The investigator is recruiting subjects for the trial per the enrollment rate • The investigator is complying with the recruitment reporting requirements (e.g., medium and frequency) to the sponsor.
Source documentation and other study records:	*k)* Verifying that source documents and other trial records are accurate, complete, kept up-to-date, and maintained: • Investigator and staff are familiar with and are complying with the requirements for accurate, complete, and up-to-date source documentation and the maintenance of source documents. • The investigator or qualified delegated staff members are familiar with ALCOAC principles for good documentation practices. • The investigator provides all source documents and other study records for monitoring, audits, and inspections by authorized personnel.
Study reporting:	*l)* Verifying that the investigator provides all the required reports, notifications, applications, and submissions, and that these documents are accurate, complete, timely, legible, dated, and identify the trial. That is, the investigator provides all the required reports, notifications, applications, and submissions to the sponsor and IRB/IEC, as applicable. For example, • Submissions to the IRB/IEC for review and approval/favorable opinion of the initial and any amendments to the protocol • Submissions to the IRB/IEC for review and approval/favorable opinion of the initial and updates to the Investigator's Brochure

(Continued)

Table 25.1 (Continued)

Site characteristic or activity:	Monitor's responsibility to assess and confirm (review records, procedures, systems, and knowledge) *compliance* with the requirements of the specified study per *ICH E6(R2) 5.18.4*:
	• Submissions to the IRB/IEC for review and approval/favorable opinion of the initial and updates to the informed consent and any information, including advertising materials, to be provided to subjects
	• Submissions, at least annually, to the IRB/IEC for continuing review and renewal of approval/favorable opinion of trial information
	• Submissions of reports of study status to the sponsor
	• Submissions of safety reports to the IRB/IEC and the sponsor
	• Submissions of protocol and trial deviations to the IRB/IEC and the sponsor
	• Notification to the IRB/IEC and sponsor, as required, of the premature termination or suspension of a trial
	• Submissions of final reports of study status to the IRB/IEC and the sponsor
Case Report Form completion:	*m)* The accuracy and completeness of the CRF entries, source documents and other trial-related records are checked for:
	• The investigator or qualified delegated staff members are completing the CRFs as instructed and submit CRFs in a timely manner.
	• The Monitor is able to verify the accuracy and completeness of the CRF entries against source documents and other trial-related records.
	• The data required by the protocol are reported accurately on the CRFs and are consistent with the source documents.
	• Any dose and/or therapy modifications are well-documented for each of the trial subjects.
	• Adverse events, concomitant medications, and intercurrent illnesses are reported in accordance with the protocol on the CRFs.
	• Visits that the subjects fail to make, tests that are not conducted, and examinations that are not performed are clearly reported as such on the CRFs.
	• All withdrawals and dropouts of enrolled subjects from the trial are reported and explained on the CRFs.

Table 25.1   (Continued)

Site characteristic or activity:	Monitor's responsibility to assess and confirm (review records, procedures, systems, and knowledge) *compliance* with the requirements of the specified study per *ICH E6(R2) 5.18.4*:
CRF corrections:	*n)* The Monitor or other sponsor representative is informing the investigator of any CRF entry error, omission, or illegibility, and is ensuring that appropriate corrections, additions, or deletions are made, dated, explained (if necessary), and approved by the investigator or by a member of the investigator's trial staff who is authorized to approve CRF changes for the investigator. This authorization is documented. • The investigator or delegated qualified staff member(s) are complying with the methods for receiving and assessing CRF errors and for making corrections to the CRFs. • The authorization of delegated staff member(s) to make changes to CRFs is documented.
Adverse events reporting:	*o)* Determining whether all adverse events (AEs) are appropriately reported within the time periods required by GCP, the protocol, the IRB/IEC, the sponsor, and the applicable regulatory requirement(s). The investigator and relevant staff are aware of and are following the protocol, regulatory, GCP, and other applicable requirements for: • Assessing and identifying adverse events and serious adverse as defined in the study protocol • The collection and follow-up period for adverse events • Recording adverse events • Determining expectedness of adverse events • Expedited reporting of adverse events and providing updates on the status, treatment, and outcomes of adverse events • Providing a subject with or referring them for appropriate medical care for adverse events resulting from their participation in the trial. As necessary, the subject is undergoing appropriate clinical procedures at unscheduled site visits (that is, not on the protocol schedule) for evaluation of such events.
Essential documents:	*p)* Determining whether the investigator is maintaining the required essential documents (Chapter 29 Essential Documents): • All evidence of trial conduct (records and reports) are maintained as essential documents of the clinical site

(Continued)

Table 25.1 (Continued)

Site characteristic or activity:	Monitor's responsibility to assess and confirm (review records, procedures, systems, and knowledge) *compliance* with the requirements of the specified study per *ICH E6(R2) 5.18.4*:
	• All essential documents are complete, legible, and available upon request to the sponsor, IRB/IEC, regulatory or health authority(ies), or their representatives for monitoring, auditing, or inspections, as applicable • All applicable essential documents are reconciled (i.e., the same versions of required documents are present) between the sponsor's and the investigator's files • All essential documents are complete, up-to-date, and are being maintained as stated in the protocol and per other sponsor and applicable regulatory requirements
Deviations reporting and corrective and preventive actions (CAPAs):	*q)* Deviations from the protocol, SOPs, GCP, and the applicable regulatory requirements are identified and communicated to the investigator and appropriate action are taken to correct and prevent recurrence of the detected deviations. Ensuring that the investigator and staff are complying with the requirements for: • Identifying, recording, and reporting deviations from the protocol, SOPs, GCP, and the applicable regulatory requirements • Investigating, identifying the root cause, and implementing corrective and preventive actions for identified deviations.

25.2.3 How: Process for Interim Monitoring

In general, the sponsor will ensure that the investigator/institution is complying with all protocol, GCP, and applicable regulatory requirements for trial conduct during the course of the study. The sponsor may accomplish this goal via:

1) Centralized monitoring techniques (ICH E6(R2) 5.18.3).
2) Monitoring of the investigator/institution individually
3) Combination of the above

The sponsor must consider that, whatever method is employed, it assures appropriate conduct of the trial in accordance with GCP.

25.2.3.1 Centralized Interim Monitoring

As discussed in the chapter on monitoring oversight (Chapter 22 Monitoring Overview), the sponsor may employ centralized monitoring techniques to review study data and site performance while the study is ongoing. In the study-specific Monitoring Plan, the sponsor will

1) Identify the critical data to be evaluated
2) The techniques for evaluating the data
3) The methods for following up on the findings

Based on the findings, the sponsor can

1) Modify the monitoring frequency of individual sites or the study
2) Modify methods for monitoring individual sites or the study
3) Modify the protocol if deemed necessary
4) Take other actions to improve study conduct by individual sites or for the study overall

Depending on the scope of the study and as stated in the Monitoring Plan, these centralized monitoring activities will be in addition to on-site review by the Monitor.

25.2.3.2   Individual Investigator/Institution Interim Monitoring

On-site investigator/institution monitoring should occur to confirm items that can be reviewed only on-site, if remote access to source documentation is not possible; e.g., informed consent documents, investigational product accountability, the operations of facilities and equipment, study source documents. The details of the visit are described below.

Reports of the centralized monitoring and of the individual on-site investigator/institution monitoring will be filed in the sponsor's and investigator's files (ICH E6(R2) 8.2.20).

25.2.4   The Investigator/Institution Interim Monitoring Visit

25.2.4.1   The Interim Monitoring Visit Checklist

The checklist above may be modified if certain characteristics or activities are not required by the specific protocol. The evaluation of characteristics and activities may occur on- or off-site, but all relevant items must be confirmed to verify that the investigator and site staff are complying with their responsibilities, including protocol procedures, study processes, and applicable regulatory requirements. The Monitor and other sponsor's representative(s) will follow standard operating procedures and the study-specific Monitoring Plan for guidance on when and how the visit may be conducted and reported site (Chapter 22 Monitoring Overview).

25.2.4.2   Preparing for the Visit

The Monitor will confirm that the site will have the following available for the interim monitoring visit:

1) The site file, including all "regulatory documents," such as:
   - Investigator and staff qualification (i.e., CVs and licenses)
   - Laboratory qualifications (certificates and normal ranges)
   - Final executed agreements (between investigator and regulatory authority(ies), between investigator and sponsor, etc.)
   - Evidence of trial insurance
   - Approval/favorable opinion of the IRB/IEC for protocol, ICF, and other study documents

   A complete list of required documentation that must be collected and maintained during the trial are described in Chapter 29.Essential Documents
2) All source documents, investigational product accountability records, laboratory collection, processing, and testing records, and other medical records that apply to the study
3) Signed ICFs
4) CRFs
5) Investigational product supplies and accountability records
6) Other study supplies
7) Records and supplies for laboratory samples collection, processing, and testing results
8) Equipment monitoring logs

The sponsor and the investigator will decide on a time that is convenient for both parties for the interim monitoring visit. The Monitor and other sponsor representatives (such as the study Medical Monitor) who have the knowledge and expertise to assess the investigator/institution, as well as the investigator, the study coordinator, and other key site personnel who are involved in the study conduct may attend the visit. The Monitor will note:

- The status of CRF completion and outstanding queries
- The status of outstanding action and follow-up items from the previous monitoring visit
- The status of investigator and site staff qualification documentation
- Documents (and their versions) collected by the sponsor and provided to the investigator
- The status of investigational product per information and study data available to the sponsor; i.e., shipments to the site, used for administration to research subjects, and returned to the sponsor or destroyed by the investigator
- The status of other study supplies shipped to and known to be used by the site

25.2.4.3 The Visit

The interim monitoring visit is not an audit with lone and independent examination of trial related activities and documents by the auditors, but should be an active assessment of the same with interactive questioning and answering (the Monitor will ask and answer questions of the Investigator and staff), discussions, and training (when necessary) by the Monitor. The Monitor will review the study records and note, discuss, and if possible, resolve findings during the visit. All items that remain unresolved during the visit will be documented in the report. The Monitor's evaluation will include, per the study Monitoring Plan and/or standard operating procedures, characteristics, and activities such as:

1) Review of CRFs and verification of the data against the source documents
2) Accountability for the investigational product
3) Identification of safety events and review of the reporting of safety events
4) Review of records and supplies for laboratory samples collection, processing, and testing results
5) Review of the site files and reconciliation with the sponsor files
6) Identification of and CAPAs for protocol and study deviations
7) Facility tours and conversations with key study personnel to discuss study status and conduct

In practice, sponsors may request that Monitors immediately contact the sponsor for urgent or critical findings. Any finding that endangers the safety of a subject or subjects or that threatens the integrity of the trial data should be immediately reported and steps taken for corrective and preventive actions (ICHE6(R2) 5.20.1). Examples of urgent or critical findings are:

- If the Monitor identifies an unreported safety event that meets the definition for expedited reporting
- Inappropriate storage or handling of investigational product
- If the Monitor suspects fraud or misconduct

The process for reporting urgent and critical findings and for issue escalation will also be described in the Monitoring Plan and/or standard operating procedures.

25.2.4.4 The Interim Monitoring Visit Report

Once all the visit criteria have been evaluated the Monitor will complete a report that describes the items reviewed and any findings and follow-up that are necessary (Chapter 22 Monitoring Overview). The report will be reviewed by a qualified sponsor representative who is responsible for investigator oversight. This interim monitoring report will be maintained in the sponsor's files (ICH E6(R2) 8.3.10). A copy of the report or a summary of the visit will be communicated to the investigator/institution as evidence of the sponsor's responsibility for monitoring the investigation.

25.2.4.5 Follow-up

The Monitor will follow-up on any outstanding items to ensure continued compliance with the protocol, GCP, and applicable regulatory requirements by an investigator/institution to conduct the trial. The Monitor will ensure that protocol and study deviations are addressed with corrective and preventive actions. Noncompliance with the protocol, SOPs, GCP, and/or applicable regulatory requirement(s) by an investigator/institution, or by member(s) of the sponsor's staff should lead to prompt action by the sponsor to determine the root cause and secure compliance (ICH E6(R2) 5.20.1; Chapter 33 Quality Assurance Components; Chapter 34 Regulatory Authority Inspections).

The sponsor must immediately investigate suspected fraud or misconduct, and immediately take steps to correct chronic noncompliance or confirmed fraud or misconduct. If the monitoring and/or auditing identify(ies) serious and/or persistent noncompliance on the part of an investigator/institution, the sponsor should terminate the investigator's/institution's participation in the trial. When an investigator's/institution's participation is terminated because of noncompliance, the sponsor should notify promptly the regulatory authority(ies) (ICH E6(R2) 5.20.2).

25.2.5 Consequences of Inadequate Investigator(s)/Institution(s) Interim Monitoring

Interim monitoring of the investigator/institution initiation is a process to verify that the investigator/institution is complying with all protocol, GCP, and applicable regulatory requirements. If

- the investigator and trial staff are not complying with the protocol procedures, GCP, and applicable regulatory requirements,
- the investigator/institution does not have adequate and qualified facilities, equipment, and clinical supplies,
- the investigator and staff are not complying with the instructions for handling and use of the investigational product,
- the investigator and staff are not complying with the procedures for the collection of data,
- ALL evidence of investigator/institution qualification and trial approval documentation are not in place prior to the site consenting the first trial participant,

then the sponsor, sponsor's monitor, and/or the investigator are not complying with GCP and applicable regulatory requirements. There is also a risk to subject's rights, safety, and well-being, the quality and integrity of the data, and to the business goals of the trial.

In clinical research, we aim to prevent the site's failure to comply with the protocol, GCP, and regulatory requirements. Additionally, we want to avoid opposing effects on the business objectives. The goal of investigator/institution interim monitoring then is to carefully review all requirements, ensure that the clinical investigator and staff are complying with those requirements, ensure that the investigator and staff continue to have adequate time, resources, supplies, and motivation to conduct the study; ensure that all required study documentation are complete and up to date, and corrective and preventive actions are being taken for noncompliance.

The typical consequences of inadequate interim monitoring are similar to those of poor selection or investigator/institution initiation:

Subject:

- Violation of rights; e.g.,
- Failure to administer or inadequately administer consent to a subject
- Breach of subject confidentiality
- Misrepresentation of the investigational product as safe and/or effective
- Violation of safety; e.g.,
- Improper administration of the investigational product
- Failure to identify and treat adverse events

Regulatory:

- Violation of protocol procedures; e.g.,
  - Failure to perform protocol procedures as described and at the time they are required
  - Failure to maintain blinding or following randomization procedures
  - Failure to address protocol deviations
- Violation of IRB procedures; e.g.,
  - Failure to submit to the IRB/IEC for initial and/or continuing review
  - Inadequate communication of study status with the IRB
- Violation of regulatory requirements; e.g.,
  - Implementing the protocol and/or consent forms that are not approved by the IRB/IEC
  - Failure to maintain adequate case histories and other source documents
  - Documenting what did not happen
  - Investigator's failure to oversee the investigation
  - Unqualified personnel performing study duties
  - Failure to report safety events as required
- Misuse/mishandling of investigational product; e.g.,
  - Inadequate accountability for the investigational product
  - Improper storage of the investigational product

Business:

- No or slow enrollment at the clinical investigational site
- Increased costs of operations at the site
- Costs related to addressing issues due to negligence7

Everything perfect?!

- If the investigator site produces perfect data, and there are no protocol deviations, and no adverse events reported, this may be a sign of a "too good to be true" situation. While this situation is certainly possible, it is highly improbable, given the nature of clinical trials; i.e., they involve human beings as research participants and as conductors of the trials. It is prudent for the Monitor(s) to carefully review such circumstances, and if there are no findings, Bravo!

25.3 Summary

The sponsor is required to ensure that the investigator/institution conducting the trial in compliance with the protocol, GCP, and applicable regulatory requirements. The process of interim monitoring involves review of all site characteristics and activities to ensure ongoing compliance. Interim monitoring may be conducted via centralized evaluation and/or on-site review. Whether interim monitoring is performed via centralized and/or individual on-site evaluation, all monitoring review and findings must be documented and action should be taken to correct any identified deviations from protocol, GCP, and/or applicable regulatory procedures. The sponsor's Monitor, who will be qualified by training and experience, will review all characteristics and activities of the investigator/institution that are necessary to evaluate compliant implementation of the study protocol. This review is to ensure the *ongoing compliance* of the investigator/institution with all protocol, GCP, and applicable regulatory requirements to avoid the possible dire and costly consequences to inadequate interim site monitoring.

Knowledge Check Questions

1) When does investigator/institution interim monitoring occur?
2) What clinical trial activities, materials, and documentation are reviewed during interim monitoring?
3) Who performs interim monitoring?
4) How does the monitor determine what is to be monitored?
5) What are some consequences of inadequate interim monitoring?

Reference

1 International Council for Harmonisation of Technical Requirements for Pharmaceuticals for Human Use (ICH), Integrated Addendum to ICH E6(R1):Guideline for Good Clinical Practice, E6(R2) (2016). Current Step 4 version dated 9 November 2016. https://www.ich.org/page/efficacy-guidelines

26

Investigator/Institution Close-out

Karen A. Henry

GCP Key Point

*Investigator/Institution closeout is a quality control activity to assess (review records, procedures, systems, and knowledge) for **completed compliance** with the specified study requirements.*

26.1   Introduction

Investigator/Institution closeout ensures that the investigator/institution has complied with the protocol, GCP, and applicable regulatory requirements of the specified study. It is the fourth monitoring phase of the trial (Chapter 22 Monitoring Overview; Plate 7 Monitoring): investigator/institution closeout takes place at the end of the study; i.e., when the investigator/institution is no longer conducting the study, having either completed the study or terminated from the study (Chapter 14 Trial Management; Start-up, On-Study, and Close-Out). The investigator/institution may discontinue participating in study conduct for many reasons and the sponsor will determine when is the most appropriate time after the investigator/institution's completion or termination of the trial to close out the trial site.

Investigator/institution closeout usually refers to the final reconciliation of study activities and compilation and archiving of essential documents at the investigator's site. A final closeout of a trial can only be done when the monitor has reviewed both investigator/institution and sponsor files and confirmed that all necessary documents are in the appropriate files (ICH E6(R2) 8.0) [1]. By the time of the closeout visit, all interim monitoring activities should have been completed. If the closeout visit will be used to perform both interim monitoring and closeout activities, then the firm's standard operating procedures may require

The Fundamentals of Clinical Research: A Universal Guide for Implementing Good Clinical Practice, First Edition. P. Michael Dubinsky and Karen A. Henry.
Companion website: www.wiley.com/go/dubinsky/clinicalresearch

both types of visit reports to be completed. Here, we are assuming that all interim monitoring review (Chapter 25 Investigator/Institution Interim Monitoring) was completed and we are presenting only closeout activities in this chapter.

26.2 Objectives

The objectives of this chapter are to describe:

1) What is the purpose of investigator/institution closeout?
2) When does investigator/institution closeout occur?
3) What are reviewed during investigator/institution closeout?
   a) Regulatory
   b) Protocol
   c) Administrative
4) The investigator/institution closeout visit
5) Follow-up after investigator/institution closeout

26.2.1 The Purpose of Investigator/Institution Closeout

The goal of investigator/institution closeout is to confirm and ensure the investigator(s), staff, and facilities *have complied* with the protocol, GCP, and applicable regulatory requirements in accordance with the study-specific monitoring plan to meet the scientific and ethical objectives of the trial:

1) Protect the rights and well-being of human subjects.
2) Maintain data integrity.
3) Compliance with the currently approved protocol, GCP, and applicable regulatory requirement(s).

This is the time to ensure that essential documents at the investigator/institution completely and accurately reflect the conduct of the trial at the investigator/institution.

26.2.2 When Does Investigator/Institution Closeout Occur?

Investigator/institution participation in study conduct may end for any of many reasons; for example,

1) Investigator met enrollment goals, and follow-up for the last subject in the study is completed, and interim monitoring is complete (Chapter 25 Investigator/Institution Interim Monitoring)
2) Institution/investigator terminates the participation of the investigator
3) Sponsor prematurely terminates the participation of an investigator for reasons such as:
   a) Lack of enrollment

    b) Misconduct or noncompliance

4) Sponsor prematurely terminates the study for reasons such as:

    a) Lack of overall enrollment

    b) Interim analysis results indicate acceptable efficacy and safety, lack of efficacy, or safety concerns

    c) Issues with investigational product supply

    d) Business or financial reasons

The sponsor will determine when the most appropriate time is for the closeout visit after the investigator/institution's completion or termination of the trial. The primary concern for determining the timing for closing out a clinical site is that the sponsor needs to ensure that the investigator/institution records and site staff remain available until the sponsor has obtained all necessary information for close out of the study (see Chapter 14 Trial Management; Start-up, On-Study, and Close-Out). If there is any anticipated need for the sponsor to have access to study documents and/or investigator/site staff, the sponsor will delay investigator/institution closeout until the completion of all anticipated access. Since investigator/institution closeout involves final payments and archiving of trial documents, premature closeout of an investigator/institution may result in motivational and time challenges to obtain access to investigator/institution staff and/or trial data. Often, final cleaning of the data and reconciliation of databases for database lock may require additional inquiries to individual sites so the sponsor may delay closeout until after database lock to ensure continued access to investigator/institution staff and/or trial data. The sponsor will consider one or more of many factors; for example,

1) A final closeout of a trial can only be performed when the monitor has reviewed both investigator/institution and sponsor files and confirmed that all necessary documents are in the appropriate files (ICH E6(R2) 8.0).

2) If the trial is a single-site study, the site could be closed after all study activities are completed, including writing of the clinical study report.

3) If the trial is a multicenter study, each individual site may be closed prior to the completion of the entire trial if the sponsor is confident that all trial data and essential documents have been monitored at the investigator/institution and are accurate and complete; else, final closeout of all trial sites may be delayed until after the database is closed.

4) If the study was initiated at an investigator/institution but no subjects received the investigational product, then final monitoring and closeout may occur prior to database lock.

26.2.3 What: Items that are Reviewed for Investigator/ Institution Closeout

Clinical trials are governed by regulatory and ethical requirements, protocol requirements, and business objectives. The general items that are reviewed to ensure that the investigator/institution has complied with the requirements for study conduct can therefore be grouped into the following:

a) Regulatory and ethical – the applicable regulations and GCP
b) Protocol – the trial-specific procedures
c) Administrative – the constraints of timelines, personnel resources, and finances

26.2.3.1 The Investigator/Institution Closeout Checklist
The checklist for investigator and site closeout includes final reconciliation of study activities and verification of all study characteristics and activities to demonstrate that the investigator and site have complied with the protocol, SOPs, GCP, and applicable regulatory requirements. These characteristics and activities are largely driven by the investigator responsibilities (see Chapter 9 Investigator and Sponsor Roles and Responsibilities) and responsibilities of the Monitor (see Chapter 22 Monitoring Overview) (Figure 26.1):

A checklist ensures that there is systematic review and reconciliation of study activities at the investigator/institution. The Monitor's responsibilities for investigator closeout are shown in Table 26.1.

1) Regulatory and GCP requirements – i.e., requirements for investigator qualifications and responsibilities that are laid out by GCP and local regulations:

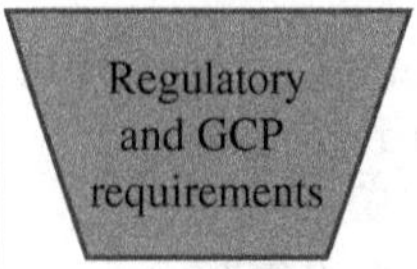

Regulatory and GCP requirements

• ICH E6(R2) 4: The investigator is responsible for:

o Investigator qualification and agreements
  • Provide evidence of education, training, and experience to assume the responsibility for the proper conduct of the trial and to meet applicable regulatory requirement(s)
  • Complying with GCP and applicable regulatory requirements
  • Permit monitoring, auditing, and inspection
o The investigational product
o Maintaining adequate resources:
  • Demonstrate ability to recruit the subject population;

Figure 26.1 Investigator/institution responsibilities to review for closeout.

- Have sufficient time to conduct the trial;
- Have adequate staff and facilities, including specialized expertise, equipment, facilities, or laboratories;
- Informing all persons assisting with the trial of the protocol, IP, and their trial duties

o The medical care of trial subjects

o Communication with institutional review board (IRB)/independent ethics committee (IEC)

o Compliance with the protocol

o Complying with randomization and unblinding procedures

o Informed consent of trial subjects

o Maintaining records and reports of the investigation

o Submitting progress reports as required

o Reporting safety events

o Complying with procedures in the event of premature termination or suspension of a trial

o Submitting final reports to the IRB/IEC and sponsor

Protocol requirements

2) Protocol requirements – i.e., clinical and operational procedures that are required by the specific protocol

Administrative requirements

3) Administrative requirements – i.e., business or non-regulatory:

- Timelines
- Personnel resources
- Data collection media and processes
- Financial
    o Sponsor's budget
    o Investigator's budget
    o Contract issues

Figure 26.1 (Continued)

Table 26.1 Investigator/institution closeout checklist.

Site characteristic or activity:	Monitor's responsibility to reconcile and confirm (review records, procedures, systems, and knowledge) *compliance* with the requirements of the specified study per *ICH E6(R2) 5.18.4*:

Appropriate investigator and site selection and continued participation:	*b)* Verifying that the essential documents demonstrate that the investigator had adequate qualifications, resources, facilities, including laboratories, equipment, and staff to safely and properly conduct the trial:
	
	• Qualification and experience of the investigator, subinvestigators, and all staff who will be delegated study tasks:
	
	  – Evidence (e.g., a current curriculum vitae) of education, training, and experience with knowledge of the therapeutic area under study
	  – Evidence of applicable regulatory qualification; e.g., current license
	  – GCP knowledge (experience conducting clinical investigations is always preferred).
	  – Adequate and appropriate communication with the sponsor and sponsor's representatives; i.e., there were no language or physical barriers that hinder communication
	
	• The investigator personally conducted the trial or supervised qualified staff who were delegated trial duties
	
	• Study duties were delegated to only qualified individuals.
	
	• A list of trial staff and their assigned duties was maintained.
	
	• All facilities and equipment were adequate and operational (e.g., capacity, temperature monitors, backups) and calibration records where applicable were maintained.
	
	• Laboratory facilities were adequate and operational and certification records were current and staff members were qualified.
	
	• Foreseen and unplanned personnel and facilities or equipment changes were managed appropriately to maintain their adequacy during the course of the trial.

Investigator compliance with investigational product requirements:	*c)* Verifying, for the investigational product(s): • Investigator(s) and relevant staff members were familiar with the investigational product(s) properties and class of the investigational product(s). • Qualified individuals were receiving, preparing, and administering the investigational product.

Table 26.1 (Continued)

Site characteristic or activity:	Monitor's responsibility to reconcile and confirm (review records, procedures, systems, and knowledge) *compliance* with the requirements of the specified study per *ICH E6(R2) 5.18.4*:
	• Investigational product was stored for times and conditions as required.
	• The investigator was retaining sufficient supplies of investigational product
	• Administration of the investigational product(s) was only to eligible subjects and at the protocol specified dose(s).
	• Subjects were provided with necessary instructions on proper use, handling, storage, and return the investigational product(s).
	• The receipt, use, and return of the investigational product(s) at the trial sites were controlled and documented adequately.
	• The disposition of unused investigational product(s) at the trial sites complied with applicable regulatory requirement(s) and was in accordance with the sponsor procedures.
Investigator compliance with the approved protocol:	*d)* Verifying that the investigator was following the approved protocol and all approved amendment(s), if any.
	• The investigator and staff members were implementing only a protocol or its amendments that had received the approval or favorable opinion of the IRB/IEC.
	• The investigator and staff members were following the approved protocol and all approved amendment(s), if any.
Subject informed consent:	*e)* Verifying that written informed consent was obtained before each subject's participation in the trial. The investigator and staff members were familiar with and were complying with the requirements for:
	• A study participant to be consented only with an informed consent form that had been reviewed and approved by the IRB/IEC
	• Specific information (required elements) to be contained in the informed consent form
	• Subject information and the administration of consent to be in a language understandable to the subject
	• Administration of and the signed and dated consent of a subject prior to their participation in the trial
	• The person administering consent to sign and date the consent form
	• Providing the subject with a copy of their signed and dated consent
	• The process for administering consent
	• Documentation of the process of consent for each study participant

(Continued)

Table 26.1 (Continued)

Site characteristic or activity:	Monitor's responsibility to reconcile and confirm (review records, procedures, systems, and knowledge) *compliance* with the requirements of the specified study per *ICH E6(R2) 5.18.4*:
	• The person administering consent to sign and date the consent form
	• Providing the subject with a copy of their signed and dated consent
	• The process for administering consent
	• Documentation of the process of consent for each study participant
	• Updating the informed consent form with new information that may influence the subject's decision to continue participating in the trial
	• Specific consenting procedures for minors, patients with cognitive impairment, vulnerable populations, emergency situations, and other trial circumstances, as applicable to the trial or clinical site location
	• Complying with local and other regulatory requirements
Investigator receives all trial information:	*f)* Ensuring that the investigator received the current Investigator's Brochure, all documents, and all trial supplies needed to conduct the trial properly and to comply with the applicable regulatory requirement(s). The investigator had received:
	• The current Investigator's Brochure
	• The current protocol
	• The current informed consent form and all information to be provided to subjects
	• CRFs and instructions for completion of CRFs and for making corrections to CRFs
	• Instructions for reporting of adverse events
	• Instructions for randomization and maintaining study blinding and conditions and instructions for unblinding
	• Instructions for reporting the study status to the sponsor
	• Instructions for reporting protocol and trial deviations to the sponsor
	• Laboratory procedures and instructions for the receipt of laboratory supplies, as applicable
	• Instructions for the receipt of investigational product supplies and instructions for storage, handling, administration and return or destruction of the IP
	• Other trial instructions, supplies, and equipment, as needed

Table 26.1 (Continued)

Site characteristic or activity:	Monitor's responsibility to reconcile and confirm (review records, procedures, systems, and knowledge) *compliance* with the requirements of the specified study per *ICH E6(R2) 5.18.4*:
Investigator and staff knowledge of the trial:	*g)* Ensuring that the investigator and the members of the investigator's trial staff were adequately informed about the trial and the trial supplies. • The investigator and staff members were familiar with and had knowledge of all trial information and trial supplies that were received.
Investigator and staff compliance:	*h)* Verifying that the investigator and the members of the investigator's trial staff were performing the specified trial functions, in accordance with the protocol and any other written agreement between the sponsor and the investigator/institution, and these functions were delegated to only unauthorized individuals. • Investigator(s) and staff members were performing the specified trial functions according to the protocol and any other written agreement between the sponsor and the investigator/institution • Investigator(s) and staff members were performing only duties for which they are qualified • Subinvestigator(s) and other site staff members were performing only duties that were delegated by the investigator
Subject eligibility:	*i)* Verifying that the investigator was enrolling only eligible subjects: • The investigator was aware of and understood the enrollment eligibility criteria for the trial • The investigator and staff had the evidence to support the eligibility (i.e., meeting all inclusion criteria and eligibility) of each subject enrolled in the trial (i.e., randomized, if applicable, or received investigational product).
Subject recruitment:	*j)* Reporting the subject recruitment rate: • The investigator was recruiting subjects for the trial per the enrollment rate • The investigator was complying with the recruitment reporting requirements (e.g., medium and frequency) to the sponsor.
Source documentation and other study records:	*k)* Verifying that source documents and other trial records were accurate, complete, kept up-to-date and maintained: • Investigator and staff members were familiar with and were complying with the requirements for accurate, complete, and up-to-date source documentation and the maintenance of source documents. • The investigator or qualified delegated staff members were familiar with ALCOAC principles for good documentation practices. • The investigator provided all source documents and other study records for monitoring, audits, and inspections by authorized personnel.

Table 26.1 (Continued)

Site characteristic or activity:	Monitor's responsibility to reconcile and confirm (review records, procedures, systems, and knowledge) *compliance* with the requirements of the specified study per *ICH E6(R2) 5.18.4*:
Study reporting:	*l)* Verifying that the investigator provided all the required reports, notifications, applications, and submissions, and that these documents are accurate, complete, timely, legible, dated, and identify the trial. That is, the investigator provided all the required reports, notifications, applications, and submissions to the sponsor and IRB/IEC, as applicable. For example,
	• Submissions to the IRB/IEC for review and approval/favorable opinion of the initial and any amendments to the protocol
	• Submissions to the IRB/IEC for review and approval/favorable opinion of the initial and updates to the Investigator's Brochure
	• Submissions to the IRB/IEC for review and approval/favorable opinion of the initial and updates to the informed consent and any information, including advertising materials, to be provided to subjects
	• Submissions, at least annually, to the IRB/IEC for continuing review and renewal of approval/favorable opinion of trial information
	• Submissions of reports of study status to the sponsor
	• Submissions of safety reports to the IRB/IEC and the sponsor
	• Submissions of protocol and trial deviations to the IRB/IEC and the sponsor
	• Notification to the IRB/IEC and sponsor, as required, of the premature termination or suspension of a trial
	• Submissions of final reports of study status to the IRB/IEC and the sponsor
Case Report Form completion:	*m)* The accuracy and completeness of the CRF entries, source documents and other trial-related records were checked for:
	• The investigator or qualified delegated staff members were completing the CRFs as instructed and submitting CRFs in a timely manner.
	• The Monitor was able to verify the accuracy and completeness of the CRF entries against source documents and other trial-related records.
	• The data required by the protocol were reported accurately on the CRFs and were consistent with the source documents.
	• Any dose and/or therapy modifications were well documented for each of the trial subjects.
	• Adverse events, concomitant medications, and intercurrent illnesses were reported in accordance with the protocol on the CRFs.

Table 26.1 (Continued)

Site characteristic or activity:	Monitor's responsibility to reconcile and confirm (review records, procedures, systems, and knowledge) *compliance* with the requirements of the specified study per *ICH E6(R2) 5.18.4*:
	• Visits that the subjects failed to make, tests that were not conducted, and examinations that were not performed were clearly reported as such on the CRFs. • All withdrawals and dropouts of enrolled subjects from the trial were reported and explained on the CRFs.
CRF corrections:	*n)* The monitor or other sponsor representative was informing the investigator of any CRF entry error, omission, or illegibility, and was ensuring that appropriate corrections, additions, or deletions were made, dated, explained (if necessary), and approved by the investigator or by a member of the investigator's trial staff who was authorized to approve CRF changes for the investigator. This authorization was documented. • The investigator or delegated qualified staff member(s) were complying with the methods for receiving and assessing CRF errors and for making corrections to the CRFs. • The authorization of delegated staff member(s) to make changes to CRFs was documented.
Adverse events reporting:	*o)* Determining whether all adverse events (AEs) were appropriately reported within the time periods required by GCP, the protocol, the IRB/IEC, the sponsor, and the applicable regulatory requirement(s). The investigator and relevant staff were aware of and were following the protocol, regulatory, GCP, and other applicable requirements for: • Assessing and identifying adverse events and serious adverse as defined in the study protocol • The collection and follow-up period for adverse events • Recording adverse events • Determining expectedness of adverse events • Expedited reporting of adverse events and providing updates on the status, treatment, and outcomes of adverse events • Providing a subject with or referring them for appropriate medical care for adverse events resulting from their participation in the trial. As necessary, the subject is undergoing appropriate clinical procedures at unscheduled site visits (that is, not on the protocol schedule) for evaluation of such events.

(Continued)

Table 26.1 (Continued)

Site characteristic or activity:	Monitor's responsibility to reconcile and confirm (review records, procedures, systems, and knowledge) *compliance* with the requirements of the specified study per *ICH E6(R2) 5.18.4*:
Essential documents:	*p)* Determining whether the investigator was maintaining the required essential documents (Chapter 29 Essential Documents): • All evidence of trial conduct (records and reports) are maintained as essential documents of the clinical site • All essential documents are complete, legible, and available upon request to the sponsor, IRB/IEC, regulatory or health authority(ies), or their representatives for monitoring, auditing, or inspections, as applicable • All applicable essential documents are reconciled (i.e., the same versions of required documents are present) between the sponsor's and the investigator's files • All essential documents are complete, up-to-date, and are being maintained as stated in the protocol and per other sponsor and applicable regulatory requirements
Deviations reporting and CAPAs:	*q)* Deviations from the protocol, SOPs, GCP, and the applicable regulatory requirements were identified and communicated to the investigator and appropriate action were taken to correct and prevent recurrence of the detected deviations. Ensuring that the investigator and staff were complying with the requirements for: • Identifying, recording, and reporting deviations from the protocol, SOPs, GCP, and the applicable regulatory requirements • Investigating, identifying the root cause, and implementing corrective and preventive actions for identified deviations.

26.2.4 How: Investigator/Institution Closeout Visit

In general, the sponsor will ensure that the investigator/institution has complied with all protocol, GCP, and applicable regulatory requirements for trial conduct. The closeout visit refers to the completion of all closeout activities for an investigator/institution, whether the review and completion of the activities are on- and/or off-site. The sponsor's monitor and or other representatives will complete the visit and the applicable reports to ensure documentation of the closeout activity.

26.2.4.1 The Closeout Visit Checklist

The checklist above may be modified if certain characteristics or activities are not required by the specific protocol. The evaluation of characteristics and activities may occur on- or off-site, but all relevant items must be confirmed to verify that the investigator and site staff were complying with their responsibilities, including protocol procedures, study processes, and applicable regulatory requirements. The sponsor may accomplish this goal via:

- On-site review of items that contain confidential subject identification information or that do need hands-on review of original sources or materials; e.g., informed consent documents, subject identification codelist, investigational product accountability, the operations of facilities and equipment, study source documents (if remote access to source documentation is not possible). The details of the visit is described below.
- Off-site review of items that do not compromise the research subject's confidentiality or that do not need hands-on review of inaccessible original sources or materials; e.g., investigation and staff qualification and delegation of study duties, IRB/IEC communication and approval documents, CRF completion.

The Monitor and other sponsor's representative(s) will follow standard operating procedures and the study-specific Monitoring Plan for guidance on when and how the visit may be conducted and reported (Chapter 22 Monitoring Overview).

26.2.4.2 Preparing for the Visit

The Monitor will confirm that the site will have the following available for review at the closeout visit:

1) The site file, including all "regulatory documents," such as:
   - Investigator and staff qualification (i.e., CVs and licenses) and delegation
   - Laboratory qualifications (certificates and normal ranges)
   - Final executed agreements (between investigator and regulatory authority(ies), if applicable; between investigator and sponsor; etc.)
   - Evidence of trial insurance
   - Approval/favorable opinion of the IRB/IEC for protocol, ICF, and other study documents

   A complete list of required documentation that must be collected and maintained after completion or termination of the trial are described in Chapter 29 Essential Documents.
2) All source documents, including safety reporting records, laboratory collection, processing, and testing records, and other medical records that apply to the study

3) Signed ICFs
4) CRFs
5) Investigational product supplies and accountability records
6) Other study supplies
7) Logs for recording and tracking protocol and study deviations
8) Records and supplies for laboratory samples collection, processing, and testing results
9) Equipment monitoring logs

The sponsor and the investigator will decide on a time that is convenient for both parties for the closeout visit. The Monitor and other sponsor representatives (such as the study Medical Monitor) who have the knowledge and expertise to assess the investigator/institution, as well as the investigator, the study coordinator, and other key site personnel who are involved in the study conduct may attend the visit. The Monitor will note:

- The status of CRF completion and outstanding queries
- The status of outstanding action and follow-up items from the previous monitoring visit
- The status of investigator and site staff qualification documentation
- Documents (and their versions) collected by the sponsor and provided to the investigator
- The status of investigational product per information and study data available to the sponsor; i.e., shipments to the site, used for administration to research subjects, and returned to the sponsor or destroyed by the investigator
- The status of safety reports
- The status of CAPAs for protocol and study deviation
- The status of other study supplies shipped to and known to be used by the site

26.2.4.3 The Visit
As previously mentioned, all interim monitoring review would have been completed by the time of the closeout visit. The closeout visit, therefore, is a general review, reconciliation, and confirmation of the characteristics and activities of study conduct. The Monitor will review the records, perform final reconciliation, and remind the investigator of any continued obligations after the site has been closed. All items that remain unresolved during the visit, and there should not be any at this type of monitoring visit, will be documented in the report. The Monitor's evaluation will include, per the study Monitoring Plan and/or standard operating procedures, a review of characteristics, and activities such as (Plate 16 Investigator/Institution Closeout):

1) Confirmation of subject case histories (Chapter 19 Informed Consent and Other Human Subject Protection):

a) Signed informed consent forms and evidence of the process for informed consent for each subject who signed consent
b) Source documents for protocol procedures and unscheduled study assessments or evaluations
c) Laboratory testing reports
d) Evidence of eligibility for the trial for subjects who enrolled in the study
e) Reason(s) for lack of eligibility for subjects who signed consent but were not enrolled in the study
f) Reason(s) for subject's discontinuation from study treatment or from the trial
g) Evidence that the subject received or was referred for medical care for study-related adverse events
h) Other medical records that reflect conduct of the study
i) Complete and accurate subject identification code list (ICH E6(R2) 8.4.3).
j) All payments have been made to research subjects per the IRB/IEC-approved amounts and methods

2) Review of safety data (Chapter 21 Safety Monitoring and Reporting):
a) All adverse events have been identified and reported per the protocol, GCP, and applicable regulatory requirements
b) Identification of ongoing safety events that must be monitored beyond site closeout

3) Review of CRF data (Chapter 20 Data Collection and Data Management):
a) All CRF data have been verified against source documents, as applicable
b) All CRFs are complete and submitted to the sponsor
c) All data queries have been addressed and all changes have been appropriately documented
d) The investigator/institution and the sponsor have copies of the final CRFs and any changes made to CRFs

4) Accountability of investigational product(Chapter 17 The Investigational Product (Clinical Supplies)):
a) All investigational product from receipt at the investigator/institution, through dispensing, administration, and destruction or return have been accounted for (ICH E6(R2) 8.4.1).
b) All used and unused investigational product have been destroyed and/or returned to the sponsor per the protocol and applicable local regulatory requirements (ICH E6(R2) 8.4.2).

5) Review of biological specimens collected from subjects:
a) All biological specimens from research subjects have complete tracking records that will be retained in the essential documents.
b) If laboratory samples must be traced for future use, then a system for their monitoring and maintenance must remain in place and specimen stored as appropriate.

6) Review of randomization and blinding records
    a) Treatment allocation and decoding documentation have been provided to the sponsor (ICH E6(R2) 8.4.6)
7) Review of documentation of protocol and study deviations (Chapter 22 Monitoring Overview; Chapter 33 Quality Assurance Components; Chapter 34 Regulatory Authority Inspections)
    a) All CAPAs for identified deviations have been completed
    b) All CAPAs for audit findings have been completed (ICH E6(R2) 8.4.4).
8) Review of investigator qualification, oversight, and delegation of responsibility (Chapters 22 Monitoring Overview; Chapter 9 Investigator and Sponsor Roles and Responsibilities)
    a) Compilation of evidence of investigator oversight of the trial; e.g., meeting minutes
    b) Complete records of investigator delegation of study duties showing who was assigned what duties
    c) Complete records of investigator qualification and training
    d) Complete records of investigator/institution staff qualification and training for assigned duties
9) Final list of the SOPs that were in effect during the course of the trial (Chapter 32 Standard Operating Procedures)
10) Essential documents (Chapter 29 Essential Documents):
    a) Essential documents have been reconciled for presence and versions between the sponsor and investigator/institution files
    b) All essential documents are in the investigator/institution's files as required
    c) A system is in place for appropriate storage and archiving of essential documents
    d) The investigator/institution has agreed to retain essential documents as required by the sponsor and applicable GCP and regulatory requirements
11) Final notifications of study status to IRB/IECs (Chapter 8 IRB/IEC Roles and Responsibilities)
12) Finances (Chapter 15 Trial Resourcing and Outsourcing):
    a) All finances between the investigator/institution and the sponsor have been reconciled.
    b) The contract between the sponsor and investigator/institution has been terminated

Final payments and termination of the contract may occur immediately following the closeout visit or during study closeout.

Additionally, the monitor will remind the investigator of their obligations beyond site closeout:

1) The investigator and site staff will be available for resolution of any issues that arise prior to close out of the overall trial

2) The investigator will notify the IRB/IEC of the trial's closure and its final status (ICH E6(R2) 8.4.7).
3) The investigator will follow-up and report on adverse events as required by the protocol
4) Site study records must be retained according to GCP, applicable regulations, and sponsor's policy
5) The sponsor's policy for preparation and review of publications based on the study results
6) Procedures for audits by the sponsor
7) Procedures for notifying the sponsor if the investigator receives notification of a regulatory inspection or audits other than by the sponsor
8) Other applicable regulatory obligations

26.2.4.4 The Investigator/Institution Closeout Visit Report

Once all the visit criteria have been evaluated the Monitor will complete a report that describes the items reviewed and any findings and follow-up that are necessary (Chapter 22 Monitoring Overview). The report will be reviewed by a qualified sponsor representative who is responsible for investigator oversight. Reports of the on-site and off-site investigator/institution closeout will be filed in the sponsor's files (ICH E6(R2) 8.4.5). A copy of the report or a summary of the visit may be communicated to the investigator/institution as evidence of the sponsor's responsibility for monitoring the investigation.

26.2.5 Follow-up After Investigator/Institution Closeout

The Monitor will follow-up on any outstanding items to ensure continued compliance with the protocol, GCP, and applicable regulatory requirements by an investigator/institution beyond site closeout. Items for follow-up after investigator/institution closeout may include but are not limited to:

- Data queries; e.g., during database lock if the site is closed prior to database lock
- Safety events follow-up, such as serious adverse events with follow-up ongoing after site closeout and pregnancies
- Sponsor audit of the investigator/institution
- Regulatory authority inspection of the investigator/institution
- Analysis of retained biological samples for subject safety follow up

When an investigator's/institution's participation is terminated because of non-compliance, the sponsor should notify promptly the regulatory authority(ies) (ICH E6(R2) 5.20.2).

26.2.6   Consequences of Inadequate Investigator/
Institution Closeout

As mentioned in Section 26.2.2 above, careful consideration should be given to the *timing* of the closeout of the clinical trial site. The sponsor wants to ensure that the site remains available and motivated for follow-up of any data or trial issues, and a clinical trial site that is closed before the sponsor has monitored, collected, and cleaned all date, may have little motivation to cooperate for sponsor follow-up data queries or review of trial records.

Additionally, the sponsor will want to ensure that the investigator/institution is ready for any *post closeout audit or inspection*. The investigator and site staff will be informed on what to do when notified of and how to handle audits or inspections after the closeout. In addition to the investigator and site staff being prepared to host an audit or inspection, all study records must be complete, reconciled, and easily accessible in the event of an audit or inspection. If the investigator/ institution is not prepared, audit and inspections may result in significant findings if staff members are not able to adequately answer questions or trial records are not complete or readily accessible.

26.3   Summary

The sponsor is required to ensure that the investigator/institution has conducted the trial in compliance with the protocol, GCP, and applicable regulatory requirements. The process of site closeout involves review of all site characteristics and activities to ensure that the essential documents at the investigator/institution accurately and completely reflect the conduct of the trial at that trial site. Site closeout may be conducted via off- and/or on-site review while ensuring access to original source documents or materials and maintaining confidential subject identification information. The sponsor's Monitor, who will be qualified by training and experience, will review all characteristics and activities of the investigator/institution that are necessary to evaluate compliant implementation of the study protocol and ensure the final reconciliation of study activities and documentation. This review is to confirm the *compliance* of the investigator/institution with all protocol, GCP, and applicable regulatory requirements to avoid the possible dire and costly consequences to inadequate site closeout.

Knowledge Check Questions
1) When does investigator/institution closeout occur?
2) What is the purpose of investigator/institution closeout?
3) What trial activities, materials, or documentation are reviewed during investigator/institution closeout?
4) What may the investigator be responsible for after investigator/institution closeout?
5) What are some consequences of inadequate investigator/institution closeout?

Reference

1 International Council for Harmonisation of Technical Requirements for Pharmaceuticals for Human Use (ICH), Integrated Addendum to ICH E6(R1):Guideline for Good Clinical Practice, E6(R2) (2016) Current Step 4 version dated 9 November. https://www.ich.org/page/efficacy-guidelines

27

Study Design and Data Analysis

Karen A. Henry

GCP Key Point

The scientific integrity of the trial and the credibility of the data from the trial depend substantially on the trial design (ICH E6(R2) 6.4).

27.1   Introduction

This chapter will present a general overview of study design and data analysis as they pertain to primarily 3 principles of GCP:

1) The rights, safety, and well-being of the trial subjects are the most important considerations and should prevail over interests of science and society (ICH E6(R2) 2.3)
2) Clinical trials should be scientifically sound, and described in a clear, detailed protocol (ICH E6(R2) 2.5)
3) All clinical trial information should be recorded, handled, and stored in a way that allows its accurate reporting, interpretation, and verification (ICH E6(R2) 2.10)

   The design of a clinical trial is determined by the trial protocol objectives, which are entirely influenced by the phase of development of the investigational product. The design of the trial will take into account protection of the safety of trial subjects, scientifically sound applications for clinical trials, and considerations for ensuring the integrity of the trial data that will be analyzed for the clinical study

The Fundamentals of Clinical Research: A Universal Guide for Implementing Good Clinical Practice, First Edition. P. Michael Dubinsky and Karen A. Henry.
© 2022 John Wiley & Sons, Inc. Published 2022 by John Wiley & Sons, Inc.
Companion website: www.wiley.com/go/dubinsky/clinicalresearch

report (Chapter 28 The Clinical Study Report). The analysis of the trial data will continue to follow these 3 main principles so that there may be assurance that the data included in an application for marketing the investigational product are true, accurate, and complete.

This chapter will discuss the above largely at a conceptual level and refer the reader to ICH E8 guideline for General Considerations for Clinical Trials [2] and ICH E9 guideline for Statistical Principles for Clinical Trials [3]. Technical details for principles and procedures for statistical design and data analysis are beyond the scope of this book.

27.2 Objectives

The objectives of this chapter are:

1) Describe clinical trial phases in drug development and describe these phases as they relate to study protocol objectives and study design
2) Discuss GCP concepts as they relate to study design
3) Describe the Statistical Analysis Plan
4) Describe preparation of the study data for analysis
5) Describe general processes for analyzing and reporting the study data

27.3 Clinical Trial Phases and Study Designs in Drug Development

Given the historical marketing and use of drug products and the resulting ethical guidelines and regulatory requirements (Chapter 1 History), a medical product must go through testing in phases before sufficient information may be garnered to prove its safety and efficacy in humans. These phases largely guide the development of the product since a proposed clinical trial protocol must adequately be supported by available nonclinical and clinical information on the investigational product (ICH E6(R2) 2.4). The phases of clinical trial testing are conventionally categorized as Phase 1 to 4 and each phase is typically characterized by the scientific objectives (pharmacokinetics, pharmacodynamics, safety, tolerability, efficacy), number of subjects, study population, statistical controls of the trial.

27.3.1 Phase 1 to 3 Studies

The hierarchy of a phase factor as a protocol objective generally evolves through the development process (phases 1 to 3) as more information is accumulated about the investigational product from each completed trial. For example:

- Assessment of pharmacokinetics:

PHASE 1 ------------*1b*----------------*2*-----------*2b*-------------- PHASE 3

Primary -- Exploratory

Pharmacokinetics is the characterization of a drug's absorption, distribution, metabolism, and excretion and help to guide dose finding and dose regimen. These assessments are usually the primary objective in a phase 1 study and may be collected as exploratory objectives by phase 3.

- Assessment of pharmacodynamics:

PHASE 1 ------------*1b*----------------*2*-----------*2b*-------------- PHASE 3

Exploratory ----------------------------- Primary/Secondary/Exploratory

Pharmacodynamic assessments provide drug response data using drug blood levels or other biomarker and help to guide dose finding and dose regimen in early studies and confirm efficacy in later studies. These assessments may be exploratory objectives in a phase 1 study and may be collected as primary, secondary, or exploratory objectives by phase 3.

- Assessment of safety and tolerability:

PHASE 1 ------------*1b*----------------*2*-----------*2b*-------------- PHASE 3

Primary -- Secondary

Assessment of safety and tolerability is usually derived from the analysis of adverse events, changes in clinical laboratory parameters, and other measures of safety and tolerability. These assessments will be primary objectives in a phase 1 study and may be collected as secondary objectives by phase 3.

- Assessment of efficacy:

PHASE 1 ------------*1b*----------------*2*-----------*2b*-------------- PHASE 3

Exploratory --- Primary

Assessment of efficacy or effectiveness of a drug using surrogate markers is usually derived from the analysis of adverse events, changes in clinical laboratory parameters, and other clinical or laboratory measures. As dose finding and dose regimen and assessment of safety are the primary objectives in phase 1, assessment of efficacy will be exploratory and graduate through phase 2 to be primary objectives by phase 3.

- Number of subjects:

PHASE 1 ------------*1b*----------------2-----------*2b*------------- PHASE 3

Few -- Numerous

The number of subjects to receive the investigational product in a first-in-human trial should be at a minimum and dosing should be staggered based on the anticipated half-life and toxicity of the investigational product in humans derived from nonclinical studies. For example, the first 6 subjects in a cohort of 12 subjects in a first-in-human study may be dosed one at a time and spaced 2 days apart for a half-life of 12 hours, followed by dosing 2 at a time, and so on. As more safety information is obtained from subsequent studies and efficacy becomes the primary objective, the sample size may be statistically determined based on anticipated therapeutic effect. Larger samples will therefore be necessary by phase 3 trials which have statistical controls.

- Study population and eligibility criteria:

PHASE 1 ------------*1b*----------------2-----------*2b*------------- PHASE 3

Broad -- Target for the product label

The subjects enrolled in phase 1 studies are usually healthy volunteers since no safety profile in humans has yet been ascertained and one of the goals for phase 1 studies is to determine pharmacokinetics in humans. However, depending on the known potential toxicity of the investigational product and the risk-benefit of using healthy volunteers, subjects with the targeted disease may be the first to receive the test product. The eligibility criteria for healthy volunteers will be strict to ensure that volunteers are indeed healthy and are not at increased risk for complications because of other underlying disease conditions, and to avoid confounding of the study results (e.g., excretion for a subject with renal insufficiency will differ from subjects with normal renal functioning). If subjects with the targeted disease are enrolled in phase 1 studies (e.g., in oncology trials where the test product may be too toxic for healthy volunteers), the eligibility criteria may be broadened to cover a class of disease, e.g., subjects with metastatic solid tumors. The study population for the phase 2 trials will consist of the target population and the eligibility criteria may narrow to include a specific indication, such as subjects with metastatic non-small cell lung cancer. By phase 3, the study population and eligibility criteria will reflect the target population intended for the product label.

- Statistical controls:

  PHASE 1 ------------*1b*----------------2-----------*2b*------------- PHASE 3

  None -- Randomized and blinded

Statistical controls refer to measures to control bias in a study. The term "bias" describes the systematic tendency of any factors associated with the design, conduct, analysis, and interpretation of the results of clinical trials to make the estimate of a treatment effect deviate from its true value (ICH E9). The most important design techniques for avoiding bias in clinical trials are blinding and randomization, and these should be normal features of most controlled clinical trials intended to be included in a marketing application (ICH E9). Phase 1 studies may employ no statistical controls; i.e, they will be open-label (the full identity, including dose levels, of the test product is known) and all subjects will receive the same treatment. Phase 2 studies may employ one or both measures to control bias and phase 3 trials will most often employ both. The comparator treatment in a phase 3 trial will most often be a placebo if ethically appropriate; else the standard of care will be selected as the comparator. Procedures should be implemented to maintain any level of blinding that is possible and appropriate for a trial to ensure the scientific integrity of the trial.

- Other study design factors:
  Cross-over, parallel cohorts, factorial or other design configurations, and hypothesis testing, and other study design factors are also employed depending on the phase of the trial. We refer the reader to consult external sources for further details which are not addressed in this book.

So, to summarize the above,

- Phase 1 studies consist of the first-in-human trial and other early open-label and uncontrolled phase studies that are conducted to determine pharmacokinetics, safety and tolerability, and dose-finding in small numbers of subjects (typically less than 25) who are either healthy volunteers or subjects with target disease, depending on the potential toxicity and risk-benefit of the investigational product.
- Phase 2 studies consist of semi-controlled (may have blinding and/or randomization) trials that are conducted to determine or confirm safety and the preliminary efficacy of an investigational product in medium to large numbers of subjects (typically approximately 200).

- Phase 3 studies consist of controlled (blinded and randomized) trials that are conducted to determine and confirm the efficacy and safety of an investigational product large to extra-large numbers of subjects (typically approximately 1,000) and are also known as registration or pivotal trials intended to serve as basis for marketing approval.
- Trials that bridge characteristics and objectives between these discreet phases may be designated *Xb*.

However, it should be noted that these factors may overlap through phases, or even skip phases depending on the type of product and the medical need it is expected to serve. For example, investigational products with orphan drug generic designations may require testing per specific phases or to meet a subset of protocol objectives per applicable regulatory requirements.

27.3.2 Phase 4 Studies

Phase 4 studies are performed as necessary to meet regulatory requirements or as desired by the sponsor for continued product development after a product has been approved by the regulatory authorities. They seek to obtain information about drug-drug interactions, dose-response, or long-term safety, epidemiological, or other information that optimizes the drug's use studies (ICH E8). These studies are considered phase 4 if their use is in alignment with the approved label for the product. Any study that contains unapproved use of the product will be categorized as phase 1, 2, or 3, or other depending on the objectives for the trial and the product's use will be considered investigational.

27.4 GCP Considerations for Study Design and Analysis

In this section we will describe the key GCP considerations of ensuring safety, scientific and data integrity as they relate to study design and analysis. The considerations included in this chapter are examples to be addressed when designing a clinical trial and may overlap with Quality-by-design concepts that are described throughout the book.

27.4.1 Safety Considerations

Examples of safety considerations for designing a clinical trial are:

1) Benefit-risk assessment: Before a trial is initiated, the foreseeable benefits risks and inconveniences must be weighed against the anticipated benefit for the individual clinical trial subject and society. A trial should be initiated and

continued only if the anticipated benefits justify the risks (ICH E6(R2) 2.6). Examples of questions to answer are:

a) Is there sufficient medical need to justify initiating this experiment in humans using the investigational product?

b) Are we able to design a trial where the benefits to be gained from conducting the trial and the subject participating in the trial outweigh the potential risks? Are we able to test the investigational product to obtain adequate information to ascertain therapeutic benefit versus risk?

c) Are we able to implement procedures to collect relevant data on benefit and risks to continuously make the benefit-risk assessment during the course of the trial?

d) Are there sufficient resources to adequately control and mitigate risks for the trial and maintain compliance with written procedures, the trial protocol, GCP, and applicable regulatory requirements?

e) Are there resources and procedures implemented to monitor, review, and report all safety findings during the trial?

2) Justification for phase and design elements that affect safety: The available nonclinical and clinical information on an investigational product should be adequate to support the proposed clinical trial (ICH E6(R2) 2.4). Some examples of questions to be answered to justify design elements of a trial are:

a) Is there sufficient information about the properties and mechanism action of the investigational drug to justify the selection of the investigational product for use in the study population for the proposed indication?

b) Is there an unmet medical need for the proposed indication to warrant exposure of the investigational product to humans?

c) Is there sufficient nonclinical and clinical information to justify the proposed initiation of minimum and maximum dose levels and dosing regimen(s) of the investigational product in the trial?

d) Is it safe to expose the number of subjects needed to meet the statistical sample size criteria? Are staggering and other spacing controls needed to test the investigational product in the study population, based on known nonclinical and clinical information about the product?

e) Does the study design require a control comparator? Is it ethical to treat controls with a placebo and deprive them of the standard of care? Do the known and anticipated risks of the selected comparator justify the anticipated benefits of using the selected comparator?

f) Are the eligibility criteria appropriate for the study population to ensure that study subjects do not have medical histories or current medical conditions that will increase their safety risk? Does the study protocol include safety criteria for discontinuing study treatment or the trial but ensuring that subjects continue to have safety follow up?

g) Do investigators have adequate and appropriate information about the investigational product (e.g., in the protocol and/or the investigator's brochure) to guide them on expected adverse events and how to clinically manage those events?

h) Do the study assessments (types, amount, and timing) needed to measure the study endpoints bear undue burden and risks to trial subjects? Are all of the assessments absolutely necessary to measure the study endpoints? Are any study assessments unessential to evaluating the study endpoints?

27.4.2 Scientific Considerations

An example of scientific considerations for designing a clinical trial is the GCP principle that clinical trials should be scientifically sound and described in a clear, detailed protocol (ICH E6(R2) 2.4). Examples of questions to answer are:

a) Is the study design so complex and complicated that it cannot be clearly described in a protocol or is not operationally viable? Are there adequate resources to follow the operational procedures necessary to conduct the trial to ensure its scientific integrity (e.g., randomization, blinding)?

b) Does the statistical design of the trial meet scientific standards for the study phase, population, and indication?

c) Are the selected endpoints reliable, valid, and clinically and scientifically acceptable measures to adequately evaluate the study objectives?

d) Is the study sample size sufficient to satisfy the statistical needs of the study? Is the number of stratification and/or randomization factors appropriate enough to enable evaluable samples sub-populations for analysis? Is the study sample size realistic for enrollment, given the availability of the study population and resources for conducting the trial?

e) Are the eligibility criteria appropriate for the study population and the study objectives? Are the eligibility criteria such that they will hinder study enrollment?

f) Is the plan for statistical analysis stated *a priori* in the trial protocol and/or in the statistical analysis plan (SAP); i.e. before the trial commences or at least prior to locking the trial database?

27.4.3 Data Integrity Considerations

Examples of data integrity considerations for designing and analyzing a clinical trial are similar to the scientific considerations, with a few additions:

a) Are the methods for controlling bias adequate and appropriate for the trial? Are there sufficient resources to effectively manage and monitor the procedures for maintaining study blinding?

b) Are the systems and operational procedures for source data recording, and data entry, verification, review, analysis, and reporting adequate to ensure compliance with written procedures, the trial protocol, GCP, and applicable regulatory requirements?

c) Are all data findings, favorable and unfavorable, reported in the clinical study report? Are unanticipated safety outcomes also analyzed in the clinical study report? Are any changes to the *a priori* statistical plan described in the clinical study report? Are missing data handled per the statistical plan?

27.5 Statistical Analysis Plan

ICH allows for some of the contents or details of some information required to be included in a protocol to be described in separate documents (ICH E6(R2) 6). Typically in practice, the clinical trial protocol will contain high level information of the statistical information required in a protocol (ICH E6(R2) 6.9) and a Statistical Analysis Plan (SAP) is created to provide a more technical and detailed elaboration of the principal features of the analysis described in the protocol, and includes detailed procedures for executing the statistical analysis of the primary and secondary variables and other data (ICH E9). The protocol may provide high level descriptions of the statistical rationale for the study sample size, the analysis populations, the analytical methods to be used to measure the protocol endpoints, and any planned interim analyses (Chapter 18 The Clinical Trial Protocol and Amendments). The SAP will contain greater detail of what is provided in the protocol and additional information such as procedures for accounting for missing, unused, and spurious data, procedures for reporting deviations, procedures for randomization and unblinding, and descriptions of systems for and procedures for compiling and analyzing the data.

The individual clinical trial protocol will contain objectives (which guide the study design), and endpoints (which guide the study assessments). The data generated from the study assessments will be recorded on study source documents and transcribed to the study case report forms (CRF). CRF data will be verified and entered into the study database, then cleaned to prepare for locking the database (Chapter 20 Data Collection and Data Management). Cleaned data will be translated into datasets for statistical analysis. The SAP will describe the methods and procedures for analyzing the data (Plate 8 Individual Study – Data Framework/ Information Flow among Key Trial Documents and Plate 12 Statistical Analysis Plan – Contents). In general, the following will be described in the SAP:

- Methods of subject allocation: A description of the procedures used to allocate study treatment(s) to the trial subjects. When the design of a study calls for measures to control bias, such as in late phases, randomization and/or a range of blinding methods may be deployed. When no measures of control are critical, such as in early phase studies, all subjects will be receiving the same treatment and no blinding measure will be deployed.

- Measurement methods of response variables: A description of how each protocol endpoint will be assessed and measured. The protocol will include the study assessments to be conducted to generate the data for evaluation of safety, tolerability, efficacy, and other protocol objectives. The variables that are typically used to analyze safety and tolerability include vital signs, in physical exam findings, laboratory test results, results from other study-specific clinical safety testing procedures, and clinical adverse events, which include diseases, signs, and symptoms that arise or worsen during the study. Safety data are usually analyzed by treatment assignment and demographics. The variables that will be used to assess and measure efficacy of an investigational product will depend on the therapeutic area being studied, for example, tumor size for an oncology trial or levels of antibodies to measure immunogenicity in a vaccine study. Statistical approaches that are accepted as appropriate by the scientific community will be used to analyze the efficacy of the data. Other approaches may be applied if proven and deemed appropriate.
- Specific hypotheses to be tested: The hypothesis to be tested depends on the type of study and its objectives. Late phase trials may be designed to show superiority, equivalence, or non-inferiority. Trials in all phases of development may include an objective to determine dose-response relationship.
- Analytical approaches to common problems including early study withdrawal and protocol violations.

An example of the sections in an SAP is:

1) Version History: A record of the versions and descriptions of change from each approved version of the SAP
2) Study Description: A description of the study design, treatments, objectives and endpoints, power and sample size justification, and descriptions of randomization and blinding procedures
3) Analysis Populations: Definitions of the analysis populations (e.g., intent to treat, safety population, per protocol population)
4) Definitions and Conventions: Definitions for endpoints, study periods and (e.g., screening, treatment) timepoints (e.g., baseline, end of study); how missing and partial data will be handled;
5) Changes to Planned Analyses: How changes to the planned analyses will be handled and reported
6) Study Population Summaries: Details of how the data for the study population will be analyzed and presented, e.g., subject disposition in the trial (i.e.,

screened, randomized, treated, discontinued, completed), demographics and baseline characteristics, medical history.

7) Study Treatments and Medications: Details of how the data for the study treatments (e.g., exposure, modifications, dosing errors) and concomitant medications and procedures will be analyzed and presented.

8) Efficacy Analyses: Description of the study hypotheses, and details of how the variables for each endpoint will be analyzed and presented.

9) Safety Summaries: Details of how the safety variables will be analyzed and presented, e.g., adverse events, deaths, vital signs, laboratory results

10) Identification and Summary of Protocol Deviations: Definitions of protocol deviations and descriptions of how protocol deviations will be identified and summarized.

11) Data Quality Assurance: Descriptions of systems and quality controls used to compile and analyze the data.

12) Tables, Figures, and Listings: Lists of and mock displays of the planned tables, figures, and listings.

27.6 Preparation of Study Data for Analysis

Some considerations for preparing study data for analyses are:

- Study data for analysis should have been verified against source documents, "cleaned" (i.e., reviewed, queried, and resolved), and approved as complete and accurate (Chapter 20 Data Collection and Data Management).

- Datasets that are prepared for analysis prior to database lock (e.g., for safety data monitoring, informal or formal interim analyses) should be identified with their cutoff dates. The sponsor may perform informal analysis of the data to provide study updates (e.g., for scientific meetings, in protocol amendments or updates to the investigator's brochure) that are not the protocol-prescribed interim analyses. These data should be considered "preliminary" if the data were not completely monitored, verified, cleaned, and approved.

- The data in the locked database will be transcribed into datasets that are compatible with the statistical tools that will be used to perform the statistical analyses.

- The statistical datasets (in practice, often separate datasets for adverse events, efficacy data, etc.) will be generated in standardized data structures and with definitions for variable names to facilitate merging and analysis of multiple datasets within a study and across multiple studies. The standardized structures may also be guided by regulatory requirements and best practices (ICH E9).

27.7 Analyzing and Reporting Study Data

Some considerations for analyzing and reporting study data are:

- Data analysis will be conducted per the protocol and SAP by qualified individuals.
- Changes from the planned analyses as described in the protocol and SAP should be made only if absolutely necessary and must be justified and reported in the CSR.
- Data analysis may occur during the course of the study to monitor data (e.g., in centralized monitoring (Chapter 22 Monitoring Overview) or for informal or formal interim analyses. The sponsor may perform informal analysis of the data to provide study updates (e.g., for scientific meetings, in protocol amendments or updates to the investigator's brochure) that are not the protocol-prescribed interim analyses. Reports for these types of analyses must include the data cutoff date and the data must be identified as "preliminary" if the data were not completely monitored, verified, cleaned, and approved.
- Data results will be summarized and reported in a CSR (Chapter 28 The Clinical Study Report). Data results may also be summarized and reported in formal Interim Study Reports, safety update reports for regulatory reporting (Chapter 21 Safety Monitoring and Reporting), publications, for scientific meetings abstracts and posters, or other presentations.
- All study results should be reported, whether favorable or unfavorable. Unanticipated outcomes, especially of safety information, should be analyzed and reported as necessary.
- Conclusions for data results should address statistical significance versus clinical significance, and correlation versus causality.
- An investigational product should not be claimed as safe or effective in any report or presentation until sufficient data are available to prove such claims. Applicable regulatory requirements should be consulted before making such claims.

27.8 Summary

How studies are designed and analyzed have a direct effect on the data results for a clinical trial. Many factors are to be considered regarding the principles, and processes and procedures that are related to study design and data analyses. An investigational product typically goes through 3 clinical developmental phases to confirm safety and efficacy prior to approval for marketing and additional information about the approved product may be obtained through phase 4 studies. The design for a specific trial will largely depend on the stage of development of the investigational product; i.e., how much is known about its pharmacological properties, and safety and efficacy profiles. Several quality-by-design factors that affect the key GCP concerns of safety and scientific and data integrity should be considered when determining study design and analyses. All study analysis methods should be described *a priori* of database lock and deviations from the plan should be justified, explained, and reported in the Clinical Study Report. Study data prepared for statistical analyses should be structured in standardized formats and be compatible with the statistical tools that will be used to conduct the analyses. Scientifically acceptable statistical methods should be employed for data analyses. Any data that are analyzed prior to database lock should be identified with a cutoff date and reported as preliminary if the data have not been thoroughly monitored, verified, cleaned, and approved as complete and accurate. All study results should be reported, whether favorable or unfavorable. Conclusions for data results should address statistical significance versus clinical significance, and correlation versus causality. An investigational product should not be claimed as safe or effective in any report or presentation until sufficient data are available to prove such claims. ICH Guidelines and applicable regulatory requirements should be consulted and followed when determining study design and data analysis methods reporting.

Knowledge Check Questions

1) What are the characteristics of the 4 phases of clinical development?
2) What are some safety considerations for study design and analysis?
3) What are some scientific considerations for study design and analysis?
4) What are some data integrity considerations for study design and analysis?
5) What are the purpose and content of the statistical analysis plan?
6) What are some considerations for preparing study data for analysis?
7) What are some considerations for analyzing study data and reporting study results?
8) Overheard:

   Let's add these two subjects to the per protocol analysis population. They each missed only one study visit but we can infer their results from the other visits.

   Principal researcher regarding two subjects who almost but did not quite fit the definition for the per protocol population but who had consistent treatment response and about 20% of the subjects had not completed the study.

Comment and discuss:
   a) Was this an appropriate decision?
   b) What are some of possible consequences to taking this action?
   c) What aspects of study design and the SAP are involved in this scenario?
   d) What precautions could have been taken to ensure having an appropriate number of evaluable subjects for data analysis?

References

1 International Council for Harmonisation of Technical Requirements for Pharmaceuticals for Human Use (ICH), Integrated Addendum to ICH E6(R1): Guideline for Good Clinical Practice, E6(R2) (2016). Current Step 4 version dated 9 November 2016. https://www.ich.org/page/efficacy-guidelines (accessed 19 July 2021).
2 International Conference on Harmonisation of Technical Requirements for Registration of Pharmaceuticals for Human Use, ICH Harmonised Tripartite Guideline: General Considerations for Clinical Trials E8 (1997). Current Step 4 version dated 17 July 1997. https://www.ich.org/page/efficacy-guidelines (accessed 19 July 2021).
3 International Conference on Harmonisation of Technical Requirements for Registration of Pharmaceuticals for Human Use, ICH Harmonised Tripartite Guideline: Statistical Principles for Clinical Trials, E9 (1998). Current Step 4 version dated 5 February 1998. https://www.ich.org/page/efficacy-guidelines (accessed 19 July 2021).

28

The Clinical Study Report

Karen A. Henry

GCP Key Point

All clinical trial information should be recorded, handled, and stored in a way that allows its accurate reporting, interpretation and verification (ICH E6(R2) 2.10)

28.1 Introduction

This chapter will focus on what goes into a clinical study/trial report (CSR). This focus not only refers to the actual required elements (ICH E3 Guideline for Structure and Content of Clinical Study Reports) [2,3] but also provides the reasoning for and the sources for the content of the CSR. Personnel involved in trial conduct should be aware that all information about a clinical trial, from the actual protocol document through trial implementation and the analysis of trial results are presented in the CSR. To this end, trial conduct personnel should recognize the interdependences of the various documents and activities that comprise a clinical trial. They will therefore design, organize, and execute the trial ensuring that all clinical trial information are recorded, handled, and stored in a way that allows its accurate reporting, interpretation and verification (ICH E6(R2) 2.10 Principles [3]. ICH E3 and regulatory authorities [4] may also provide detailed templates for presenting trial data in the CSR so it is recommended that trial systems are set up to collect and maintain trial information accordingly to facilitate availability and transfer of the information to the CSR. Since the ultimate use of the clinical trial data for the CSR is for integration with other trials in the clinical development process for an investigational product, it is also prudent that, as much as is possible, standards are established for the uniform recording, handling, and storage of trial information for all clinical trials to be included in the application dossier.

The Fundamentals of Clinical Research: A Universal Guide for Implementing Good Clinical Practice, First Edition. P. Michael Dubinsky and Karen A. Henry.
© 2022 John Wiley & Sons, Inc. Published 2022 by John Wiley & Sons, Inc.
Companion website: www.wiley.com/go/dubinsky/clinicalresearch

In this chapter, we will focus on the contents of and the operational activities involved in developing a CSR to meet the regulatory requirements. In this chapter, a clinical study report is synonymous with clinical trial report.

28.2 Objectives

The objectives of this chapter are:

1) Define a clinical study report
2) Describe the purpose of a clinical study report
3) Describe the context for a clinical study report in an individual clinical trial and in clinical development
4) Describe the types of clinical study reports
5) Describe the contents of a clinical study report
6) Describe the process for developing a clinical study report
7) Describe typical deficiencies of a clinical study report
8) Discuss changes to a clinical study report
9) Discuss quality-by-design considerations for the contents of the CSR

28.2.1 Definition of a Clinical Study/Trial Report

A Clinical Trial/Study Report (CSR) is a written description of a trial/study of any therapeutic, prophylactic, or diagnostic agent conducted in human subjects, in which the clinical and statistical description, presentations, and analyses are fully integrated into a single report (ICH E3 Guideline for Structure and Content of Clinical Study Reports) (ICH E6(R2) 1.13). The CSR is the description of how a trial was conducted and the results and interpretation of the trial and is written at the conclusion of the trial.

28.2.2 Purpose of a Clinical Study/Trial Report

Whether the trial is completed or prematurely terminated, the sponsor should ensure that the clinical trial reports are prepared and provided to the regulatory agency(ies) as required by the applicable regulatory requirement(s) (ICH E6(R2) 5.22). The CSR documents the results and interpretation of the trial (ICH E6(R2) 8.4.8).

The CSR is intended to describe the methods used for conducting a trial and the results and the interpretation of the results for a trial. This information allows regulatory authorities and other interested parties (such as clinical investigators, drug development partners) the opportunity to review and assess the clinical experiment for its scientific integrity and for the new information it contributes regarding the safety, efficacy, clinical pharmacology, of the investigational product, the class of products, or therapeutic area under study. The trial information in the CSR may also facilitate the production of post-trial publications and other data summaries to be issued for general public viewing.

28.3 Context for a Clinical Study/Trial Report in a Clinical Trial and in Clinical Development

The CSR is one of the key documents for a clinical trial. It is the culminating document that contains all trial inputs (Plate 14 Clinical Study Report – Contents):

- The clinical trial protocol
- Statistics and data analysis: methods and reports
- Trial management: study conduct and study administrative structure
- Clinical supplies: identity and batch(s), allocation of treatment to subjects
- IRB/IEC and regulatory authority communication: IRB/IECs used and IRB/IEC or RA issues
- Data collection and data management: trial data and sample case report forms
- Laboratory testing: testing procedures, results, and standardization of normal ranges
- Trial monitoring: protocol and trial deviations
- Quality assurance: quality assurance procedures and audits and findings
- Regulatory inspections: inspections and findings
- Publications of study results

All inputs will be recorded as essential documents and included in the study files (Chapter 29 Essential Documents). Inputs for the CSR may be grouped as reporting of study design and conduct (i.e., the study methods) and study results as follows:

- Study methods:
  - Study protocol
    - o Study objectives
    - o Study endpoints
    - o Study assessments
    - o Ethical and regulatory requirements
  - Informed consent forms templates
  - Case report forms templates
  - Statistical analysis plan (SAP)
  - Study administrative structure, including transfer of research obligations to contract research organizations (CROs)

– Study operating procedures, such as quality assurance and control methods, as they pertain to the trial data, e.g. monitoring, informed consent procedures.
– List of investigators
– List of IRBs/IECs
– Investigational product identity and batches
– Planned changes to the investigation; i.e., changes and amendments to any of the above

Study results:

• Subject screening and eligibility data
• Subject enrollment (including randomization) and treatment
• Study assessments results
  – Safety, pharmacology, and efficacy laboratory testing results
  – Results of all other assessments

• Adverse events and narratives of safety events
• Completed case report forms for significant adverse events
• Statistical reports (i.e., tables, listings, and figures) generated from the statistical analyses
• Protocol deviations
• Deviations from the pre-database lock SAP
• Audits and inspections results
• Publications on the study pre-finalization of the CSR

Recall that a single clinical trial protocol is only one of the set of various protocols that will be executed as part of the general clinical development or investigational plan that supports the target product profile for a product (Chapter 3 GCP in Context; Plate 1 Clinical Development and Trials Process). Also, each individual clinical trial protocol is designed to obtain specific information that will enhance knowledge of the safety and efficacy of the use of the product in the target patient population. Consequently, the CSR for an individual trial provides information that is specific to that trial and the addition of the results from each clinical trial accumulate safety, pharmacological, and efficacy information about the investigational product. This cumulative knowledge base of the investigational product will help to inform the sponsor and the regulatory authorities of the scientific needs for the next trial in the development program.

When a sponsor is submitting an application for approval for marketing a product, the sponsor will integrate all data from the collection of individual supportive and pivotal trials that are relevant to support the claim(s) for safety and efficacy of the product for the proposed indication. It is helpful if there have been established standards that were consistently used for the trial design and structure of the databases for each trial from phase 1 to phase 3 to facilitate combining the data from the various trials. This is not to say that all trials will have the same research design and objectives, but it is saying that each trial will employ similar properties for design and structure, such as, similar testing procedures (e.g. assays for laboratory testing), similar assessments for measuring safety and efficacy (e.g., scales or instruments), have similar definitions for analysis populations, and similar data definitions for study variables (e.g., groupings for categorical variables).

28.3.1 Types of Clinical Study/Trial Reports

Regulatory authorities may have different requirements for the reporting of clinical trial results depending on the type of study, terminating status of the study and the intended use of the study results. There are generally three types of final and complete CSRs and other subtypes of partial information for a CSR:

1) A full report
   The full report contains complete and comprehensive descriptions of study design, conduct, analyses, results, and interpretation of all study results and generally conforms to the requirements of the ICH E3 Guideline. The full report is usually required for controlled studies and for studies that will be used in support of the effectiveness evaluation of an investigational product in an application for marketing approval.
2) An abbreviated report
   An abbreviated report contains summarized study methods, comprehensive safety results and interpretations, and summarized efficacy. The report may be written for uncontrolled studies, seriously flawed or aborted studies, or for controlled studies that examine conditions clearly unrelated to those for which a claim for approval for marketing is made. An abbreviated report should contain sufficient detail of design and results to allow the regulatory authority to determine whether a full report is needed. (ICH E3 Guideline). The sponsor should consult with the governing regulatory authority for guidance on content and the acceptability of an abbreviated report for a specific trial.
3) A report synopsis
   A synopsis (ICH E3 Guideline has an example of the format and content of the synopsis) may be prepared and submitted as a stand-alone document to a regulatory authority for a study. The regulatory authority may require the synopsis in advance of the full report, or may accept the synopsis alone in an application for approval for marketing if the study is needed to contribute toward the safety evaluation of a product but is not needed for the product's evaluation of efficacy or clinical pharmacology. (FDA Guidance for Industry, Submission of Abbreviated Reports and Synopses in Support of Marketing Applications, U.S. Department of Health and Human Services, Food and Drug Administration,

Center for Drug Evaluation and Research (CDER), Center for Biologics Evaluation and Research (CBER), August 1999, Clinical). The sponsor should consult with the governing regulatory authority for guidance on the acceptability of a synopsis report for a specific trial.

4) Subtypes with partial information

a) Supplemental

A CSR may be updated with supplementary information if new study information becomes available after the CSR is finalized. For example, survival data collected after a trial is completed may be analyzed and prepared as a supplemental report to the original CSR.

b) Interim

An interim CSR would be generated for data analysis prior to the completion of a trial and would be updated with the final data for the final CSR.

c) Erratum

An *erratum* to a final CSR may be provided for *ad hoc* errors found after a final CSR has been submitted to the regulatory authority (Section 28.3.5).

d) CSR amendment

A final CSR may be amended in extreme circumstances (Section 28.3.5).

28.3.2 Contents of a Clinical Study/Trial Report

The discussion in this section pertains to a full CSR. Information in the CSR may be added or reduced depending on the type of CSR as described above.

The ICH E3 Guideline outlays sections for the general contents and format of a clinical study report as follows:

- **Administrative**
  - Sections 1–4
- **Study Conduct** (includes planned investigation and changes from the planned investigation)
  - Sections 5–9, and some in 16
- **Study Results** (includes protocol deviations)
  - Sections 10–15, and some in 16

The contents of a CSR, except for the interpretations of trial results, must be traceable to the evidence of trial conduct; i.e., the essential documents in the study files.

Below are the contents of the various sections. Please refer to ICH E3 for details. However, here are some considerations for compiling information for the sections.

28.3.2.1 Administrative

- Section 1.0 Title Page

Much of the title page information will be in the protocol.

The study initiation date is the date of first patient consent, or any other verifiable definition (e.g., data the first subject was randomized).

The date of study completion or date of early study termination is the date of the last subject study visit or contact.

All dates should be verifiable in the listings provided with the CSR.

- Section 2.0 Synopsis (see Section 28.3.3.3.1)
- Section 3.0 Table of Contents
- Section 4.0 List of Abbreviations and Definitions of Terms

28.3.2.2 Study Conduct

- Sections 5 (Ethics), 7 to 9 (Introduction, Study Objectives, Investigational Plan)
- These sections describe how the study was planned to be conducted. It will also describe any changes to the planned study conduct. The discussion should provide the reader with a clear and complete description of the development context for the trial, the planned investigation, and what, when with respect to unblinding of the data, and the implications of changes to the planned investigation, if any, occurred. Per ICH E6(R2) 5.0.7, the sponsor should describe the quality management approach implemented in the trial and summarize important deviations from the predefined quality tolerance limits and remedial actions taken in the clinical study report.

The following sources should be considered for such relevant information:

- Original protocol
- Protocol amendments
- Changes in study conduct communicated via:
    o Administrative letters/Letters to investigators
    o Newsletters to investigational sites and CROs
    o Relevant trial communication (emails, telephone contacts)
    o Project and study team meetings (meeting minutes)
    o Written agreements with investigators
    o Written agreements with CROs or other vendors
    o Written Charters and minutes of meetings for data monitoring committees
- Case report form amendments
- Changes in randomization procedures
- Changes in data collection procedures
- Changes in subject screening procedures (e.g., rescreening)
- Changes in, e.g., drug storage requirements, packaging, labeling as described in the protocol
- Changes in, e.g., pharmacology testing procedures, assays
- Changes to the SAP
- Changes to, e.g., investigator assessment of endpoints, definitions for analysis sets, new analyses, changes in Ns
- Changes to, e.g., safety collection and follow-up periods, committees procedures
- Quality assurance pre-study qualification and on- and post-study auditing activities
- All other media used for communicating study information or documenting study information

- Section 6.0 Investigators and Study Administrative Structure
  This section provides the reader with the identities, roles, and responsibilities for those who were involved in the execution of the trial. For each trial function, it will describe:
  - If the sponsor, CRO, and/or other third party/vendor was responsible
  - Name, address. and contact name of responsible party
  - Detailed summary of obligation if delegated to CRO/third party
  The responsible party(ies) for the following trial functions will be identified:
  - Medical oversight and safety
  - Pharmacovigilance (relevant staff including the medical reviewer and the location and "ownership" of the database)
  - Biometry/statistics
  - Data management and the clinical trial database
  - Medical writing
  - Trial files maintenance and management system
  - Other databases (please specify)
  - Project-/trial management (key/lead) and sponsor oversight
  - Clinical trial monitoring
  - Randomization
  - CRO selection and qualification
  - Auditing
  - Central laboratory testing and analysis services (e.g. ECG, specimen testing, imaging)
  - Randomization process and the randomization list generation and management
  - Investigational product supply, packaging, labeling, shipment, tracking, returns, disposition (Manufacturer of the investigational product should be indicated in Section 9.4 Treatment)
  - Data monitoring/evaluation committees
  - Other activities

28.3.2.3 Study Results

These sections will include a report of important study deviations from the planned trial procedures (including planned changes to the trial), and presentation of trial data (tables, figures, and listings) and discussions and interpretations of the trial data. Clinical data are presented as tables, which are the data summarized for frequencies or other descriptive or inferential statistical results, figures, with graphical depictions (e.g., bar charts, data plots) of the data, and listings, which are lines of individual datapoints. It is typical for summary data presented in tables to be supported by listings showing the individual datapoints. For example, a summary table of subject demographics may depict frequencies and descriptive statistics of demographic characteristics by treatment groups for all subjects who were administered the investigational product (the safety population). A corresponding listing will display rows of the demographic characteristics for each individual subject, grouped by treatment group.

The following are sections related to trial results:

- Section 10 Study Patients
This section describes the disposition of study subjects and important protocol deviations.
  - 10.1 Disposition of Subjects
  This section includes summary tables, listings, and accountability of all subjects from consent to the end of study, to describe subjects who:
    - o Consented and screened
    - o Screen failed, including reason(s) for screen fail
    - o Enrolled: randomized, treated, discontinued treatment and/or study (including reason), completed the study
  - 10.2 Protocol Deviations

  This section includes a summary table, listing, and discussion of important deviations related to study inclusion or exclusion criteria, conduct of the trial, patient management, or patient assessment. Important deviations may be committed by the investigator, sponsor, or their representatives, or by the research subject.
- Section 11.0 Efficacy Evaluation
This section includes summary tables, listings, and discussions of planned analyses (per the protocol, protocol amendments, and the SAP) and unanticipated necessary analyses related to efficacy of the investigational product.

  Note, data and discussions for efficacy endpoints may be omitted from this section for studies that contain only pharmacological testing and be presented in a separately titled section.

  This section will address the following, as applicable:
  - 11.1 Data Sets Analyzed
  - 11.2 Demographic and Other Baseline Characteristics
  - 11.3 Measurements of Treatment Compliance
  A method for ensuring treatment compliance should be established for the study and the method may be a documented process or measurable. For example, a process is that study drug will be administered by qualified study site personnel and this will be documented; whereas, the collection of laboratory data to determine the pharmacological levels of study drug may be used as a measure of compliance for study treatment that is self-administered at home by study subjects.
  - 11.4 Efficacy Results and Tabulations of Individual Patient Data
    - o 11.4.1 Analysis of Efficacy
    - o 11.4.2 Statistical/Analytical Issues

- 11.4.2.1 Adjustments for Covariates
- 11.4.2.2 Handling of Dropouts or Missing Data
- 11.4.2.3 Interim Analyses and Data Monitoring
- 11.4.2.4 Multicentre Studies
- 11.4.2.5 Multiple Comparison/Multiplicity
- 11.4.2.6 Use of an "Efficacy Subset" of Patients
- 11.4.2.7 Active-Control Studies Intended to Show Equivalence
- 11.4.2.8 Examination of Subgroups
  - o 11.4.3 Tabulation of Individual Response Data
  - o 11.4.4 Drug Dose, Drug Concentration, and Relationships to Response and by demographics
  - o 11.4.5 Drug–Drug and Drug–Disease Interactions, and Relationships to Response and by Demographics
  - o 11.4.6 By-Patient Displays
  - o 11.4.7 Conclusions – pharmacology
- Section 12.0 Safety Evaluation

This section includes summary tables, listings, and discussions of planned analyses (per the protocol, protocol amendments, and the SAP) and unanticipated necessary analyses related to safety of the investigational product.

The following should be considered sources for safety information to be presented in this section:

- The clinical database (Chapter 20 Data Collection and Data Management)
- The safety database (Chapter 21 Safety Monitoring and Reporting)
- Meeting minutes from safety data monitoring, special steering, or data evaluation committees or individuals
- Submissions of individual, summary, and periodic safety reports to investigators, ethics committees, and regulatory authorities
- Safety reports and clinical chart and safety information obtained from investigators, other health care providers, or subject self-reporting for the subjects
- Other relevant and valid sources

The sponsor should determine and document the hierarchy of sourcing for the safety data; for example, whether the data in safety narratives from clinical charts override data in the clinical database (i.e., reported via the case report forms) or *vice versa*.

This section will address the following, as applicable:

- 12.1 Extent of Exposure
- 12.2 Adverse Events
- 12.3 Deaths, Other Serious Adverse Events, and Other Significant Adverse Events
- 12.4 Clinical Laboratory Evaluation
  - o 12.4.2 Evaluation of Each Laboratory Parameter

- ■ 12.4.2.1 Laboratory Values Over Time
- ■ 12.4.2.2 Individual Patient Changes
- ■ 12.4.2.3 Individual Clinically significant Abnormalities
- – 12.5 Vital Signs, Physical Findings, and Other Observations Related to Safety
- Section 13.0 Discussion and Overall Conclusions
  All conclusions must be supported by information contained within the CSR.
- Section 14.0 Tables, Figures, and Graphs Referred to but not Included in the Text
  - – 14.1 Demographic Data
  - – 14.2 Efficacy Data
  - – 14.3 Safety Data
- Section 15.0 Reference List
- Section 16.0 Appendices
  - – 16.1 Study Information
    - o 16.1.1 Appendices – Protocol and Protocol Amendments
    - o 16.1.2 Sample Case Report Form(s) (CRFs) [unique pages only]
    - o Include sample patient diary card or other data collection tools
    - o 16.1.3 List of IECs of IRBs [plus the name of the committee chair if required by the regulatory authority]
    - o Include Representative Written Information for Patient and Sample Consent Forms (can be the template developed for the study)
    - o 16.1.4 List and Description of Investigators:

Name of investigator	Site (Full address)	Country	Number of subjects screened	Number of subjects enrolled

Note: Investigator CVs of equivalent summaries of training and experience relevant to the performance of the clinical study must be in the TMF.

- – If investigator sites were located in different countries, include the total number of sites and subjects enrolled per country:

Country	Total number of sites enrolling patients	Total number of subjects enrolled

- o 16.1.5 Signatures of Principal or Coordinating Investigator(s) (must have for EU countries) or Sponsor's Responsible Medical Officer [depending on the regulatory authority's requirement]
- o 16.1.6 Listing of Subjects Receiving Test Drug(s)/Investigational Product(s) From Specific Batches, Where More Than One Batch Was Used
- o 16.1.7 Randomization Scheme and Codes (Patient Identification and Treatment Assigned)

o 16.1.8 Audit Certificates (if available)

o 16.1.9 Documentation of Statistical Methods (if not provided in the body of the report)

o 16.1.10 Documentation of Inter-Laboratory Standardization Methods and Quality Assurance Procedures if used (for pivotal studies where these represent study end-points and otherwise on request)

o 16.1.11 Publications Based on the Study

o 16.1.12 Important Publications Referenced in the Report

o 16.2 Subject Data Listings

– 16.2.1 Discontinued Subjects

o 16.2.2 Protocol Deviations

o 16.2.3 Subjects Excluded from the Efficacy Analysis

o 16.2.4 Demographic Data

o 16.2.5 Compliance and/or Drug Concentration Data [if available]

o 16.2.6 Individual Efficacy Response Data

o 16.2.7 Adverse Event Listing (each patient)

o 16.2.8 Listing of Individual Laboratory Measurements by Patient [when required by regulatory authorities

– 16.3 Subject CRFs

o 16.3.1 CRFs for Death, Other Serious Adverse Events, and Withdrawals for Adverse Events (safety reports to regulatory authorities should be in the TMF)

o 16.3.2 Other CRFs Submitted

– 16.4 Individual Patient Data Listings

28.3.3 Process for Developing a Clinical Study/Trial Report

As seen from the prescribed contents of the CSR, as is for the protocol, the information to be included are of a wide variety and, in product development, these information are generated by a variety of specialized expertise.

The development process is also similar to that for creating any document: creating an outline, drafting, review, and finalization. In the case of a clinical trial CSR, it is standard procedure for the document to also be ascribed formal signature(s) of approval.

28.3.3.1 Defining Roles and Timelines

Per ICH E6 5.4, the sponsor should utilize qualified individuals (e.g., biostatisticians, clinical pharmacologists, and physicians) as appropriate, throughout all stages of the trial process, from designing the protocol and CRFs and planning the analyses to analyzing and preparing interim and final clinical trial reports. For the collaboration, it will be necessary to identify the owner of the document's content and the writer for the document (if the individuals are different), who are the reviewers and approvers, and who will make final decisions in the event of conflicting opinions or unresolved issues. Standard operating procedures for the firm may stipulate which roles in the organization are the required reviewers and approvers.

Note: The single-center trial investigator or the multicenter coordinating investigator will at least review and approve the CSR (ICH E3).

The CSR has contributions from various subject matter experts (SMEs) and individuals, such as the medical monitor and the biostatistician, will collaborate to determine interpretations and conclusions of the study results.

Note: The analytical methods would have been determined *a priori* in the SAP, unless unanticipated results warrant additional analyses.

The SMEs may include the medical monitor, biostatistician, clinical pharmacologist (for pharmacology testing and reporting), and study team personnel responsible for trial management and operations (for investigator and ethics committee information, study operations deviations, etc.), pharmacovigilance (for safety reporting data, narratives, etc.), study drug supplies (for investigational product identity, distribution, issues, etc.), and quality assurance (for audit information). The writer will consult with the contributors to determine the discussion content, including interpretations and conclusions, for the CSR.

To facilitate the collaboration, a meeting may be organized with contributors, reviewers, and approvers to agree on interpretations of the data, CSR development timelines, expected deliverables from contributors, and the scope of review from reviewers and approvers. The timelines will include the anticipated date for delivery of the statistical outputs (tables, figures, and listings) as these are needed to discuss and prepare the study results. The CSR writer will inform each SME of the specific information needed for CSR and establish a system for receiving the information.

28.3.3.2 Clinical Study/Trial Report Structure and Content

As described above, the structure and content for the CSR are generally already stipulated by the ICH (ICH E3) and applicable regulatory requirements, which may be reflected in standard operating procedures along with additional contents specific to the firm, including writing styles and conventions. The CSR largely contains a synopsis, and administrative, study methods, and study results information. These sections comprise text, in-text tables, figures, and listings, as well as several appendices of trial documents and reports of study data.

28.3.3.3 Drafting, Reviewing, and Approving the Clinical Study/Trial Report

The CSR sections may be drafted and reviewed all at once, or in parts as a time-saving strategy. For example, the writer may prepare the administrative and methods sections using the sources presented above in advance of the delivery of the statistical reports. The results sections would then be drafted once the study results are available, and the synopsis may lastly be prepared because it contains the summarized study results and the conclusions.

The typical process for the development of a document is displayed in Plate 19 Typical Process for Document Development. For a CSR:

1) The writer uses the contributions from SMEs, the interpretations as discussed with the SMEs, and other sources of information to draft the CSR, ensuring that the required elements are included.
2) The drafted document is reviewed by assigned reviewers and approvers, and their comments are adjudicated until there is agreement on the contents. The writer will be keen to maintain version control throughout the development process.
3) To foster quality, the document should be checked for accuracy and compliance with standard operating procedures and regulatory requirements prior to being finalized, for example, a checklist may be used to ensure that all required elements are present.
   ➢ The CSR content should be checked against its sources, for internal consistency of information within the document, and for consistency with the appendices.
4) The person(s) who will take responsibility for the content of the CSR will lastly document their approval.
5) The CSR will be submitted to the regulatory authority(ies) and investigator(s), as applicable.

28.3.3.3.1 Developing the Clinical Study/Trial Report Synopsis The writer will prepare the CSR synopsis after completion of the content for the CSR but prior to approval of the CSR.

The format and content of the synopsis is per ICH E3 and applicable regulatory requirements. The content of the synopsis must stand alone from the full CSR; i.e., contain sufficient summary information and not have references to the full CSR. The synopsis is a summary of the study design, critical methodological information, study population, disposition of subjects, important protocol deviations, treatment compliance, safety and efficacy results (including numerical data and not just text or p-values), and interpretations of study results.

A synopsis of the full report is usually placed at the beginning of a full report or may be submitted to a regulatory authority as a stand-alone document (see Section 28.3.1).

28.3.4 Typical Deficiencies in a Clinical Study/Trial Report

Regulatory authority(ies) may inspect a clinical trial in conjunction with its CSR as part of their review of a sponsor's application for marketing approval of a product. The authority(ies) may employ different inspection strategies; such as reviewing the data in the database and comparing the results with the CSR, or reviewing the essential documents at investigator sites and/or at the sponsor's and comparing them with the content in the CSR. The results of the inspector's review will permit the authority to determine whether the trial data are acceptable for inclusion in the assessment of safety and efficacy for approval of the product for marketing. A sponsor's goal is to ensure that all relevant trial data are included. Forcibly excluded data means a significant loss of time and money for the sponsor and could mean unnecessary additional exposure of the investigational product if a trial has to be repeated.

Examples of inspectional findings that are related to a CSR are:

- Inaccurate reporting of administrative information regarding vendors/contractors: the CSR stated that the CRO monitored all investigational sites but the sponsor had actually independently monitored 2 of those sites
- Inaccurate reporting of randomization procedures: The CSR stated that investigators obtained randomization assignments for subjects via a specified electronic system but the sponsor had verbally provided the assignment for 4 subjects before the electronic system was launched.
- Inaccurate reporting of protocol deviations: The numbers and types of protocol deviations that were reported in the CSR did not match the essential documents at the investigational sites.
- Inaccurate reporting of subject screening procedures: The CSR omitted that some subjects were rescreened if certain laboratory screening results were outside the eligibility boundaries.
  - Definitions for analysis sets: The definition of the per-protocol population (i.e., the collection window for the acceptance of a subject's blood draw for drug concentration was widened for inclusion in the per-protocol population but this was not mentioned in the CSR
  - Changes/deviations in drug storage requirements: The parameters for acceptable temperature excursions for the storage of the investigational product administered to subjects were widened for inclusion of the subjects in the per-protocol population but this was not mentioned in the CSR.
- Unsupported safety or efficacy conclusions about the trial: The CSR claimed that the investigational product was safe and well-tolerated, but the study results contained significant adverse events that were not discussed for their relationship to the study drug. The CSR also claimed efficacy based on p-value estimation methods that were not included in the SAP nor included as changes to the planned analyses.

It is therefore important that procedures are established to ensure the accurate reporting of trial results in a CSR to avoid findings of deficiencies that may negatively impact the quality of the CSR and the information available for review of the benefit-risk of an investigational product.

28.3.5 Changes to a Clinical Study/Trial Reports

Changes to a finalized CSR, regardless of the type of CSR (Section 28.3.1) may be administrative or substantive.

If the changes to a CSR are administrative; i.e., they do not affect the understanding of the results or interpretation of the data, then an *erratum* may be created and submitted. For example, corrections may be provided for a row of data was inadvertently omitted from a table or for the contact information that was incorrect for a responsible party in the study administrative structure. Additionally, clarifications may be provided for inconsistently reported information in the report.

If the changes are substantive; i.e., the changes affect the understanding and or the results of the data, then the CSR may be amended or rewritten, depending on the extent of the changes. A CSR may be amended or rewritten under extreme circumstances, such as if an error is identified that affects the understanding of the data and/or the interpretation of the study results. For example, if an incorrect or inappropriate definition for any of the analysis populations for a trial was used for a CSR, and the new definition globally affects the study results for the changed populations, then the CSR may have to be significantly amended or rewritten.

If changes to a final approved clinical study report are required, the report must be amended via an authorized procedure.

28.3.6 Quality-by-Design Considerations for the Contents of a Clinical Study/Trial Report

A number of principles and operational considerations that promote GCP, quality, and compliance may guide the planning and contents a CSR. Data principles and trial operations considerations to foster quality for the CSR include:

- Clinical research context: The context for a clinical study/trial report in a clinical trial and in clinical development, which are key considerations for facilitating the quality of individual CSRs, integrated CSR data, and applications for marketing approval.
- Publishing: Regardless of the medium used to submit a single clinical study report or a collection of reports (e.g., printed hard copy or electronic), the publisher will be cross-referencing information within the individual report as well as externally to the report(s). It is helpful if the organization of the information is standardized across all reports to simplify the publishing. Regulatory authority(ies) may also have requirements for publishing CSRs and applications for marketing approval of a product.
- Relationship with the Trial Master File: Except for the interpretation of trial results, all study conduct and results information in the CSR must be supported by the essential documents for a trial. It is helpful for the study team to be aware

of and plan data collection and documentation of study information accordingly to ensure that the information is complete and readily available for the CSR. For example,

- The operations team may maintain documentation of the study administrative structure and a list of the investigators with all contact details, any changes to investigators, and any transfers of research subjects between investigators.
- The study team will ensure that important protocol deviations are tracked and entered into the clinical database.
- The study team will document and log all changes to the planned investigation, not only for protocol amendments, but also for inclusion in the CSR, especially if the changes are not included in protocol amendments.
- The study team will ensure that narratives of significant safety events (per ICH E3) are prepared and formatted in a standardized manner for inclusion in the appendices of the CSR.

• The CSR template per ICH E3: Following the ICH Guideline not only helps to assure that all required information are included in the CSR, but it helps to organize the information to facilitate review by regulatory authorities. Notably, the Guidance is flexible for information that is not applicable to the specific study or information about the study that needs to be added but is not addressed in the template.

The study team should establish processes that will ensure the accurate and complete reporting of trial conduct and results in a CSR. It is important for the team to plan for the reporting of the study conduct and results during study start-up and on-study management to ensure that all information for the CSR are organized and ready for implementation during the creation of the CSR.

28.4 Summary

The CSR is a written description of a trial/study of any therapeutic, prophylactic, or diagnostic agent conducted in human subjects, in which the clinical and statistical description, presentations, and analyses are fully integrated into a single report.

The CSR documents the conduct, results, and interpretation of a clinical trial. Regulatory authorities governing the location of a clinical trial and investigators participating in the conduct of a clinical trial will want to receive a report of the conduct and results of the trial. Additionally, sponsors may want to report trial results in publications and may be required to report trial results in public registries for clinical trials.

The CSR is the reporting of study conduct and results for a single trial but consideration should be given to the fact that the information for a single trial will be combined with the information from multiple trials in an application for approval for marketing a product.

Study conduct and results may be reported in a full, abbreviated, or supplemental CSR, depending on the status of the trial and the intended use of the report. Interim study results may be reported in an interim report, which will be followed by a complete report upon conclusion of the trial.

The contents of a CSR are prescribed by the ICH E3 Guidance or applicable regulatory requirements. A CSR generally contains administrative information, study conduct or methods (i.e., a description of the planned investigation and planned changes from the planned investigation), and study results (i.e., important protocol deviations and presentation and interpretation of the study data, including study conclusions). The sponsor will determine which ICH sections are applicable to the specific trial and may also add sections as appropriate for the specific trial. All CSR information, except for interpretation of trial results, should be supported by sources contained in the essential documents for a trial.

A CSR is developed similarly to other clinical technical documents with assigned owners, writers, reviewers, and approvers. Minimum approvers are stipulated by regulatory requirements. Administrative changes to a CSR may be communicated via an erratum but substantive changes, i.e., those that affect the understanding and/or interpretation of the study results, may necessitate an amended or rewritten CSR.

Several considerations to enable quality-by-design principles can be factored into the preparation of information for a CSR to avoid typical and potentially costly deficiencies. To ensure highest quality, all trial SMEs should be aware of their required contribution for a CSR and should plan for the reporting of the study conduct and results during study start-up and on-study management to ensure that all information for the CSR are organized and ready for implementation during the creation of the CSR.

Knowledge Check Questions

1) What is a CSR?
2) What is the purpose of a CSR?
3) What are the contents of a CSR?
4) What are the types of CSRs?
5) What are some of the triggers for changing a CSR?
6) What are the key quality-by-design considerations for planning for a CSR?
7) Overheard:

   Absence of evidence is not evidence of absence.

   Regulatory affairs executive referring to conclusions about the performance of the investigational drug in the drafted clinical study report based on analyses that were not performed because the data were not collected as it was deemed unnecessary based on theoretical assumptions.

Comment and discuss:

a) What are some of the typical deficiencies of a CSR?
b) What aspects of the CSR are linked to the essential documents?

References

1 International Council for Harmonisation of Technical Requirements for Pharmaceuticals for Human Use (ICH), Guideline for Structure and Content of Clinical Study Reports, E3 (1995). Current Step 4 version dated 30 November 1995. https://www.ich.org/page/efficacy-guidelines

2 E3 Implementation Working Group ICH E3 (2012). Guideline: Structure and Content of Clinical Study Reports Questions & Answers (R1) Current version dated 6 July 2012. https://www.ich.org/page/efficacy-guidelines

3 ICH E6(R2): International Council for Harmonisation of Technical Requirements for Pharmaceuticals for Human Use (ICH), Integrated Addendum to ICH E6(R1):Guideline for Good Clinical Practice, E6(R2) (2016), Current Step 4 version dated 9 November 2016. https://www.ich.org/page/efficacy-guidelines

4 United States Food and Drug Administration Guidance for Industry, Submission of Abbreviated Reports and Synopses in Support of Marketing Applications, U.S. Department of Health and Human Services, Food and Drug Administration, Center for Drug Evaluation and Research (CDER), Center for Biologics Evaluation and Research (CBER), August 1999, Clinical. https://www.fda.gov/media/71125/download

29

Essential Documents

Karen A. Henry

GCP Key Point

Essential documents are the evidence of trial conduct: If it is not documented, it did not happen; and if it did not happen, it should not be documented.

29.1 Introduction

All clinical trial information should be recorded, handled, and stored in a way that allows its accurate reporting, interpretation, and verification (ICH E6(R2) 2.10). The essential documents are all that exist of evidence of trial conduct. As is often said in the industry: *If it is not documented, it did not happen; and if it did not happen, it should not be documented.*

Trial information comprises not only study data collected via the CRFs, but also the records of all trial procedures and GCP and regulatory compliance processes. These records of trial information are known as essential documents. A reviewer of trial conduct (e.g., monitor, auditor, inspector, or other authorized individual) should be able to analyze or reconstruct, at any time during the course of the trial or after the trial has completed, exactly how the trial was executed based on the records. A reviewer should readily be able to access any important information of a trial with confidence that such information is accurate and true. It is therefore important that ALCOAC principles are used to generate records and essential documents are current, organized, accessible, and legible at all times per the protocol, GCP, and applicable regulatory requirements. There is no trial if there are no essential documents of the trial.

In this chapter, we will review the list of essential documents and describe their attributes, including how they should be structured, maintained, monitored, and retained.

The Fundamentals of Clinical Research: A Universal Guide for Implementing Good Clinical Practice, First Edition. P. Michael Dubinsky and Karen A. Henry.
© 2022 John Wiley & Sons, Inc. Published 2022 by John Wiley & Sons, Inc.
Companion website: www.wiley.com/go/dubinsky/clinicalresearch

29.2 Objectives

The objectives of this chapter are to:

1) Define essential documents and their purpose
2) Describe essential documents
3) Describe important attributes for essential documents
4) Describe practices for good documentation
5) Describe the structure and location of files
6) Describe written procedures for managing essential documents
7) Describe retention and archiving of documents
8) Describe access to essential documents

29.2.1 Definition and Purpose

Essential Documents are those documents which individually and collectively permit evaluation of the conduct of a study and the quality of the data produced (ICH E6(R2) 1.23, 8.1).

> ➢ Essential documents are the evidence of trial conduct.

29.2.2 List of Essential Documents

The ICH has provided a comprehensive list of the minimum essential documents that should be maintained as evidence of the trial along with the purpose for each document (ICH E6(R2) 8.2-4). The files for a trial may have more or fewer documents, depending on applicable regulatory requirements and the protocol design. The list groups and displays the documents according to the stage of the trial during which they will normally be generated:

1) Before the clinical phase of the trial commences:
   Essential documents that are generated and secured before the clinical phase of the trial commences include those that pertain to qualification and set up of all trial resources (personnel, firms, facilities, equipment, and systems) and to trial authorization by ethics committee(s) and regulatory authority(ies).
2) During the clinical conduct of the trial:
   Those documents that are generated and secured during the clinical conduct of the trial pertain to the evidence of implementation of the trial, such as, protocol procedures to evaluate the study protocol objectives; handling, use, and accountability of the investigational product; informed consent, safety reporting, ethics committee continuing review, and other GCP and regulatory processes.

3) After completion or termination of the trial:

Once the trial is completed or after early termination, Essential Documents that pertain to the closeout of each investigator/institution and closeout of the entire trial will be added to the files, such as, documents that reflect final trial status (e.g., final investigational product accountability, the clinical study report), and informing ethics committee(s) and regulatory authority(ies) of the final status of the trial.

Plate 6 Individual Clinical Trial – Essential Documents also depicts the Essential Documents by clinical trial activity or key clinical trial document.

29.2.3 Attributes of Essential Documents

Essential documents are the evidence of trial conduct; i.e., they serve to demonstrate the compliance of the investigator, sponsor, and monitor with the standards of Good Clinical Practice and with all applicable regulatory requirements (ICH E6(R2) 8.1). Additionally, they are governed by the principle that all clinical trial information should be recorded, handled, and stored in a way that allows its accurate reporting, interpretation, and verification (ICH E6(R2) 2.10). In practice, therefore, we apply a core set of attributes for essential documents in order that they meet these requirements. In this book, we have created an acronym to facilitate remembering the important attributes, which are QATIC:

- **Q**uality review: records and files will undergo periodic and final quality review of document content and versions for compliance with standard operating procedures (SOPs), good documentation practices (GDPs), any Essential Documents Filing Plan, GCP, and applicable regulatory requirements, and for alignment with the inventory of records.
- **A**LCOAC principles and other GDPs: every record (originals or certified copies) should bear the properties of ALCOAC principles to ensure GDPs (Section 29.2.4.1)
- **T**imely filing: files will always be inspection ready!
- **I**nventory: a searchable current list of all records contained in the files with their version history and the location of the records will be maintained.
- **C**hange control: controlled access and audit trails to reflect who filed or changed, what, when, and why.

29.2.4 Good Documentation Practices

29.2.4.1 ALCOAC Principles

All personnel who are participating in the preparation and execution of a trial should be trained on and employ GDP for creating records for the trial to ensure that trial information is accurate and true. In practice, the principles that apply to source documentation are carried through for all essential documents: *Source data should be Attributable, Legible, Contemporaneous, Original, Accurate, and Complete. Changes to source data should be traceable, should not obscure the original entry and should be explained if necessary (e.g., via an audit trail)* (ICH E6(R2) 4.9.0).

A record should have an owner, a clear subject matter, be complete, and have a date and/or version of generation. Consideration should also be given to institutional and local applicable regulatory requirements for acceptable documentation.

All of the following quality characteristics should be applied when creating or changing records:

Attributable: It is clear who created the record or how (e.g., report from an instrument) the record was created. Initials for persons should be traceable to their full names, and records from instruments should also be traceable to an operator. The record should reflect the subject matter of the record; e.g., the research subject's ID, training procedures.

Legible: The information in the records is readable, intelligible, and decipherable, and is not defaced, faded, or obliterated. Consideration should be given to ensuring that the "ink" used will be permanent and is not erasable and that the medium is of sufficient quality to withstand handling and environmental changes over time.

Contemporaneous: The information was recorded and completed at the time as it happened and not in advance or retrospectively of its occurrence. Retrospective documentation should be noted as such and signed with the current date.

Original: The record is the first documentation of the event.

Accurate: All the information in the record are correct and true.

Complete: All pages and parts (e.g., appendices) are contained within or attached to the record. No information is cut off or missing from the record. It is advisable to indicate "page x of y" on all documents to be able to account for all pages. The reason for any missing information should be noted on the record; e.g., if the information is not available, not applicable, not done.

29.2.4.2 Changes to Records

Any change or correction to a study record, including CRFs, should have an audit trail; i.e., the original entry should not be obscured, the date the change was made, an identification of who made the change, a clear entry of the new information, and the reason the change was made (if necessary). Audit trails of changes should be maintained for both written and electronic changes and corrections. (ICH E6(R2) 4.9.3). ALCOAC principles also apply when making changes or corrections to records.

29.2.4.3 Certified Copies of Records

Copies may be used to replace an original document in the files of essential documents, but the copy must be certified as being an exact and true copy. That is, a copy (irrespective of the type of media used) of the original record that has been verified (i.e., by a dated signature or by generation through a validated process) must have the same information, including data that describe the context, content, and structure, as the original (ICH E6(R2) 1.63). Consideration should also be given to the necessity for copies to reflect all color used in originals.

29.2.5 Structure and Location of Files

29.2.5.1 All Trial Files

The sponsor and investigator and their respective representatives are maintaining and retaining records that they each generate and records that they each collect. In practice, the collection of essential documents for a trial are typically called the Trial Master File (TMF). The TMF encompasses all essential documents for the trial, including that of the sponsor and its representatives, and at the investigator(s) and their representatives. The term "TMF" sometimes more narrowly refers to the files housed by the sponsor and the files housed by the investigator are referred to as the Investigator Site File (ISF). The sponsor and investigator/institution will determine the terminology and structures for organizing essential documents in order to facilitate trial operations while maintaining compliance with GCP and applicable regulatory requirements.

The following are considerations for developing file structures and where essential documents for the trial will be located:

- Plate 18 Example of Structure of Files for Essential Documents offers examples of the structure of files containing essential documents at the sponsor/CRO and investigator/institution, respectively. The ICH E6(R2) Section 8 outlays a list of all the documents that should be retained for a trial by the sponsor and the investigator/institution. This list is a helpful start to creating a structure to house all records for the trial. Plate 6 Essential Documents displays essential documents collected by the sponsor/CRO and investigator/institution before the study starts, during the study, and at the end of the study.
- As displayed in ICH E6(R2) Section 8, both the sponsor and investigator are retaining records, and many of the same records are retained by both. Therefore, the file structures at all locations can use similar order and numbering systems. Use of ICH E6(R2) Section 8 as a base for file structures also facilitate monitoring, auditing, and inspections since the monitors, auditors, and inspectors are already familiar with the ICH E6(R2) Section 8 guidance so the records can be easily identified and located.
- The filing structure may also be grouped by when essential documents are collected; i.e., during the three general implementation phases of a trial:
  - Before the Clinical Phase of the Trial Commences
    During this planning stage the documents should be generated and should be on file before the trial formally starts (ICH E6(R2) 8.2).

- During the Clinical Conduct of the Trial
  In addition to having on file the documents collected before the trial started, documents generated during the trial should be filed as evidence that all new relevant information is documented as it becomes available (ICH E6(R2) 8.3).
- After Completion or Termination of the Trial
  After completion or termination of the trial, all of the documents collected before and during the trial should be in the file together with additional site and study closeout documents (ICH E6(R2) 8.4).

- When setting up filing systems, sections should be added for essential documents that are necessary to supplement trial information or sections may be reduced, where justified (the justification must be documented), based on the importance and relevance of the specific documents to the trial. It is also acceptable to combine some of the documents, provided the individual elements are readily identifiable. (ICH E6(R2) 8.1). Additional documents that are related to trial conduct may also be included in the TMF and ISF; e.g., checklists and documentation that support written processes and procedures.

- When a trial is conducted in multiple regions or countries, the records and files should be in conformance with the applicable regulatory requirement(s) of the country(ies) where the sponsor and investigator sites are located.

- Establish files both at the investigator/institution's site and at the sponsor's office (ICH E6(R2) 8.1). When third parties are used (e.g., CROs or vendors by the sponsor or vendors by the investigator), files will also be established in their locations.

- If tasks are delegated or contracted, the sponsor and investigator are each obligated to ensure that they have written agreements for their access to all the records that are related to the delegated or contracted duties or functions. Generally, the sponsor and investigator may not have access to each other's files. However, wholly or partially integrated systems may be established to facilitate files maintenance and sharing. For example, in an electronic filing system used for a multiregional trial, the sponsor may load key trial documents, such as the protocol (Chapter 18 The Clinical Trial Protocol and Amendments), investigator's brochure (Chapter 16 The Investigator's Brochure), and informed consent template (Chapter 19 Informed Consent and Other Human Subject Protection), onto a central location for all sites and the sponsor to access. At the same time, the investigator will load documents, such as their IRB/IEC approvals (Chapter 24 Investigator/Institution Initiation) and investigator qualification documents (Chapter 23), for the sponsor's access.

  ➢ Note that whenever files are shared, the systems and processes will be designed and established such that only authorized personnel may have access to information that must have limited viewership; e.g., personal identification for trial subjects (Chapter 19 Informed Consent and Other Human Subject Protection), randomization decodes (Chapter 27 Study Design and Data Analysis).

- A file index; i.e., a matrix that lists the name and description of each record to be filed and the name of the file where the record is located, will be created and maintained for the full course of the trial and archived with the final trial documents. This index allows for quick identification of the records that are in the files and the location of records for the trial team's access during the trial and for retrieval during audits and inspections.
- Since the TMF is a collection of all the records for a trial and many different players participate in the generation and collection of documents, records and/or their locations may be cross-referenced or pointed to avoid duplication or to preserve confidentiality of or facilitate preferential access for specific records. That is, a file in one physical location may point to a file in another physical location via notes in the file folder and/or the trial file index. For example, written agreements with financial information may be housed by the firm's department for legal affairs and may not be maintained with other study records. The index will then contain a note explaining where these records are maintained.

29.2.6 Sponsor Files

The sponsor is the generator and distributor of documents that pertain to multiple levels of drug development information, for example:

- the investigational product, for which there can be multiple indications
- the indication, for which there can be multiple studies
- a single study, for which there can be multiple investigators in multiple world regions (e.g., South America, Europe)
- a world region, in which there can be investigator sites in multiple countries
- a country, in which there can be multiple investigator sites
- each individual investigator/institution.

A sponsor may also employ CROs to carry out study-related activities or duties (ICH E6(R2) 5.2). The sponsor is therefore possibly retaining documents at many levels of information:

1. Related to the investigational product; e.g., investigator brochure, investigational product release
    1.1 Related to an indication; e.g., oncology, vaccines
        1.1.1 Related to the individual study protocol; e.g., study protocol, study informed consent template
            1.1.1.1 Related to world regions, if applicable
                1.1.1.1.1 Related to individual countries within regions, if applicable
                    1.1.1.1.1.1 Related to a site management organization (SMO) (Chapter 15 Trial Resourcing and Outsourcing), if applicable.

1.1.1.1.1.1.1 Related to the individual investigator/investigational site; e.g., investigator CVs, IRB/IEC approval

  1.2 Related to CROs and vendors; e.g., agreements, product/service information, if applicable

The sponsor files may therefore be organized by investigational product, indication, study protocol, and investigator/institution. If records are generated by region or country, then the structure may include levels for regions, within which are countries (e.g., for submissions to regulatory authorities to each country), then the investigator/institutional levels would be contained within each region or country. An SMO could oversee some or all investigators and these files would precede the files for the individual investigators. Separate files are better created for CRO agreements, contracts, etc. but the records for the delegated duties are better filed under the respective file topic; e.g., interim monitoring visit reports for an individual investigator. Some records (e.g., serious adverse event reports) can be organized by the individual site, by study protocol, by country, by region, or by the investigational product, and the sponsor will decide which works best for its operations. All grouping of trial files may be subdivided into smaller subsets to facilitate identification of documents.

29.2.6.1 CRO Files

When a sponsor transfers trial-related duties and functions to a CRO, the CRO is responsible for maintenance and retention of their records (ICH E6(R2) 5.2.4; 5.5.6). However, since the ultimate responsibility for the quality and integrity of the trial data always resides with the sponsor (ICH E6(R2) 5.2.1), the sponsor will oversee those records, including records for tasks that are subcontracted to another party by the sponsor's contracted CRO(s). The sponsor will have agreements with the CROs for accessing those records for review and for transferring those records to a central location for retention and archiving.

29.2.6.2 Investigator Files

Each investigator/institution will maintain essential documents to reflect how the trial is carried out at the clinical site. Investigator/institution files should/will include all records, as applicable, as displayed in ICH E6(R2) 8. The ISF will be organized to facilitate operations at the clinical site while ensuring compliance with institutional and applicable regulatory requirements. For example, all documents that pertain to the IRB submissions and oversight, investigator and trial site qualifications, and study information from the sponsor, may be stored together, source documents (Chapter 20 Data Collection and Data Management) that pertain to trial subjects may be stored by trial subject, and documents pertaining to pharmacy activities (e.g., investigational product handling, storing, preparation, and dispensing) may be stored at the pharmacy. When a trial has partial blinding, all blinded documentation may be organized and managed together and unblinded materials may be maintained separately to ensure integrity of the blind.

29.2.7 Written Procedures Pertaining to Essential Documents

Essential documents for the conduct of a trial amount to numerous individual records that are generated and collected by many different parties. These documents must also be retained for a certain period of time as required by regulatory requirements or longer as desired and must be made available to monitors, auditors, and inspectors at any given time. A firm's SOPs may provide guidance that applies to all studies but each study may also have trial-specific requirements due to the nature of the study (e.g., phase, design) or the infrastructure in place for conduct and management of the specific study (e.g., the use of CROs) (Chapter 31 Quality Responsibilities). It is advisable, therefore, to describe the procedures for the structure, collection, maintenance, retention, access, and archiving of essential documents in writing and train all who are involved on the procedures.

29.2.7.1 The Essential Documents File Index

Written procedures should clearly identify who is responsible for which document and the location of the documents. The file index is a written matrix that lists the name and description of each record to be filed and the corresponding responsible party (sponsor, CRO, and investigator) and location for the record; the index reflects the TMF structure and location of documents. Considerations for creating a filing structure and determining the locations of files are presented above (Section 29.2.5). This index should be created when the files are set up for a trial and will be a comprehensive list of all essential documents required for the trial. The index may also include other records that support the evidence of trial conduct, such as checklists (e.g., protocol contents checklist (Chapter 18 The Clinical Trial Protocol and Amendments) and documentation of processes associated with SOPs. The index may be updated or modified as necessary during the trial via controlled processes and stored with final archived trial documentation.

- Generally, the party who has regulatory responsibility for an essential document is responsible to ensure that it is in their files; e.g.,
  - The sponsor is responsible for providing the investigator's brochure to the investigator (ICH E6(R2) 5.6.2); therefore, the sponsor maintains a copy of the IB that was provided to the investigator, the investigator maintains a copy of what they received from the sponsor, and the sponsor also maintains documentation of the investigator's receipt of the IB.
  - The investigator is responsible for submitting the IB to the IRB/IEC for review (ICH E6(R2) 4.4.2); therefore, the investigator maintains evidence that they submitted the IB to the IRB/IEC.

– If a CRO is used for interim trial monitoring of investigational sites, the CRO will maintain copies of the monitoring reports (ICH E6(R2) 5.2.4). Additionally, the sponsor will also maintain copies of the monitoring reports as they will receive copies of the reports for review as part of their responsibility for oversight of the trial (ICH E6(R2) 5.2.2).

29.2.7.2 Inventory of Essential Documents

A file inventory may be created to indicate the documents are actually collected against the documents that are planned for collection in the index. The versions and dates of final filing of a document into the TMF may be recorded along with any comments, such as a reason for missing or incomplete records. Sponsors, CROs, and/or investigators may assign an individual or team of individuals who will be responsible for maintaining the file inventory.

29.2.7.3 Essential Documents Filing Plan

A written plan for managing essential documents (Plan) for a trial may be established by the trial management team. The Plan may describe procedures for the structure, collection, maintenance, retention, and archiving of essential documents. The purpose of the Plan is to help all persons involved in the conduct of the study to know what, when, and where documents will be filed, and who is responsible for which document. In practice, sponsors will typically describe these procedures in a written trial-specific Plan that can be used to guide all sponsor representatives who are responsible for the creation, collection, filing, maintenance, and retention of essential documents for the trial. The sponsor's Plan may also provide guidance for the structure and management of investigator/institution files, but the investigator/institution may have their own Plan for systems and procedures. The Plan includes descriptions of processes and systems for:

- What records will go into the files; i.e., the list of essential documents and other records that will be collected and maintained as evidence of trial conduct
- How the files will be organized; i.e., the structure for the files and a description for how cross-references or pointers may be used
- Where the files will be located; i.e., identification of which files will go into which location
- The timing for setting up files for a study and who will set up the files; e.g., will files be set up with the creation of the protocol, or on first IRB/IEC approval of a protocol?
- The establishment and maintenance of the file index, showing the file structure and the location or responsible party for each document
- The flow of documents from origination to final file destination
- The originality of records:

- In practice, generally, the original version of the document (the "wet ink" version) is maintained by the party generating the document (see ICH E6(R2) 8.1); however, electronic generation and maintenance of records may render this practice irrelevant in some instances. For example, the traditional "wet ink" versions of paper records may not be maintained but "certified" copies are maintained electronically. Additionally, if all records are generated and maintained electronically, then audit trails will identify which records are "original" versus which are copies. Users may also sign documents via electronic procedures. Whatever system is used, the written procedures for the organization should be clear on the process and all users should be trained and follow the processes.
- When a copy is used to replace an original document (e.g., source documents, CRF), the copy should fulfill the requirements for certified copies. (ICH E6(R2) 8.1) (Section 29.2.4.3).
- Generally, all documents used for official submissions or as official documentation of trial conduct should be retained as essential documents. In practice, it is recommended that drafts of documents are maintained in the official files only if those drafts were actually officially used in trial conduct; e.g., submitted to a regulatory authority or an IRB/IEC. If the retention of other working drafts of documents are deemed necessary by the firm, they should be maintained in unofficial file locations.
- The responsibilities for transmittal (i.e., transfer or submission) of records:
  - Which records are transmitted by whom; i.e., the list of records that are to be transmitted to for filing by their responsible parties as described in the index
  - Who transmits to whom; i.e., Sponsors, CROs, and/or investigators may assign an individual or team of individuals who will be responsible for receiving documents for review prior to submitting the documents to the filing system. For example., one individual on the sponsor team may be assigned to receive all documents for centralized review and processing before they are transmitted to the filing team; another sponsor representative may be assigned to specifically receive and review documentation of investigator qualifications from the clinical site before transmitting to the centralized reviewer; a coordinator at the investigator may be responsible for the filing of all trial subject source records while another individual may be responsible for the collection, review, and filing of IRB/IEC and sponsor documents.
  - How are individual and/or groups of electronic and/or hard copies of essential documents records transmitted; e.g., requirements for protecting the content of the document(s) and for the security of transmittal medium.
  - How to communicate transmittal and receipt of an essential document; e.g., transmittal procedures may include instructions to identify the document(s), the section in which the record is to reside, the date, and sender of a

lll

document(s), as well as the receiver's acknowledgement and date of receipt of the document(s).
- How documents are reviewed for quality; e.g. the individuals transmitting and receiving a document for filing reviews the document for completeness and other characteristics of GDPs (Section 29.2.7.4).
- When are records transmitted; i.e., the timing of transmitting records, whether they are individually created, periodically in batches, and/or at the end of the trial:
  - Essential documents should be filed as soon as they are generated so that files remain current. Filing essential documents at the investigator/institution and sponsor sites in a timely manner can greatly assist in the successful management of a trial by the investigator, sponsor and monitor (ICH E6(R2) 8.1).
  - Current files enable quick access to records for monitors, auditors, and inspectors, in addition to trial execution and management personnel who need to have trial information at any given time as part of the process to confirm the validity of the trial conduct and the integrity of data collected (ICH E6(R2) 8.1).
  - Having current information about the status of documents allows monitors and study managers to address any issues with collection or transmittal of documents.
  - Study status can also be quickly determined for business purposes.
  - As trial documentation should be inspection ready, it is recommended that the sponsor and investigator ensure that documentation for any outsourced or delegated duties are carefully overseen and tracked. Given that a sponsor or investigator indeed has final regulatory responsibility for the evidence of trial conduct, the safest course of action is for trial-required documents to be transmitted to them and in their possession as soon as the documents are created and ready for filing in order to reduce the risk for missing or lost documents at the time of an audit or inspection.
- Processes and timing for review and reconciliation of records:
  - The sponsor and investigator and their respective representatives are maintaining and retaining records that they each generate and records that they each collect. As displayed in ICH E6(R2) 8, both the sponsor and investigator are retaining records, and many of the same records are retained by both. Given that the sponsor and investigator have overlapping records, both investigator/institution and sponsor files should be reviewed periodically to confirm that all necessary documents are reconciled across the various files locations (ICH E6(R2) 8.1). Reconciling files means that files will be reviewed to ensure that:
    o Documents that are required to be in both locations, should be of identical content and version, e.g., protocol/amendment(s) (ICH E6(R2) 8.3.2), curriculum vitae for new investigator(s) and/or subinvestigator(s) (ICH E6(R2) 8.3.5)

o Documents that are required to be only in investigator files should not appear in the sponsor files, e.g., records with subject personal identification, such as the subject identification code list (ICH E6(R2) 8.3.21)

o Documents that are required to be only in the sponsor files should not appear in the investigator files, e.g., the master randomization list, which should be with a sponsor's third party if applicable (ICH E6(R2) 8.2.18)

The Plan may be updated or amended as necessary, but it is prudent to retain all previous versions because they reflect how the procedures were to be carried out when each version was effective.

29.2.7.4 Quality Review of Files

Files should be reviewed periodically at all locations for completeness and any deficiencies should be addressed immediately to ensure readiness for audits and inspections.

Sponsors, CROs, and investigator/institutions may review their own files as part of their quality control procedures (ICH E6(R2) 2.13). The quality of a document may be reviewed as it is handled and channeled through the submission and filing process and batches of records may be reviewed periodically. Additionally, a final review of each investigator files and of the sponsor's and CRO files should be performed prior to closing out a clinical site or the trial, respectively (ICH E6(R2) 8.1). Individual records and files may be reviewed by:

- A member of the study team who is familiar with the study conduct to confirm,
  - Document content, ensuring that it is relevant, true, and complete, given the known information about the status of the study
  - Document versions, given the known information about the status of the study
  - The list of records in the inventory, given the known information about the status of the study
  - That records are filed in the appropriate location(s)
- A records control team member or other quality control representative to confirm,
  - The application of ALCOAC principles to each record
  - Alignment between the index and the inventory
  - Complete audit trails for system control
- A sponsor's monitor during monitoring of the investigator files (ICH E6(R2) 5.18.4 (p)).
- Files may be audited periodically by a sponsor representative or investigator/institution representative to review:
  - Compliance with the firm's written processes and procedures, the protocol, the Plan, ICH E6(R2), and applicable regulatory requirements

29.2.8 Retention of and Continued Access to Essential Documents

All essential documents for a trial will be retained during the course of the trial and archived for a specified period after trial completion or termination. The sponsor and the investigator should have ready access to certain documents at all times during the trial as well as after completion or termination of the trial.

29.2.8.1 Requirements for Retention
The sponsor and investigator and their representatives will maintain trial records according to the Plan and applicable regulatory requirements. Written agreements between the parties will also include requirements for record retention and access to documents.

The sponsor has obligations to inform the investigators, CROs, and vendors of requirements. These requirements may be placed in the protocol (Chapter 18 The Clinical Trial Protocol and Amendments) and/or other written agreements (e.g., Chapter 15 Trial Resourcing and Outsourcing) between the sponsor and the investigator and the investigator may acknowledge the requirement via signing the protocol and/or other written agreements with the sponsor.

The investigator also has obligations to inform vendors and other third party participations of the requirements. The agreements will include, as applicable:

- Informing the party of the need for record retention (e.g., ICH E6(R2) 5.5.12)
- Obtaining acknowledgement from the party of their responsibility to retain essential documents (e.g., ICH E6(R2) 5.6.3 (d)
- Requirements for the party to retain records as specified in the trial Plan and applicable regulatory requirements (ICH E6(R2) 8)
- Requirements for the party to take measures to prevent accidental or premature destruction of these documents (e.g., ICH E6(R2) 4.9.4)
- Requirements for the party to maintain a record of the location(s) of their respective essential documents including source documents.
- Requirements for the party to ensure that the storage system used during the trial and for archiving (irrespective of the type of media used) provides for document identification, version history, search, and retrieval. (ICH E6(R2) 8.1).
- Specifications for the duration for retaining essential documents as described below (Section 29.2.8.2).
- Specifications that a party will be informed when the trial-related records are no longer needed. (ICH E6(R2) 5.5.12).
- Requirements for access to essential documents as described below (Section 29.2.8.3)

29.2.8.2 Retention Period
Essential documents for a trial must be retained and archived for a specific period and the length of the period may vary:

- Per ICH E6(R2), the investigator should retain essential documents until at least 2-years after the last approval of a marketing application in an ICH region and until there are no pending or contemplated marketing applications in an ICH region or at least 2 years have elapsed since the formal discontinuation of clinical development of the investigational product (i.e., for any or all indications, routes of administration, or dosage forms (ICH E6(R2) 5.5.8)); however, documents should be retained for a longer period, however, if required by the applicable regulatory requirement (ICH E6(R2) 4.9.5). These durations also apply to the sponsor (ICH E6(R2) 5.5.11).

- World regions or countries may have the same or different retention periods from the ICH Guidelines. A country or region may require as many as 25 years or longer for essential documents to be retained.
- Additionally, the sponsor may request a longer period than is mandated by governing regulatory authorities for records retention (e.g., ICH E6(R2) 5.5.11). A sponsor may request longer retention periods, for example, in case review of or access to files are necessary for long-term study of an investigational product.

29.2.8.3 Access to Essential Documents

All essential documents for a trial will be retained during the course of the trial and archived after trial completion or termination so that they are accessible at any given time during the trial or as required after the trial:

- The sponsor should obtain the investigator's/institution's agreement to permit monitoring, auditing, and inspection (ICH E6(R2) 4.1.4 and 5.6.3(c))
- Any or all essential documents may be subject to, and should be available for, audit by the sponsor's auditor and inspection by the regulatory authority(ies) (ICH E6(R2) 8.1)
- The sponsor should ensure that the investigator has control of and continuous access to the CRF data reported to the sponsor. The sponsor should not have exclusive control of those data (ICH E6(R2) 8.1)
- The investigator/institution should have control of all essential documents and records generated by the investigator/institution before, during, and after the trial (ICH E6(R2) 8.1)

Essential documents should also be retained and archived in a format that is readily accessible and legible. Considerations should be given to:

- Changing technologies for storing data and study information to ensure that they are translatable as needed
- Security of essential documents to ensure access is restricted to only authorized individuals
- Security of essential documents to guard against destruction or loss of records
- Maintaining backup copies of essential documents

29.3 Summary

Sponsors and investigators are required to document trial conduct and retain and archive the evidence of trial conduct (i.e., essential documents) for a required duration so that they are readily accessible to monitors, auditors, and regulatory inspectors as part of the process for verification of the validity of the trial conduct and the integrity of data collected. The structure and procedures for collection, quality review, and maintenance of trial files may be described in study-specific plans to ensure that all involved in the trial conduct are informed and trained on how what documents will be collected and how those documents will be transmitted, filed, retained, and archived.

Essential documents are all that exist of evidence of trial conduct. As is commonly said in the field: *If it is not documented, it did not happen; and if it did not happen, it should not be documented.*

Knowledge Check Questions

1) How can you determine who is responsible for which essential document?
2) What is the purpose of essential documents?
3) What principles apply to the creation of an essential document?
4) Which essential documents must be present before the study starts?
5) Which essential documents are collected while the study is on-going?
6) Which essential documents must be present when the study ends?
7) For how long must essential documents be retained?
8) What are some of the requirements for access to essential documents during the study and after the end of the study?
9) *Overheard*:
   I can't believe I am going to lose my job over the Trial Master File!
   Corporate executive, responsible for clinical operations functions that included essential documents management and storage, saying when the findings from the audit of the Trial Master File for a phase 3 pivotal trial included critical findings of missing, incomplete, and inappropriate filing of documents.
   Comment and discuss:
   a) The importance of the Trial Master File, which is a commonly used term for the collection of the sponsor's essential documents for a trial.
   b) What does the sponsor have to lose if their essential documents are missing, incomplete, or inappropriate?

Reference

1 International Council for Harmonisation of Technical Requirements for Pharmaceuticals for Human Use (ICH), Integrated Addendum to ICH E6(R1):Guideline for Good Clinical Practice, E6(R2) (2016). Current Step 4 version dated 9 November 2016. https://www.ich.org/page/efficacy-guidelines

Part V

Quality in Clinical Trials

30

Quality Systems in Clinical Research

P. Michael Dubinsky

GCP Key Point

GCP principle 2.13 calls for the implementation of systems with procedures that assure the quality of every aspect of the trial. By embracing quality systems we position our study and our research team to implement this principle.

It is a fundamental tenant of GCP that clinical trial sponsors are specifically charged with implementing and maintaining quality control (QC) and quality assurance (QA) systems to ensure that trials are conducted and reported in conformance with the protocol, applicable regulations and GCP. That said each of the key players in the clinical trial endeavor have a responsibility to apply and integrate a quality systems approach into their areas of trial activity.

30.1   Introduction

Quality systems have not always been a stated and visible element of the clinical research endeavor. It originated in the world of pharmaceutical and medical device manufacturing (good manufacturing practice/quality system regulation – GMP/QSR) and has logically and appropriately been extended into the world of clinical research. Regulations and Directives governing clinical trials do not specifically use the terminology – quality system – except through indirect references and by adopting or supporting guidelines such as the ICH E6(R2) support given to the 2016 revision of the ICH E6(R2) guideline which speaks to quality management expectations certainly sets the tone for adoption of the quality system mentality. The emergence of quality system applications is in part a function of the scientific

The Fundamentals of Clinical Research: A Universal Guide for Implementing Good Clinical Practice, First Edition. P. Michael Dubinsky and Karen A. Henry.
© 2022 John Wiley & Sons, Inc. Published 2022 by John Wiley & Sons, Inc.
Companion website: www.wiley.com/go/dubinsky/clinicalresearch

and regulatory initiatives which stress the prevention of recurring problems in the conduct of clinical research. The effectiveness of a quality systems approach is dependent upon having quality management in place. While not interchangeable, the terms quality systems and quality management are inextricably intertwined. From an ethical standpoint one could opine that if a human biomedical study is not conducted in a quality manner it would be a violation of ethical principles because performing the study otherwise would expose the subjects to experimental products and procedures in a manner whereby data and/or subject safety is at risk of being compromised and the purpose of their participation is questionable.

30.1.1 Objectives

To learn about the:

1) concept and definition of quality systems;
2) to learn why quality systems are being integrated into the clinical trial arena;
3) what constitutes or makes up quality systems; and
4) how the quality systems approach is implemented.

30.1.2 Advent of Quality Systems in Clinical Research

Despite being mentioned in many written articles and industry publications quality systems are not specifically defined in regulations governing clinical trials such as the FDA's IND regulations at 21 CFR 312 or the EU's recent regulation No 536/2014 of 16 April 2014 on clinical trials on medicinal products for human use which repealed Directive 2001/20/EC (1) – the Clinical Trial Directive.

Two sources which define quality systems in a manner which fits for GCP is the definition used by the FDA in their Quality Systems Regulation governing the manufacture of medical device products – 21 CFR 820. That definition is: *Quality system means the organizational structure, responsibilities, procedures, processes, and resources for implementing quality management.* The other definition comes from the WHO Handbook for GCP: *"Quality systems" for clinical trials are formalized practices (e.g. monitoring programs, auditing programs, complaint handling systems) for periodically reviewing the adequacy of clinical trial activities and practices, and for revising such practices as needed so that data and process quality are maintained.*

The application of QC and QA steps has roots that extend initially from the manufacturing sector. Quality approaches were extended into the healthcare and other industries in the twentieth century and were built into regulatory requirements as part of cGMP for regulated drug and medical device products. There is no specific year or event which can be held up as the seminal one for the emergence of quality in human clinical research matters. If we were to suggest a seminal event in terms of when quality migrated to human clinical trial matters as an expectation it would probably be the publication of the Good Clinical Practice Guideline by the International Conference on Harmonization (ICH) c. 1996. The regulatory authorities who oversee the manufacturing of drug and medical device products and their industry counterparts were the founders of the ICH and it is reasonable to expect that they brought their experiences with quality and quality systems into the discussion about guidelines for conduct of clinical trials in humans. Publication of the World Health Organization's Handbook for Good Clinical Research Practice in 2005 shows further integration of the quality systems concept as the term is specifically defined (as mentioned earlier) for the conduct of human clinical trials. There has also been a long standing goal of regulatory authorities to put in place measures which would reduce the recurrence of significant nonconformances in the conduct of clinical trials such as failure to follow the protocol (trial plan) by investigators and failure to adequately monitor clinical trials by sponsors and monitors. These types of nonconformances have been present since the advent of regulatory controls over the trials by FDA began c. 1962. The quality systems approach is geared to prevent such nonconformity.

Most recently the ICH-GCP was amended E6 (R2) in 2016 whereby the sponsor will be expected to establish a quality management system. The system is all encompassing and is expected to focus on subject protections and data integrity. Risk assessment and management throughout the trial is a part of these recent expectations. This newly revised ICH guidance goes a long way toward solidifying the axiom that quality is everybody's business in the conduct of a clinical trial, not just the QA or quality group.

The concept of establishing and implementing quality systems is founded on the ISO standard for quality management systems ISO 9001 [1]. That standard recognizes that there are several systems operating in an organization such as management, financial and environmental. The quality system has the overarching objective of directing and controlling the organization's systems from a quality standpoint.

So why integrate the quality system concept into clinical trials if it is an approach which originated in the manufacturing arena and regulations may not specifically require it? The reasons are the same as for implementing good clinical practice – ensuring data integrity and subject protection. By applying a quality systems approach goals such as performing procedures correctly the first time and avoiding costly repeat steps due to nonconforming processes are realized. The addition of the risk assessment process furthers the expectation that designing quality into all aspects of a trial eliminates many if not all opportunity for failure or discrepancy.

Over the last several years regulatory authorities have come to expect that sponsors, investigators, contract research organizations and the other players in the clinical research community will have adopted a quality systems approach and mindset to their conduct of clinical trials. One explanation for why quality systems are expected even though they are not specified in regulation is the notion that "current good clinical practice" requires it. In the pharmaceutical and medical device manufacturing arena GMP is almost always preceded by the word *current*. The term *current* is found in the Federal Food Drug and Cosmetic Act at Sec 501(a) (2) (B) which defines current Good Manufacturing Practice (cGMP). From a manufacturing standpoint regulators knew when they wrote the regulations that the technology and capabilities of the manufacturing community would change over time so they drafted general requirements which could evolve along with industry, technology, and science. The only difference for GCP is that the words do not show up in the governing statute. Current good clinical practice is a reflection not of regulatory "creep" but of recognizing that technology and science have matured over time. Including quality systems approaches in clinical research is a logical part of that maturation.

30.1.3 Quality Systems Building Blocks

Establishing the foundational building blocks that need to be in place for the quality systems approach to be successful is the first step. The building blocks are not unique to clinical trials and can benefit almost every professional discipline. The building blocks underpin the structure of every process applied in the clinical trial endeavor and demonstrate that management has a culture of quality as they approach the conduct of the trial. The building blocks are: written procedures; change control; qualification of people, supplies and vendors; training; record keeping systems and documentation; management involvement; corrective and preventive action (CAPA); and risk assessment and management. Figure 30.1 depicts a Quality Management System.

30.1.3.1 Written Procedures
Having written procedures, better known as Standard Operating Procedures is not only an expectation for ensuring quality it is a stated requirement for regulated drug development including clinical trial activities conducted internationally. ICH E6(R2) mentions procedures (SOPs) numerous times across the eight sections. The presence of written procedures especially for all regulated activity ensures that all personnel are on the same page and that work is accomplished in conformance with regulations, organizational policy, and in a uniform manner. SOPs must be maintained via a controlled documentation system.

30.1.3.2 Change Control
The term *Change Control* originates in the drug manufacturing arena and refers to a systematic approach to making changes in procedure, process, or materials. Some call it an ordered approach to moving from one controlled state to another.

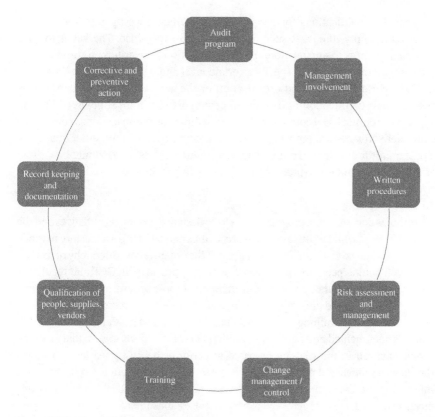

Figure 30.1 A quality management system.

In terms of clinical trial activities we often think of changes to the protocol or informed consent. The important factor is to have a controlled approach to implementing change which involves all pertinent players and sign offs by those who need to know. The pertinent players include the regulatory authorities who may need to be notified of change and if so in what time frame. The objective of change control is not just to ensure everyone knows, but to ensure that all effective elements have a heads-up on an impending modification and can provide their input – be it support or concern – before the change is implemented.

30.1.3.3 Qualification of People, Supplies, Vendors

Qualification of people, supplies (things), and vendors (service providers) is an integral building block of a quality system because it allows for selections to be made on sound criteria with the objective of those people, things and service providers doing the assigned work in a manner that is accountable and of high quality.

In terms of qualifications for people such as clinical investigators a sponsor is expected to apply standards such as training and experience. The key is to have criteria/standards to apply before making a selection. The criteria for investigator selection for example might specify a certain level and type of licensure, participation in a certain professional organization or the achievement of certain quality goals such as certification by a standard setting organization. Supplies (things) to support the clinical trial could be as basic as sample collection kits or as complex as computer software programs to collect and analyze trial data. Whether qualifying a trial monitor or a supplier of data management services there should be written criteria and a standard written process in place to be followed.

30.1.3.4 Training

An organization's training program needs to be designed around its initiatives and the risks associated with failure to perform procedures and tasks in a satisfactory manner. Training should be given an important place in the organization's hierarchy of responsibilities. Training personnel and if need be service providers in GCP and regulatory responsibilities should be given the full attention of those sponsoring and conducting trials. Training should encompass the applicable procedures, protocol and as appropriate update GCP training. Training should be conducted as a prospective activity which is documented and part of an overall program to actively ensure that all of the people engaged in the trial are prepared to perform their assigned tasks. Trainers should be qualified and proficient even if the training assignment is a collateral duty. Integrating the QA staff into the training program where applicable sends a strong message that quality cuts across all aspects of the establishments' activities.

30.1.3.5 Record Keeping Systems and Documentation

Record keeping will always be an integral part of the quality systems in large measure because the record of what was done, who did it, when they did it and whether any changes were made in the process or outcome are as integral to the validity of clinical trial data as it is to the data documenting the manufacture of a drug product. The records must be available for review and verification at a later time. The systems used for record maintenance must be controlled and if electronic be validated as to their reliability and reproducibility. Quality practices must be put in place to address aspects such as content, accessibility, retention, terminology, review and approval as appropriate, audit trails, controls, physical protections, and/or backup. As noted in Part 8 of the ICH E6(R2)-GCP documentation is the key to evaluating whether a clinical trial was conducted in conformance with regulatory and scientific parameters and whether the data produced is of high quality. The record never forgets!

30.1.3.6 Corrective and Preventive Action (CAPA)

Having a systematic approach to dealing with failures, mistakes, incorrect implementation as well as nonconformances in general is the mark of a quality-oriented organization. The application of the CAPA principles is not really new to clinical trial activity but the terminology and full acceptance of the concept has been evolving since the mid-2000s. The terminology comes from medical device arena where manufacturers have a regulatory manufacturing requirement to evaluate or analyze data from a variety of sources such as audits and defect reports and institute corrective action steps to avoid identified mistakes or noncompliance in the future. To be true CAPA the analysis has to look beyond an individual report for the root cause and examine the system as well as similar systems to ensure the cause of the mistake or non-compliance is resolved completely. In addition the CAPA approach includes taking proactive steps to prevent nonconformances from occurring. In clinical trials the requirement to have a monitoring system (see Chapter 22 Monitoring Overview) in place was never called either a quality system or a CAPA but that was prior to the terms being used in the clinical trial venue. Monitoring is a step whereby the implementation of process steps are examined to ensure they are occurring as planned. If nonconformity is identified it is examined individually and hopefully across all sites to determine if it is systemic. Corrective actions are instituted and if appropriate modifications to a process are made to avoid future non-conformance.

30.1.3.7 Management Involvement

Management's role as a foundational building block in a quality system approach cannot be overemphasized. Absent the people who are in a position to effect change through decision-making, delivery of needed resources and removal of stumbling blocks to progress, the system would be subject to going off course or becoming noncompliant at any time. Setting organizational or institutional policies that are clearly understood and practiced is a key first step and staying in touch through communication is a manifestation of management's exercise of responsibility and leadership. In the FDA's Investigations Operations Manual [2] the topic of evidence development includes a discussion on how to document the individual (s) at an organization who have the duty and power to detect, prevent, and correct violations. That person(s) is the one with the responsibility. The point being that FDA wants their inspectors (investigators), during the course of an inspection, to document who at the firm can effect change so that if violations are documented the appropriate management official can be called to answer for it. In the quality system approach, management is expected to be taking or overseeing proactive steps to detect, prevent, and, if present, correct circumstances which represent a deviation from the regulations, protocol or GCP. The types of communications might include participation during meetings where trial status is discussed among the team members and sticky wickets are described and solutions developed.The management's role that is now defined in revisions to the GCP as well as in the minds of regulators is that *quality management* must be in place. Quality management means, that the sponsor should implement a system to manage quality throughout the design, conduct, recording, evaluation, reporting, and archiving of clinical trials. While this may sound like something new, as with quality systems, quality management is a logical evolution of management's role in trial oversight. It does however call for management to utilize a risk management approach throughout the stages of the trial's life cycle.

30.1.3.8 Risk Assessment and Management

Since there is a Chapter 13 Risk Assessment and Quality Management being devoted to Risk Assessment and Management we will not go into detail here. Briefly it is imperative that risk be, identified, evaluated, controlled, communicated, reviewed, and reported based on a tangible plan. The ICH E6(R2) specifically calls for a sponsor to establish a program of risk assessment and management which incorporates the elements of risk identification, evaluation, control, communication, review, and reporting. One key objective of having a risk assessment program is identifying ways that quality can be designed into the trial.

30.1.4 Quality Control vs. Quality Assurance

There are many available definitions for the terms QC and QA. For the purpose of this text we will utilize the ones provided in the ICH E6(R2) at Section 1.46 and 1.47. They are reproduced in our glossary. QC is generally understood to be the day to day steps that are taken to ensure that an activity is occurring as planned. QA is often thought of only as audits and in fact an audit is a QA activity but the ICH definition demands we think a bit broader than just audits.

QA encompasses the entire set of plans and actions which collectively are established and performed to ensure that the trial meets the standards in the regulations, the plan laid out in the protocol and the practices described in GCP. In the simplest terms QA means ensuring that all activities supporting the clinical trial are operating in a manner which embodies the use of the quality system building blocks. That would include the performance of audits (examinations) of internal and external operating systems to ensure they are operating according to plan. QA is also an operating system within the overall plan that prospectively examines other systems to ensure they are operating as planned, according to written procedures, and in conformance with requirements. The goal of a sound QA program is to prevent nonconformance. The trial sponsor is usually tasked with the QA responsibility either through their own organization or by contracting with an outside QA consultant. QA is organizationally separate from the clinical operations activities to avoid any bias or conflict of interest.

QC in clinical trials is comprised of two elements both of which are considered operational in nature. The first is internal QC performed by the clinical operations staff and/or by site personnel involved in the trial. Having an organizational group called QC is not required and might only cause confusion if it were present. A classic example of operational QC is the ongoing assessment of essential trial documents to be certain they are complete, consistent in content and in conformance with regulatory requirements. So if an evaluation of the trial CRF is being performed using a checklist approach to ensure consistency with the Protocol that would be a QC activity. QC activities must be defined in written procedures and documented in appropriate records. Much of the QC responsibility will fall to the study sponsor but not necessarily all of it. For example conducting a check of the site regulatory binder to ensure completeness or verifying the completeness of the monitoring log would be performed by site staff and considered a QC task. The second part of the QC equation for clinical trials is monitoring. Why regulators did not just title monitoring a QC activity in their regulations, directives and guidelines always escaped me because that is what it was from day one. In reading over *ICH E6(R2) 5.18.4 Monitor's Responsibilities* it is clear that the intent is performing QC activity when words such as verifying, ensuring and checking are utilized. It is clear that while GCP does not use the wording QC it expects that QC will be implemented by clinical trial sponsors, investigators, and all involved players.

Both QA and QC activities are expected to integrate use of the quality system building blocks into their procedures and processes.

30.1.5 Quality Systems Approach

Quality systems are both a way of doing business and a mindset that is achievable at the managerial, operational, and personal level. If the fundamental building blocks are in place and the organization, i.e. the people adopt and adapt those fundamentals, then over time quality becomes built in from the beginning of each task or assignment. The primary objectives of applying the quality systems approach is to prevent nonconformance; detect non-conformance early on when it does occur; and to correct nonconformance from a systematic standpoint. The prevention of nonconformance is a function of having the building blocks in place and being used as well as an active QA program to ensure systems are operating as planned. The detection of nonconformance is accomplished via a QC program that is designed to identify nonconformances in real time. CAPA seeks to make effective and lasting fixes of nonconforming activity as well as improve processes and procedures.

It is generally seen as management's responsibility to establish the presence of the quality system building blocks in the organization and the processes. By doing so quality management will be realized. It is the responsibility of all employees and staff to utilize these quality attributes to create and nurture a quality culture.

30.1.6 Summary

The application of a quality systems approach to human biomedical clinical trials has become a *de facto* regulatory expectation if not requirement. The quality systems approach calls for implementing a number of building blocks – written procedures; change control; qualification of people, supplies and vendors; training; record keeping systems and documentation; management involvement; CAPA, and risk assessment in an active and purposeful manner. If these basic building blocks are implemented and adopted by the players in the clinical trial arena then they become a way of doing business and a mindset. Quality systems are meant to prevent non-compliance and when detected to affect corrective action. QA and QC are part of the quality systems approach.

Knowledge Check Questions

1) The description of quality systems can be found in the ICH E6(R2). True or False? False ICH E6(R2) does not define quality systems however the WHO handbook of GCP does define quality systems. Principle 2.13 of ICH E6(R2) does however call for the implementation of systems with procedures that assure the quality of every aspect of a trial.

2) The goals of implementing a quality systems approach in clinical trials are to ensure data quality and protect human subjects. True or False? True.

3) Having written procedures and training staff using those procedures are some of the quality system building blocks. Does the quality systems approach dictate how often that training needs to occur? If so where would you expect to find the details? If not how often would you perform the training? What might motivate the need for re-training?

4) Qualifying people, services, supplies (things) and processes is a practice that fits into the quality systems approach, correct? If you agree do you think that the QA unit must be the ones who do the qualifying? Or can it be done by others? Who might those others be?

5) Do you agree with the following description? QA and QC differ in that QA is implemented by management and QC is performed by staff assigned to perform the day-to-day activities associated with running a trial. An example of a QC activity is a CRA who conducts monitoring of a clinical trial site.

References

1 ISO 9001:2015 (2015). *Quality Management Systems – Requirements*. Geneva, Switzerland: International Organization for Standardization.

2 US FDA (2019). Investigators Operations Manual (IOM). Chapter 5 Establishment Inspections – Subchapter 5.3 Evidence Development, Responsible Individuals 5.3.6. https://www.fda.gov/media/76769/download (accessed 21 January 2020).

31

Quality Responsibilities

P. Michael Dubinsky

GCP Key Point
GCP delineates specific responsibilities for each of the key players in a clinical trial- IRB/IEC, Investigator and Sponsor. Integrating quality into the framework of executing those responsibilities is expected per ICH Principle 2.13

Implementing a clinical trial involves a large number of people, disciplines, business decisions, scientific and technical assessments, timelines, ethical considerations and often complex project management challenges. Integrating quality thinking, systems, and practices into all of these matters represents a challenge. ICH E6(R2) provides many specifics as to the responsibilities that the key players in the trial need to address. Among those responsibilities are ensuring that the quality aspects of trial implementation are addressed.

31.1 Introduction

Building quality into all aspects of a clinical trial calls for each of the key players to accept responsibility for ensuring conformance to the regulations, protocol and GCP. By adopting quality system approaches, establishing QC practices and integrating a QA program the likelihood of conformance with regulations, directives and principles is significantly enhanced. Under ICH E6(R2) the sponsor of a clinical trial is assigned QA and QC responsibilities in Section 5.1 as well as numerous quality related tasks throughout Section 5. That said the investigator and IRB also have a responsibility for building in quality pursuant to ICH E6(R2)

The Fundamentals of Clinical Research: A Universal Guide for Implementing Good Clinical Practice, First Edition. P. Michael Dubinsky and Karen A. Henry.

Principle 2.13. In this chapter we will examine the quality related tasks assigned to the key players as part of ICH E6(R2).

31.1.1   Objectives

The objectives of this chapter are to:

- Pinpoint quality and quality related responsibilities/tasks described in ICH E6(R2).
- Examine how the organizational structure, communication, and operational aspects play a key role in effecting quality.
- Comment on how quality fits into performance of the tasks for which each player has responsibility.
- Offer some examples of how quality can be integrated into the areas of responsibility in a manner whereby it becomes part of the operating mindset.

31.1.2   Sponsor

The sponsor of a clinical trial, whether a commercial organization, educational institution, or individual sponsor-investigator has responsibility for most of the trial related duties and functions described in regulation and ICH E6(R2). In addition, the sponsor is expected to plan the entire set of trial related activities. Sponsors may delegate or transfer responsibilities to other organizations, e.g. vendors and CROs, however the responsibility for the protection of the human subjects and the integrity of the data will always track back to the sponsor.

The specific responsibilities related to quality are found throughout ICH E6(R2) Section 5. Section 5.1 outlines the QA and QC expectations. The specific quality actions that are described are to have SOPs, written agreements and apply some level of quality control over all steps of data handling. Table 31.1 depicts in a condensed manner quality and quality related expectations which fall to the sponsor.

The current ICH E6(R2) does not describe or allude to preparing a written quality plan for each trial however certain prepared plans, e.g. the monitoring plan, risk management plan, adverse experience reporting plan and the statistical plan are part of an overall quality effort. A quality systems approach to conducting clinical trials is in itself a living quality plan.

Based on experience it is our view that quality responsibilities are best met when a firm organizes itself to support quality, communicates internally and externally in a manner whereby nonconforming situations can be prevented and/or addressed and establishes QC and QA programs that are administered and documented by qualified personnel. Sustainable quality is found in a three part framework: the organizational structure, the lines of communication and the operating practices that are built using the quality system building blocks.

Table 31.1 Overview of expectations which fall to the sponsor.

Section from the ICH GCP	Statement of sponsor's responsibilities
5.0	Quality Management – This is an addendum to the ICH E6(R2) which calls for the sponsor to manage quality throughout all stages and aspects of the trial. The risk assessment and management expectations are outlined in it.
5.1	QA and QC. Implement and maintain QA and QC systems including SOPs, apply QC to all aspects of data management, develop written agreements
5.2	Sponsors may transfer in writing responsibilities to contract research organizations but the ultimate responsibility lies with the sponsor. The 2016 addendum calls for the sponsor to apply oversight to CROs and fully document subcontracting of responsibilities.
5.3	Designate qualified medical personnel
5.4	Utilize qualified individuals
5.5	Utilize qualified individuals, consider an independent data monitoring committee, make sure systems meet standards, maintain security over data, maintain backup of data, retain essential documents. The 2016 addendum calls for the sponsor to document that computerized systems be validated based on a risk assessment that includes the potential impact on human subject protection and data integrity. In addition; SOPs for the computerized systems must be maintained and those SOPs must contain specified elements such as documenting data changes and maintaining adequate backup.
5.6	Select qualified investigators, obtain investigator's agreement to allow monitoring, inspections, etc.
5.7	Define, establish and allocate duties and functions
5.11	Confirm review and approval by IRB/IEC
5.13	Ensure that INV product is manufactured in conformance with applicable GMP
5.16	Conduct ongoing safety evaluation
5.18	Plan and execute trial monitoring that includes qualified monitors with specific responsibilities and an overall plan to ensure conformance of trial activities to the protocol, regulations, SOPs and GCP. The 2016 addendum calls for development of a risk based approach to monitoring that includes on site and centralized elements. Also a monitoring plan is specifically mentioned and expected to be in place.
5.19	Consider audits as part of the QA activities. Select qualified auditors, follow written procedures and deal with non-compliance. The 2016 addendum calls for root cause analysis of serious noncompliance and implementation of corrective and preventive actions.

31.1.3 Contract Research Organization (CRO)

The ICH E6(R2) specifically outlines CRO responsibilities under the Sponsor Section 5.2 (see Sections 5.2.1–5.2.4). The baseline premise is that if the sponsor transfers any trial related tasks to the CRO the CRO must also implement the necessary QA and QC systems and responsibilities as if they were the sponsor. All such responsibility transfers must be documented in writing, i.e. written contracts. One approach that is used to ensure that the quality expectations of the sponsor are clearly stated and that the CRO clearly understands those expectations is by including a quality agreement as part of the contract. A quality agreement would specifically address topics such as regulatory requirements, good clinical practice, and SOPs from the standpoint of which ones apply, which party has the lead responsibility and how communication on these items are to occur. Depending upon the tasks transferred to the CRO quality indicators which might be tracked and discussed as part of the agreement are: number and type of monitoring findings; turnover rate for key personnel assigned to the trial; number of protocol deviations/violations; number and type of data corrections required.

31.1.4 Clinical Investigator (CI)

Is there a definitive set of quality responsibilities for the clinical investigator at a site? In reviewing the ICH E6(R2) and regulations (e.g. FDA regulations at 21 CFR 312) the investigator is not specifically directed to apply quality procedures or practices other than the general quality principle found at GCP 2.13. In reviewing the ICH E6(R2) the following quality or quality related responsibilities are found. They are presented in the table below in a condensed manner.

Section of ICH GCP	Clinical investigator quality responsibilities
4.1.4	Permit monitoring and auditing
4.1.5	Maintain a list of qualified persons to whom duties have been assigned.
4.2.2–4.2.4	Investigator should have sufficient time and qualified staff to complete the trial. The 2016 addendum calls for the investigator to supervise any individual or party to whom the investigator delegates trial related duties. If such arrangements are made the person(s) to whom the duties are delegated must be qualified to perform those duties/functions. Appropriate record keeping to document such arrangements is expected.
4.4	Investigator should have IRB/IEC written approval for all appropriate trial related documents, e.g. protocol and informed consent forms

4.5.2	Deviations or changes from the protocol should not be implemented without sponsor or IRB/IEC documented approval.
4.6.3	Complete all INV product record keeping responsibilities
4.8.2	Written ICF and any other information provided to subjects should be reviewed for necessary changes when new information becomes available.
4.9.0	This provision added per the 2016 Addendum – Calls for the investigator/institution to maintain accurate and adequate source documents and records.
4.9.1	Investigator should ensure the accuracy, completeness, legibility, and timeliness of the data reported to the sponsor
4.9.3	Changes to data should be dated, initialed, and explained and should not obscure the original entry.

There are other opportunities for the CI to identify and act on quality initiatives. Inspiration for quality related steps might for example be drawn from the types of non-compliances which are documented during inspections of clinical trial investigator sites by regulatory authorities.

Key areas of noncompliance reported by regulatory authorities include:

- Failure to follow the investigational plan and/or regulations
- Protocol deviations
- Inadequate recordkeeping
- Inadequate accountability for the investigational product
- Inadequate communication with the IRB
- Inadequate subject protection – failure to report AEs and informed consent issues

Using these somewhat general statements of noncompliance we can create a list of quality steps that if instituted/implemented and overseen at the trial site by the clinical investigator can mitigate noncompliance risks. Such an activity would be in agreement with the risk assessment steps directed at avoiding or mitigating noncompliance. Being in charge of the site's conformance to the protocol and exercising trial oversight by the CI cannot be overemphasized. The steps could include the following.

31.1.4.1 Follow the Investigational Plan

The CI should ensure that all site staff associated with performing protocol steps are trained using the protocol and have a full understanding of their specific role and its importance. Establishing a periodic meeting of key staff which would discuss the protocol, potential, and real noncompliances which arise as well as solutions is a sound practice. Documenting such meetings as well as any decisions made about corrective actions is essential.

31.1.4.2 Avoid Protocol Deviations

Adherence to all aspects of the protocol should be a given in a trial however it does not always happen. Protocol deviations, i.e. situations where either data reliability or patient safety are of concern, must be avoided so deciding early on- prior to enrolling the first subject that such deviations are unacceptable is in keeping with GCP. If deviations are considered then there needs to be in place an SOP to guide the decision process. Having records of the decision making especially the rationale provided by key decision makers, e.g. the sponsor's medical director is essential for accountability at a later time. From the standpoint of documentation having an original signature from the key decision makers available is appropriate. Most SOPs would provide a form to use which includes spaces for the key information and signatures. Engaging the IRB/IEC for their opinion may also be appropriate, e.g. if the study population is considered vulnerable, and if a pattern of deviations emerges then protocol changes must be considered. It is useful to note that some competent authorities consider allowing "waivers" from the protocol as potentially noncompliant with GCP on their face and if a flaw is found in the protocol then a change/revision ought to be pursued through the appropriate channels [1].

31.1.4.3 Documentation

Decide on the trial record keeping responsibilities at the outset and include that as part of the protocol training process. Establishing the official record set for a trial will include defining the source documents for the data and how they will be maintained. The site's Trial Master File (sTMF) represents a primary location for documentation. Many records of a trial will be electronic whether they are directly entered into an electronic data capture system or transposed into an electronic system by site staff. Site staff should create a list all of the records which are expected to be maintained and define how they will be created, who is the most responsible party for each one and where the record can be located for review. It is possible the sponsor may initiate such an effort themselves but defining the record keeping plan for the study is a quality step that enhances the sites' trial master file process and prevents misunderstanding from occurring.

31.1.4.4 INV Product Accountability

Issues with investigational product accountability can be avoided by applying quality practices in several key risk areas. The first is ensuring that the procedures for receipt, storage, dispersal, and disposition are clear and in keeping with the protocol requirements. If a pharmacist/pharmacy is involved (and many times they are) ensuring that the personal in the pharmacy are trained/informed as to their role from the standpoint of receipt, storage, distribution and return of unused IMP. If the institution/organization has an Investigational Drug Service (IDS) (pharmacy) then utilizing the services of that unit is a wise choice (it may be the only choice!)

since they have developed processes and procedures to ensure compliance with all investigational drug accountability expectations. Most of the drug accountability deficiencies reported are clearly the result of carelessness, poor documentation practices and lack of sound record systems. Drawing on the support of experienced pharmacy professionals is a quality step that should be pursued.

31.1.4.5 Communication

The topic of establishing sound communication procedures and practices was discussed as a sponsor responsibility but it is not confined to the sponsor as a skillset. The investigator ought to be communicating with the other players, e.g. the IRB as well as the site staff assigned to the study. Whether the IRB/IEC is local or central in nature the investigator must establish effective lines of communication so that when the situations demanding IRB/IEC review arise the pathway is understood and advanced planning can be implemented. Failing to obtain ongoing IRB/IEC approval for a study is an example of a deficiency which is easily avoided. Investigators should establish at the time of study start up, the plan/timetable for when a request for continuing review of a study is needed. The ownership of that task should be assigned to the appropriate staff member if not the investigator. An effective project planning scheme and/or adding IRB/IEC continuing review to the sites study schedule of events might be useful.

31.1.4.6 Subject Protections

Subject protections are one of the two key reasons underpinning the development and implementation of GCP. The failure to report adverse events and/or administer informed consent in strict conformance with the applicable regulations, written procedures, protocol and GCP must be avoided. In terms of quality responsibility, these two aspects of trial conduct must be described in written procedures. Training against those procedures must occur and the importance of adhering to the procedures should be emphasized among the entire study team. Since the primary responsibility for reporting adverse events resides with sponsors, ensuring that the procedural steps for the site to assemble information and communicate it to the sponsor in a timely manner are well understood. Engaging in a mock practice situation for reporting a serious unexpected adverse event would be a good quality practice. In terms of informed consent arranging for a seasoned representative from the IRB/IEC, to conduct training of staff on ethical practices and witness a subject undergoing informed consent as part of ongoing training should be meaningful. Most IRB/IECs develop and conduct training programs which are geared to promote compliant practices by the site staff conducting the trial. If the IRB is central in nature such steps might not be as doable but using the available communication technology most of the important elements of hands on training can still be accomplished.

31.1.5 Institutional Review Board/Independent Ethics Committee (IRB/IEC)

The IRB/IEC's should organizationally be separate from the other research groups which conduct/perform the clinical trial activities. Avoiding any appearance of conflict of interest based on who can influence the IRB/IEC's approach to its work as well as the decisions it makes, is a key aspect of maintaining its independent judgment role. Specific quality or quality related responsibilities drawn from ICH E6(R2) are listed in a truncated manner in the table below.

Section of ICHGCP	IRB/IEC quality responsibility
3.1.3	IRB/IEC should review and evaluate the qualifications of the CI for the proposed trial.
3.1.4	IRB/IEC should conduct continuing review of each trial at appropriate intervals or at least 1 X/year.
3.2.2	The IRB/IEC should conduct work according to SOPs and keep records of performing the work
3.2.6	Non-members may be contacted for specific expertise
3.3	IRB/IEC should establish, document in writing, and follow SOPs.
3.4	IRB/IEC should retain all relevant records

From the standpoint of building quality into its functional responsibilities the IRB/IEC should consider becoming accredited by a professional group such as the Association for Accreditation of Human Research Programs, Inc. [1], which offer an assessment process directed at determining whether certain standards are met. Other quality related steps the IRB/IEC might arrange are an investigator self-assessment program where the CI is provided a self-assessment tool for use and a protocol assessment program where protocols are randomly selected and assessed for completeness.

31.1.6 Additional Quality Factors

In addition to the specific or implied quality responsibilities of the players in the clinical trial process there are three factors which contribute to the success of implementing a quality systems approach. Those factors are addressed in the following topic narratives.

31.1.6.1 Organizational Structure

Organizationally does the sponsor have a central control point for quality assurance activities and if so what influence does it have? Sponsors must have an organizational focal point for quality functions and decisions. This quality assurance focal point must be at a level in the organization where it can effect change if necessary and must have an influential voice in high level decision-making. The title for the office e.g. Senior Director of Clinical Quality Assurance, given to the position is not as important as its role. The human resources allocated to quality functions are usually much less than to operational groups and this is in part because a large portion of the QC activities are actually performed by clinical operations and other staff not directly assigned to the quality unit. The presence of a high level quality position in the organization is a reflection of the organization's quality mindset and an indication of organizational commitment from the top. The placement of the quality focal point must also be separate from the Clinical Development group to avoid bias or conflict of interest.

31.1.6.2 Communication

From a communication standpoint does the sponsor have in place systems to facilitate discussion, decision making and escalation for important matters? You might be asking, Why is this important? Effective or *quality* communication is critical to the success of all undertakings. Success in establishing and conducting effective QC and QA activities is no exception. Communication must occur across groups and not be confined to management. Communication has to be two-way to be effective. In today's world of instant communications one would think that establishing a sound and effective communications network would be easy but the secret is in the transparency and trust that exists among the people involved in the trial. If an atmosphere of trust and respect exists then decisions are honored, issues can be surfaced and addressed, and pathways to resolution can be reached. Communication can occur in writing, face–to-face, via electronic means, telephone, etc., but there needs to be forums and venues for it to occur, documentation prepared and as follow up on decisions to occur. Communication is not specifically mentioned as one of the foundational building of quality systems since it is an inherent attribute of each one that is included here.

31.1.6.3 Operational

Operationally does the sponsor have the fundamental building blocks of a quality system in place and working? Asking and answering whether the fundamental building blocks of a quality system are in place and functioning efficiently is a fair step for management to take. If not then the possibility or risk of a quality failure is present. Examples of questions which could be used to frame out exactly whether the building blocks are present and robust in design follow.

31.1.6.3.1 Management Involvement

Have senior staff from medical and clinical affairs been attending and/or participating in clinical trial team meetings? If so what is the evidence supporting that participation, e.g. meeting notes.

31.1.6.3.2   Change Management/Change Control

Have any changes occurred in trial protocols or other essential documents in the recent past and if so did the change process follow a written SOP? Were IRB and, as necessary, regulatory authority approvals obtained?

31.1.6.3.3   Training

Has the organization met GCP update training in conformance with policy and procedural instructions? Is there a program in place to identify new GCP expectations and if so are regular updates provided? Have new staff members brought on because of turnover undergone training? Is the turnover rate problematic?

31.1.6.3.4   Qualifications

Does the organization have an SOP for qualification of CROs, vendors, monitors, and IRBs? Except for individual monitors, does the SOP include a prequalification visit or audit and if so, are clinical QA staff involved? Can pre-qualification visits be waived and if so why?

31.1.6.3.5   Recordkeeping and Documentation

When was the Data management group last audited and were there any issues? If so are they now resolved?

31.1.6.3.6   Corrective and Preventive Action (CAPA)

Other than follow up to monitoring findings what sources does the organization draw from to add or include items in the CAPA system? Does the organization have a CAPA system in place?

31.1.6.3.7   Written Procedures

Are the clinical SOPs maintained by a central documentation system and if so does the Development/Clinical group have a representative serving on the Document Control coordination team? Has that person been participating as expected?

31.1.6.3.8   QA

Have the internal and external audit plans been followed over the past 12 months and are all audit findings resolved?

31.1.6.3.9   QC

Does the organization employ a checklist review processes for essential documents, e.g. Protocol/CRF/ICF and are those checklists maintained or destroyed? If maintained are the checklist available for regulatory agency inspection? If not maintained then is there documentation of the review process? Who, When, What and Why?

31.1.6.3.10 Risk Assessment and Management

Did the organization conduct a risk assessment process for the trial and if so do the questions listed form the categories above fit into the areas of potential concern identified during that assessment?

31.1.7 Summary

In this chapter, we extracted from ICH E6(R2) the specific quality responsibilities and also tasks/responsibilities which are quality related based on their linkage to the quality systems building blocks. In reviewing these lists it becomes apparent that quality responsibilities are inherent in the ICH E6(R2) structure even if the term quality is not specifically used.

In addition we examined three key factors that contribute significantly to the success of the quality status of a clinical trial from the standpoint of building quality into the process. The first is the organizational structure and whether it supports and fosters a quality environment. Establishing a quality focal point in an organization and giving it some clout is a critical aspect.

The second factor is communication skills and having processes in place to effect sound transfer of information. Communications systems must be recognized, utilized, and provide documentation schemes to be effective.

Ensuring that the building blocks of a quality systems program are in place is the third factor. With the fundamentals in place the likelihood that the people performing the work will, over time, adopt a quality mindset is significantly enhanced. The integration of quality system approaches into the day to day work will prevent nonconformances and noncompliances.

Drawing on nonconformance data from site inspections conducted by regulatory authorities gives us a reference point for areas of risk in the conduct of human clinical trials. If a CI addresses those potential risk areas by applying quality practices the likelihood that noncompliance will be avoided is enhanced.

Knowledge Check Questions

1) Where in the ICH E6(R2) guidelines does it describe the quality responsibilities of the sponsor, investigator, IRB/IEC? Do you agree that there is a responsibility to build quality into a clinical trial activity? If so why?

2) Under ICH E6(R2) are trial sponsors expected to establish a written quality plan for each trial similar to the way a data management plan might be prepared? Is there any other plan that ICH E6(R2) calls for which represents quality activities called for by GCP?

3) Do you think it is appropriate as part of a quality responsibility under GCP for the sponsor to plan an audit of an investigator site and conduct it before the site has completed enrollment? If so why do you think an early audit might be useful?

4) Does ICH E6(R2) specify any communication responsibilities for the sponsor, CRO, clinical investigator, or IRB? If so, please list it (them). If not then why was a section of the chapter committed to communication?

5) One way to assess risk in terms of noncompliance at trial sites is to study findings from inspections at sites by regulatory authorities. Name two such findings and one thing you might do to mitigate the possibility of it occurring.

Reference

1 European Medicines Agency (2020). Good Clinical Practice Q&A, GCP Matters. https://www.ema.europa.eu/en/human-regulatory/research-development/compliance/good-clinical-practice/qa-good-clinical-practice-gcp#gcp-matters-section (accessed 1 June 2020).

32

Standard Operating Procedures

P. Michael Dubinsky

GCP Key Point

Throughout ICH E6(R2) references are made to establishing, in writing, the procedures to be followed by the responsible party. Written procedures represent a quality system building block which if used for training, followed, and kept current will contribute significantly to assuring quality in trial implementation.

Assuring the accuracy and reliability, i.e. the credibility, of the data developed during a clinical trial is one of the two objectives of GCP. Therefore the systems, practices, and procedures associated with performing tasks during the course of a clinical trial are essential to meeting this objective. In Chapter 30 Quality Systems in Clinical Research, written procedures were discussed as a fundamental building block of a quality systems approach. This chapter will expand that topic from the standpoint of describing written procedures, the types of issues that might be encountered and where in GCP the procedures are specifically expected.

32.1 Introduction

Written standard operating procedures are an integral part of just about every industry and discipline. They are integral in establishing a quality management system and take on special importance in undertakings which are regulated. Some people would argue that required standard operating procedures (SOPs) are simply a reference point to inspect against when inspectors and auditors arrive to do their work. That said they, the procedures, do represent a formidable tool which can, if used to the best advantage prevent errors, ensure conformance to standards, and underscore a commitment to quality.

The Fundamentals of Clinical Research: A Universal Guide for Implementing Good Clinical Practice, First Edition. P. Michael Dubinsky and Karen A. Henry.
© 2022 John Wiley & Sons, Inc. Published 2022 by John Wiley & Sons, Inc.
Companion website: www.wiley.com/go/dubinsky/clinicalresearch

32.1.1 Objectives

The objectives of this chapter are to: (i) identify the sections of the ICH E6(R2) that contain references to written procedures, in particular SOPs; (ii) describe some areas and aspects of SOPs that often become problematic and therefore are to be avoided; and (iii) to offer some thoughts on how to avoid the problematic aspects of maintaining a sound SOP program in your organization.

32.1.2 Expectations/Requirements for SOPs

It is fair to say that regulatory and competent authorities around the globe expect/ require there be written procedures in place describing the full range of trial-related activities. ICH E6(R2) places the responsibility for preparing and maintaining the majority of these written procedures squarely on the trial sponsor but the IRB and investigator also have responsibilities in this area. In order to place the expectations for written procedures in perspective the following Table 32.1 constructed from ICH E6(R2) excerpts is helpful.

32.1.3 SOPs as Part of a Document Control Program

ICH E6(R2) does not describe how to write SOPs, how they should be structured, or how to best design the overall document program at an organization and this text will not do so either. It is useful however to make several points about the system in which SOPs and other documents which are utilized in trial performance are located.

32.1.3.1 Controlled Versus Uncontrolled Documents

SOPs must be part of a controlled document system. A controlled document system is one which has the following attributes:

- Documents are approved for completeness and content prior to use by an organizational official of high standing.
- A process for updating, or obsoleting is included
- Changes follow a set pathway and a record of the changes and the reason underpinning the change is documented
- Version control is applied
- Historical copies are retained
- Obsolete versions are removed from active use and suitably dispositioned or identified to avoid them being mistaken for current versions.
- The procedure is usually associated with meeting a regulatory requirement.
- The development and updating of the document follows an SOP on SOPs.

Table 32.1 Expectations for written procedures (constructed from ICH E6(R2) excerpts).

E6 Sec No.	Text excerpt	Remarks/points/comments	Responsible party
Glossary 1.6 Audit	A systematic and independent examination of trial-related activities and documents to determine whether the evaluated trial-related activities were conducted, and the data were recorded, analyzed, and accurately reported according to the protocol, sponsor's standard operating procedures (SOPs),...	This definition indicates that the Sponsor is expected to have SOPs in place for all trial-related activities as well as data collection, management, and analysis	Sponsor
Glossary 1.38 Monitoring	...conducted, recorded, and reported in accordance with the protocol, Standard Operating Procedures (SOPs)...	This excerpt from the definition of *Monitoring* indicates that an SOP(s) Is expected to be in place for the trial-related activity.	Sponsor
Glossary 1.55 SOP	Detailed, written instructions to achieve uniformity of the performance of a specific function.	Definition of Standard Operating Procedures (SOP's).	All parties
Principles 2.13	Systems with procedures that assure the quality of every aspect of the trial should be implemented.	This GCP principle does not specify written procedures but that is the implication if they are to support systems.	All parties
IRB 3.2.2 Composition...	The IRB/IEC should perform its functions according to written operating procedures,...	This indicates that IRB/IEC functions and operations are grounded in written SOPs	IRB/IEC
IRB 3.2.3 Composition...	An IRB/IEC should make its decisions at announced meetings at which at least a quorum, as stipulated in its written operating procedures, is present.	The number of members that constitutes a quorum for the IRB is to be found in a written SOP	IRB
IRB 3.3 Procedures	Procedures – The IRB/IEC should establish, document in writing, and follow its procedures, which should include...	In items 3.3.1 through 3.3.9 specific procedures that should be in writing are listed	IRB

(Continued)

Table 32.1 (Continued)

E6 Sec No.	Text excerpt	Remarks/points/comments	Responsible party
IRB 3.4 Records	Records – The IRB/IEC should retain all relevant records (e.g., written procedures. . . for a period of at least three years after completion of the trial. . .The IRB/IEC may be asked. . . to provide its written procedures. . .	In this section, the retention period for both the written procedures as well as records associated with performing the procedures is defined.	IRB
Investigator 4.4.1 Communication with IRB	. . .dated approval/favorable opinion from the IRB/IEC. . . subject recruitment procedures (e.g., advertisements). . .	This section indicates that subject recruitment procedures shall be written and approved by the IRB. These may not be considered SOPs but rather study-specific procedures	Investigator
Randomization 4.7 Procedures	Randomization procedures and unblinding – The investigator should follow the trial's randomization procedures. . .	Written procedures describing randomization and unblinding are likely to be found in the protocol as well as in SOPs.	Sponsor, Investigator
Informed Consent 4.8.10 (d)	The trial procedures to be followed,. . .	Here and in other E6 locations trial procedures are referenced reinforcing the fact that the protocol, informed consent, and supporting materials represent trial-specific procedures that are to be followed.	Sponsor, Investigator, IRB
Records and Reports 4.9.3	Sponsors should have written procedures to assure that changes or corrections in CRFs made by sponsor's designated representatives are documented, are necessary, and are endorsed by the investigator.	This procedural expectation is focused on written directions for changing and correcting CRF entries. It represents good documentation practice instructions.	Sponsor, Investigator

Section			
Sponsor 5.0 Quality Mgt.	Quality management includes... and procedures for data collection and processing...	This section is the key part of the R2 addendum to the ICH E6(R2) from 2016. It outlines the expectation of a Risk Assessment and Management process being implemented. Procedural instructions for such an undertaking are intuitive and SOPs are mentioned, see item 5.0.2.	Sponsor
QA and QC 5.1	QA and QC systems must be implemented and maintained and have SOPs.	Written SOPs describing the QA and QC systems, e.g. monitoring are expected.	Sponsor, Investigator, IRB
Trial Mgt. 5.5.2	The Independent Data Monitoring Committee should have written operating procedures	Calls for written procedures to guide any independent data monitoring committee or data safety monitoring committee	Sponsor and the IDMC
Trial Mgt. 5.5.3 Addendum	For electronic systems SOPs for using the systems as well as SOPs for setup, installation and use.	This new section added as part of the 2016 Addendum calls for SOPs to be in place covering all aspects of computerized system operation.	Sponsor
Investigator Selection 5.6.3	The sponsor should obtain the investigator's/ institution's agreement:... (b) to comply with procedures for data recording/reporting;...	Calls for the sponsor to obtain the investigator's written agreement to follow written procedures e.g. those guiding the use of the CRF. The written procedures may be SOPs or work instructions.	Sponsor, Investigator
Compensation of subjects/ investigator 5.8.2	The sponsor's policies and procedures should address the costs of treatment of trial subjects in the event of trial-related injuries in accordance with the applicable regulatory requirement(s).	Calls for the sponsor to have in place written procedures for reimbursement of subjects who are injured as part of a trial in those jurisdictions where regulations require it.	Sponsor, Investigator

(Continued)

Table 32.1 (Continued)

E6 Sec No.	Text excerpt	Remarks/points/comments	Responsible party
Supplying/ handling IMP 5.14.3	The sponsor should ensure that written procedures include instructions that the investigator/institution should follow for the handling and storage of investigational product(s) for the trial...	This section of E6 specifically outlines the following; The procedures should address adequate and safe receipt, handling, storage, dispensing, retrieval of unused product from subjects, and return of unused investigational product(s) to the sponsor (or alternative disposition if authorized by the sponsor and in compliance with the applicable regulatory requirement(s)).	Sponsor
Monitoring 5.18.3	...however in exceptional circumstances the sponsor may determine that central monitoring in conjunction with procedures such as investigators' training and meetings, and extensive written guidance can assure appropriate conduct of the trial in accordance with GCP...	This E6 instruction indicates that the risk-based monitoring approach can be utilized if there are written procedures describing the other steps that will be taken to ensure the trial is performed according to GCP.	Sponsor
Monitoring 5.18.5	Monitoring Procedures – The monitor(s) should follow the sponsor's established written SOPs as well as those procedures that are specified by the sponsor for monitoring a specific trial.	Monitoring, as the primary QC element in trial conduct must have written procedures describing how it will be performed and whether ancillary materials such as monitoring plans will be prepared.	Sponsor
Audit 5.19.3	The sponsor should ensure that the auditing of clinical trials/systems is conducted in accordance with the sponsor's written procedures on what to audit, how to audit, the frequency of audits, and the form and content of audit reports.	This E6 section specifies that Sponsor QA audit procedures must also be in writing and be specific as to key elements.	Sponsor

Section	Description	Responsible
Trial Design 6.4.2	A description of the type/design of trial to be conducted (e.g. double-blind, placebo-controlled, parallel design) and a schematic diagram of trial design, procedures, and stages.	Sponsor
Trial Design 6.4.7	Accountability procedures for the investigational product(s).. . .	Sponsor
Subjects-Selection, Withdrawal and Treatment 6.5.3 and 6.6.3	Subject withdrawal criteria (i.e. terminating investigational product treatment/trial treatment) and procedures. . .	Sponsor
Safety 6.8.3	Procedures for eliciting reports of and for recording and reporting adverse event and intercurrent illnesses.	Sponsor

This E6 section describes the procedural expectations for the trial design found in the protocol.

Investigational product accountability must be described in written procedures (SOPs) and in the protocol.

This E6 section describes procedures which are found in the protocol

While the protocol must describe the procedures for safety reporting, the sponsor will also be expected to have in place written SOPs describing experience reporting from site to sponsor and sponsor to regulatory authority and IRBs as appropriate.

Other documents which would normally be part of the controlled document system at an organization might include organizational policies, organizational charts/diagrams labeling, and product specifications.

Uncontrolled documents are ones which have importance and significance but may not need to be controlled as rigorously because they represent daily work instructions to implement a procedure. Examples from the clinical trial arena might be monitoring plans, instructions for a clinical trial management system (CTMS), checklists for evaluating essential documents and timeline targets for submitting monitoring reports.

32.1.4 The Value of SOPs

From time to time you may hear someone comment that the reason why SOPs are required is because the regulators decided they were necessary. Whether there is truth to that point of view is not as important as placing in perspective the value that having SOPs and a sound SOP program in place at your organization. Below are outlined some of the reasons why SOPs add value to your overall trial program.

32.1.4.1 Avoids Differing Interpretation of Requirements
SOPs are supposed to reflect the policies of the organization translated into action steps. In the clinical trial GCP arena there are at times opportunities for differing points of view to arise about how to implement or fulfil a requirement. For example, the administration of informed consent. Having SOPs avoid such situations.

32.1.4.2 Personnel Turnover
Because of the range of the skillsets that the Pharma, biotech, biologics, and device industries require to successfully conduct clinical trial activities personnel changes are not uncommon for a variety of reasons. While the duties and responsibilities have similar titles each firm's culture, policies, and therapeutic targets influence how they perform certain tasks. Having a sound up-to-date SOP program allows for seamless transitions.

32.1.4.3 Differing Processes
Companies often have differing approaches to accomplish the same requirement. SOPs aid considerably in ensuring that personnel follow the correct process and not the one from the last place the person worked.

32.1.4.4 Answers are Available Even if Management Is Not
Situations do arise when a supervisor or management official may not be immediately available (even in the world of high tech it happens) to serve as a sounding board for an immediate answer to a situation which may not be encountered day

to day. Issue elevation type situations come to mind as an example. A check with the SOP can quickly provide the answer and the pathway to follow.

32.1.4.5 Organizational Transparency Is Improved
By publishing standard procedures and processes, information is shared among the organization's staff members thereby removing the potential for misunderstandings and misconceptions as to the way things are done, who does them, and why they are performed in a certain manner.

32.1.4.6 Knowledge Transfer Is Facilitated
As noted above, personnel turnover does occur and absent written procedures, standards and policies, the accumulated and historical knowledge can be lost. Written SOPs aid in avoiding those situations.

32.1.5 Issues with SOPs and How to Avoid Them

Table 32.2 depicts some of the most common issues that arise with SOPs, thoughts on common root causes for the issue being present and suggested approach to prevent or cure the issue. They are not all encompassing but the goal is not to be all encompassing but rather to tune the reader into quality thinking-prevention of issues.

32.1.6 Avoiding SOP Issues

Each firm should have in place an SOP on SOPs and following that SOP is essential. One element in the SOP on SOPs will be the mandatory review/update period. Generally a time span of once every two years for a review/update is chosen. A one year review requirement is not uncommon. The important step here is to honor that review period commitment.

Bottlenecks in the controlled documentation system can surface even in organizations/companies which see themselves as progressive and free of bureaucratic stumbling blocks. Bottlenecks can take different forms but a common one is one or two key executives who feel a need to edit every document that they are in charge of approving. Keeping the final approval level for SOP changes reasonable or ensuring delegations of authority exist to allow documents in the review scheme to move forward are useful steps to consider.

Having an SOP owner who performs responsibly in terms of ensuring the review periods are honored, substantive changes to procedures and organizational structure are adopted into the SOP(s) may not be the sure-fire way to avoid issues but it is, based on experience, way ahead of most other preventive measures to avoid SOP issues. Tying job responsibilities, performance review and awards to

Table 32.2 The most common issues arising from SOPs.

SOP issue	Likely root cause (?)	Prevention/Cure
Failure to keep SOP up to date	Could be multiple reasons, e.g. SOP owner fails to initiate change	Management oversight of documentation system via audit or review. Remove bottlenecks
SOP too detailed or too sketchy	SOP is not being written by the people who use them. SOP audience (user) is not providing review/feedback	Is the SOP on SOPs adequate in terms of responsibilities?
SOP terminology is open to interpretation thereby resulting in different implementation	Terminology used is not well defined or is not conformed to current technology, state of the art.	Are SOPs being reviewed according to a planned schedule (SOP on SOPs) if not get back on track. Are SMEs participating in the review process?
SOP too long and difficult to follow/accomplish	Process steps may need to be broken down into phases/pieces. (Rule of 10?)	May need to convene a meeting of key personnel to decide on how to best reduce size/complexity without impacting needed steps.
SOPs are not being created to match the company's growth as process and procedural steps expand	Management is not giving the quality system the attention and importance it needs	Bring in a competent QA/QC staff member or consultant to convince management of the importance of adopting quality practices early on.
SOPs are not seen as necessary because the firm is following the regulations and therefore in compliance. E.g. monitoring studies	Failure to understand the purpose of SOPs. They are in part for documenting how your processes and procedures comply with the regulations and guidelines	Send management out for some training in quality systems
Staff are not following the SOP	SOP not in sync with current practices	Have SOP waivers been documented and tracked? Is there an SOP providing an avenue for waivers? Is the SOP language understood by the audience? Do supervisors enforce the SOP expectations?

application of SOPs where appropriate sounds more management-oriented than quality-oriented but it is both. Staff find it much easier to avoid SOP issues if it links to their paycheck and employment status.

A final thought on clinical-related SOPs. Unlike SOPs directing product manufacture SOPs associated with GCP matters generally do not require that the quality assurance unit be the final sign off for approval. QA should however be in the review loop to ensure the SOP meets regulatory expectations as well as organization policies.

From the training standpoint SOPs can offer some challenges but applying some common sense prevents those challenges from becoming pitfalls. First avoid *drive by* training. Training on SOPs is very often conducted via a "read and understand" process. During an audit of a company's training program I once found that records documented that approximately 50 staff members were trained on approximately 50 SOPs within a one hour period of time. The training records were all prepared in the *read and understand* format. I termed this event *drive by* training and doubted the effectiveness of the training. In assessing organizational training events for SOP matters it is recommended that:

- Read and understand format is often used but "classroom" training ensures that most if not all questions, including the stupid ones get asked and answered and everyone who needs to, hears the full set of Q&A.
- Staff should revisit SOPs when there are important changes and/or annually. If they feel self-conscious about calling it retraining call it something else – call it a banana.
- Seriously consider giving exams/quizzes as part of the training exercise. Include a question which calls on the staff member to make a decision when some complexity arises. E.g. During monitoring serious noncompliance is identified. The SOP calls for Compliance/QA to be contacted first. However, the Head of Clinical Operations wants to try and rectify the situation him/herself. What does one do?
- Ensure that staff members know where to find/locate SOPs and that you know which SOPs are being used for a particular trial. E.g. if a CRO is being utilized are you following the CRO's SOPs, or those of the sponsor?

The points above relate to following the SOP on SOPs, avoiding bottlenecks and making SOP training effective should go a long way in terms of preventing the types of SOP issues listed in the table from occurring.

32.1.7 System Development and Configuration

The nature and scope of a company's SOP program is to a great extent decided upon as the overall documentation and record control program evolves. A key attribute of the SOP program is whether it is viewed as an integral part of the quality system approach or if it is seen as a must do in case the regulatory authorities ask for them – and they will at some point. From the GCP standpoint item 2.13 – the systems principle stands out as the overarching expectation. The principle does not specifically state that a system of written SOPs must be in place but the expectation is obvious. Absent a complete and effective SOP program it would not seem likely the principle can be met. The development of an SOP program is a function of several factors including the following:

32.1.7.1 The Status of the Organization's Regulated Activities

If you are a start up with no active human clinical trials then having SOPs describing such activity would not be required. Once a company engages in regulated activity having the written procedures describing how they are complying with the regulations, guidelines, best practices, etc. is expected. Establishing the SOP program however can and should start sooner rather than later so that the procedural steps and foundation for SOP development exist.

32.1.7.2 The Size of the Organization and the Functions that are Being Performed

A "virtual" organization (and it does exist) that outsources many or all activities associated with conducting a clinical trial will need to have a basic set of SOPs but they will need to ensure that certain ones, e.g. those governing activities such as outsourcing, vendor/CRO qualification, validation of computerized systems, and a quality assurance audit program are robust and followed. If the company relies on CROs to have SOPs available for the functions delegated to them then they need to be certain they have an approach to assessing the acceptability of the CRO's SOPs for adequacy and completeness.

32.1.7.3 Employee Experience and Qualifications

One premise of drafting SOPs is that the folks who perform the work are the best candidates to write the SOPs for their specific tasks. If the staff are seasoned veterans of the clinical trial arena they should be able to draft and deliver a sound SOP that draws on their experience but adapts it to the policies and practices of the company. Also the detail of an SOP may be governed by the experience of the staff recognizing that turnover will occur at some point in time.

32.1.7.4 Compliance History

If a firm has been active in regulated activities for some time and has been inspected by regulatory authorities they should have a real time understanding of their compliance quotient or status. If they have not fared well when evaluated by a regulatory agency inspector/investigator the need for a full range of SOPs is probably already established. If they have been judged to be in substantial compliance then it is likely they have a sound SOP program and structure in place.

32.1.8   SOP Program Configuration

Regarding program configuration and structure there are three points that stand out from a quality standpoint. The content of the SOP program, the change control element, and the scope of the program.

32.1.8.1   System Content
While SOPs themselves are the primary content most documentation programs address other documents which are integral to the Company's documentation activities. Documents such as company policies and work instructions come to mind. Policies are high-level statements of the company philosophy and culture. They cut across a range of matters including human resources, compliance with law and regulation, mission, social commitment to name a few. For clinical trials establishing a written ethical standards policy would be logical. Another would be a Quality Policy. Policies would be controlled documents as are SOPs. Work instructions are maintained as part of the document control program but are not generally treated as controlled documents needing sign off by senior management but rather are updated by the unit which uses them day to day. An example of work instructions (which are usually detailed *how to* write ups) are the user instructions for the data management system employed at the company. The data management group keeps the instructions up-to-date based on manufacturer's directions, updates, etc. and would not need to obtain high-level management approval on the details.

32.1.8.2   Change Control
If the SOPs are housed in a company's overall document control system there is likely a built in change control process that ensures all parties know about change and that necessary documentation of those changes occurs as the process unfolds. Documentation of participants, timeframes, changes, approvals and reasons for change is included, should it need to be accessed at a later time.

Program Scope – Defining the scope or reach of the SOP program and each procedure is important in terms of ensuring that all groups having a stake in the development of the procedures are engaged. E.g. does the SOP apply across the entire organization (SOP on SOPs), is it cross functional (document retention), or is focused on a single group/department (Monitoring).

32.1.9   Summary

SOPs are both a necessity and an asset to building quality into the conduct of clinical trials. They are required in many global regions from a regulatory standpoint and expected as part of fulfilling GCP compliance. SOPs support a quality approach to conduct of clinical trials in that they add value in a number of ways such as providing a blueprint for the performance of procedures in a uniform and consistent manner. They are however not without potential issues. SOPs can be too long, too short, and quickly become out of date. Therefore, having a sound SOP on SOP development and content and following it is essential for success. Developing the scope and content of an SOP program is driven by a number of factors including regulatory activity, personnel experience, and compliance history. The types of documents in the SOP development program generally include policies and work instruction in addition to the SOPs themselves because the SOPs are a reflection of company policy and the work instructions supplement specific SOPs but at the group or unit level. Ensuring that quality system building blocks such as change control are an element in the SOP program is important.

Knowledge Check Questions

1) All parties involved in the conduct of clinical trials have the responsibility/ expectation to prepare **SOPs** (written procedures) describing their roles in trial-related activity. True ___ or False ____
2) Select the attributes which apply to a controlled document system.
   - Changes are documented _____
   - Final approval for changes are given by a group leader _____
   - Documents are version controlled _____
   - The company CEO maintains the system _____
   - SOP titles/topics generally are associated with meeting regulatory requirements._____
3) SOPs are written to be open for interpretation True _____ or False _____
4) The SOP for Monitoring of Clinical trials is always the same for all companies. True ___ or False _____
5) Being out of date or inconsistent with current practices is a common issue or concern encountered with SOPs? True ____ or False _____
6) Having an _____ (owner) for an SOP helps prevent problems or issues from occurring.
7) Staff training on SOPs can benefit from quizzes which test for understanding and retention. True _____ or False _____
8) You identify what you believe is a necessary change to a company SOP. What would be a logical first step toward implementing that change?
   - E-mail the company CEO
   - E-mail the QA group
   - Call a colleague who works in another group
   - Check the SOP on SOPs for guidance

33

Quality Assurance Components

P. Michael Dubinsky

GCP Key Point
Determining whether the clinical trial was conducted according to the protocol, regulations, GCP, and SOPs is an audit function. Establishing a system of corrective and preventive action helps ensure that when audited a trial meets the expectations of each.

33.1   Introduction

Audits represent the most visible and expected component of a quality assurance function established by the trial sponsor. Audits are often misunderstood in that the primary objective is to determine whether the in place procedures and processes are being performed according to plan. The plan of course for a clinical trial embraces the protocol, the regulations, GCP, and applicable SOPs. The outcome of an audit is a reflection of the training, experience, qualifications, technical and communication skills of the people conducting the trial. Establishing a system of corrective and preventive action (CAPA) which was described in Chapter 30 Quality Systems in Clinical Research as one of the foundational building blocks of a quality system can contribute significantly to staying on plan.

The sponsor of a clinical trial has the responsibility for establishing a viable audit plan that best serves the objective of identifying whether all the trial activities and systems used to implement those activities are performed according to GCP, the applicable regulations, SOPs and the protocol. Since audits are not expected to be conducted at 100% of all activity that is occurring selecting for audit those activities that will best signal potential problems or demonstrate full

The Fundamentals of Clinical Research: A Universal Guide for Implementing Good Clinical Practice, First Edition. P. Michael Dubinsky and Karen A. Henry.
© 2022 John Wiley & Sons, Inc. Published 2022 by John Wiley & Sons, Inc.
Companion website: www.wiley.com/go/dubinsky/clinicalresearch

compliance can be as much art as science. CAPA systems are generally not managed by the QA group however QA can make contributions to the CAPA system.

33.2 Objectives

The objective of this chapter is to outline the approach taken to develop and implement audit plans for clinical trial related activities. In addition the topic of CAPA plans, which are mentioned in Chapter 30 Quality Systems in Clinical Research, will be expanded upon.

33.3 Audit Plans

ICHGCP sections 1.6 and 5.19 are the key sections of GCP to access for reference with the narrative and discussion in this chapter.

Initially there are several well-known but important axioms to keep in perspective as the topic of audits is discussed.

- Do not wait for a regulatory authority, to perform your QA audit. Regulatory authorities inspect rather than audit and the possible outcomes are significantly different than a sponsor audit.
- Quality Assurance auditors are not regulators. They are members of the company team whose goal is a successful and compliant clinical trial. Auditors take their assignments seriously and are trained to show respect for the professionals they interact with during an audit. Returning that respect is useful.
- The outcome of most audits is that the systems are working and compliance is achieved.
- Audits are expected to sample at a reasonable percentage, e.g. 10%, the ongoing clinical trial activities not to assess them 100%.
- QA must be organizationally separate from the clinical/medical operations groups in a company.

Quality Assurance audits are generally planned at three levels: Places, processes, and things. Places include trial sites, laboratories, CROs, vendors, and IRBs. Processes include monitoring, data management, investigational product accountability, trial management, and clinical investigator-trial site compliance. Things include essential documents, clinical study reports, laboratory instrumentation, regulatory document binders, and source documents.

Audits include operations external and internal to the sponsor.

Audit plans are:

- Most often prepared annually and can be modified to meet company or regulatory needs which arise.

- Transparent and are communicated so groups and activities which are scheduled for audit know early on.

Reports generated by audits are:

- Confidential and are distributed on a need to know basis.
- Are not shared with regulatory authorities except in special situations.

Support for a company's outsourcing group (if one exists) is provided either in the form of audits or QA staff who accompany outsourcing staff during visits to vendors to provide first hand audit expertise in assessing the vendor/CRO.

As with all positions associated with the clinical trial endeavor auditors must be trained in their discipline and operate in conformance with approved SOPs. Quality assurance auditing of clinical activities differs significantly from auditing the manufacturing side of the pharmaceutical and device industry therefore it is common for clinical QA auditors to receive special training not only in trial conduct and therapeutic concepts but also in approaches to interviewing professional practitioners and others who perform the work. Auditing a clinical trial site run by a thought leader in their therapeutic discipline comes to mind as a situation which may call for seasoned people skills to be at the ready to avoid misunderstandings and yet accomplish the task.

Implementing a sound and robust clinical QA audit plan/program needs not be a secret. Regulatory authorities do ask for both QA SOPs if they exist, as well as audit plans and status reports. Such information can and should be shared because it demonstrates a commitment to quality and can have a positive impact on the regulator's view about the company's commitment to compliance and quality.

Independence of the audit program from the clinical development department is critical. If the clinical QA audit program's work is influenced by others then its effectiveness is compromised. That is not to say that flexibility cannot be exercised but in order for the program to have integrity it must be able to schedule and complete work according to plan and without undue delay.

Audit plans should be guided by a risk assessment process which considers matters such as protocol complexity, size and status of the trial, experience of the location(s) to be audited, company priority, and whether issues have already arisen with the trial.

33.4 Audit Implementation

Audit implementation should not be saved for the end of a clinical trial and treated as part of the wrap up or close out for the purpose of documenting that the trial was conducted in compliance with the regulations, protocol, etc. Nor should audits be reserved for situations where significant noncompliance is identified. Applying those criteria is generally a reactionary approach and not in keeping with the first principle of QA-preventing problems. This of course is referring to the external audits of trial related activity in particular sites. For example having auditors visit several sites early on in a multisite trial should identify whether investigator/site training on the protocol was effective and if not surface those areas that may need attention across participating sites. This example is most applicable for multisite studies but can be just as important for Phase I and II studies especially if the sites do not have a proven track record with the sponsor. Communication is a key element in a successful audit program and lining up the sites and as appropriate other activities to be audited early on to ensure their cooperation is important. Sites are often engaged in several trials at a time and are being visited and/or audited by more than one sponsor. That is not to mention inspections by regulatory authorities and/or internal regulatory groups at their institution. Therefore they are reluctant to commit to unnecessary visits or audits beyond what is often defined in the site contract. Audit programs therefore have become attuned to communicating audit plans early on, sticking to those plans and being efficient in performing the work. Sites need to permit audits as expected by GCP and to have the key staff available to answer questions, provide explanations, and discuss any issues that might arise. Unlike regulatory inspections an infrequently mentioned upside of audits is that they can and do verify that the quality management systems that are supposed to be in place and working are doing just that!

33.5 Corrective and Preventive Action – CAPA

Using a centralized approach to keeping track of issues that do surface through audits, inspections, monitoring visits, complaints, etc., is called CAPA

CAPA is most often viewed as a QC process but it is being included here because the company QA function will ensure it is functioning correctly as a system and will pick up the baton if key issues in the CAPA system are being ignored.

If the audit identifies instances of noncompliance in terms of adherence to protocol, regulations, GCP or SOP those findings will be transmitted to the responsible person at the site, other facility, or organizational unit being audited. While an audit report is prepared the full report is not usually transmitted, only the findings. There are several options audit groups utilize to communicate the findings and one which is often used is to channel the communication of adverse or nonconforming findings through the clinical development department to the site. This ensures that all parties are on the same page at the same time and utilizes the established line of communications between the site (or CRO/vendor) and the sponsor. The expectation is that the site will respond by defining their corrective action steps or plan as well as a timetable for implementation. If the site has an active CAPA system then the audit findings would be tracked using it. CAPA systems are as mentioned in Chapter 30 Quality Systems in Clinical Research, one of the fundamental building blocks of a Quality System. CAPA is not confined to tracking items that are raised only by audits and should include quality improvement initiatives, monitoring findings, complaints, findings from internal department audits, IRB audits, regulatory inspections to name possible contributors (see Figure 33.1). CAPA programs are important for several reasons. First they should have the attention of management in terms of ensuring that corrective action commitments are fulfilled on time and as necessary resources are directed to support the corrections. Secondly they are meant to look beyond an individual finding to see whether there is a systemic problem or issue that needs to be addressed and if so implement the corrective steps necessary to address those situations. Thirdly the CAPA approach ensures that the commitment to correct does not unnecessarily become a victim of higher priorities and stays relevant until it is fully resolved. Fourth if the system receives input from a wide range of sources it should allow for the identification of trends.

Creating a CAPA does not require sophisticated off-the-shelf software although it is available. It does require some commitment from management and a basic approach to track the key elements of the inputs and seeing commitments to

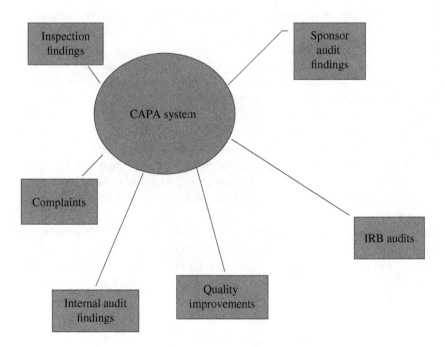

Figure 33.1 CAPA system inputs.

correct through to completion. CAPA is not a stated requirement of the applicable clinical trial regulations/requirements at least not in a specific citation or listing. The ICH E6(R2) does however mention it at section 5.20.1. It has also become however an expected approach in the clinical community and regulatory inspectors will inquire about the existence of such systems. A key question then arises- Do regulators have access to CAPA information and records? An inquiry with the FDA's Office of Good Clinical Practice (Personal communication, M.Melvin, FDA) indicates that FDA investigators will not ask for CAPA records at a sponsor or trial site. They may of course have access to some records which contribute to the content of a CAPA – e.g. monitoring reports. In at least some of the EU member states CAPA is required however the depth of review taken by inspectors is guided by current inspectional findings and whether past inspectional findings remain uncorrected. It is the sense of this author that having a CAPA system in place is a best practice but taking steps to ensure that the content is appropriately protected from inappropriate exposure is a valid risk to manage.

33.6 Summary

This chapter has outlined several QA components which are integral to meeting fundamental GCP expectations. Audits are and will likely remain the first thing that comes to mind when QA is referenced. Conducting audits may not be an FDA regulatory requirement for clinical trial sponsors but having an audit plan and implementing it is obligatory if a sponsor is to fully apply the QA expectations of ICH E6(R2) principle 2.13. It is not a best practice to wait until a trial is completed and the regulatory authorities schedule an inspection to begin thinking about the audit plan and how it will be implemented. Having a transparent, flexible audit plan, designed utilizing a risk assessment approach, and implementing it will pay dividends in terms of identifying potential noncompliance, areas of GCP weakness as well as excellence in meeting program expectations. Using a centralized approach to keeping track of issues that do surface through audits, inspections, monitoring visits, complaints, etc., is called CAPA. Whether you call it CAPA (or call it a banana) putting in place a central repository for all such inputs allows for critical examination, management awareness and most importantly no surprises if a significant or critical matter does show up on the radar of a regulator. By employing the CAPA mindset not only the issue but also the corrective action steps are clear and transparent.

Knowledge Check Questions

1) Conducting audits and having an audit plan are required by the ICH E6(R2). True ____ or False ____

2) In terms of developing an audit plan for a Phase III trial the sponsor will likely schedule. % of sites for audit. (a) 100% (b) 50% (c) 20% (d) 7%

3) Reports of site audits are most effective if posted in the company lounge or cafeteria so all employees can read through them and offer opinions. Agree_____ or disagree_____

4) GCP QA auditors are most effective if they approach the work as if they were conducting a regulatory inspection. Agree_____ or Disagree

   _____.

5) Select the true statements concerning QA audits, audit programs, and Audit Plans

   - Auditors work in conjunction with clinical development to successfully complete the trial _____.
   - Audit programs are best if coordinated by clinical development.____
   - The company's list of active trials is included when developing an audit plan. True _____ or False_____
   - Sites can deny permission to conduct an audit according to GCP. Agree____ or disagree ____
   - The company's medical monitor is the most qualified to select site locations for monitoring
   - Auditing early in the life cycle of a trial is *most or least* effective approach.

6) CAPA systems originated when the FDA's IND regulations were updated in 1987. Correct_____ or Incorrect_____?

7) Select the most accurate statement about CAPA.

   a) By having a CAPA system firms guarantee full compliance with regulatory requirements.

   b) A well designed CAPA system engages management and has their support.

   c) Regulatory agency inspectors always ask for access to a firm's CAPA system because it saves them time in terms of uncovering problems.

   d) You have to purchase special computer software in order to have an effective CAPA system.

34

Regulatory Authority Inspections

P. Michael Dubinsky

GCP Key Point

GCP requires that investigators permit regulatory agency inspections and that sponsors secure agreements from all parties allowing inspections at any time. Since inspections happen- being knowledgeable and savvy about them makes for a manageable and productive experience.

34.1 Introduction

Once a clinical trial application has been submitted and received approval by a regulatory/competent authority the possibility that an inspection may be scheduled and occur becomes reality. Inspections of clinical trial activities, in particular the investigator site and the sponsor are important facets of the oversight/compliance programs that regulators have in place to ensure that if human clinical trials are underway subjects are protected and applicable requirements are being met. In theory if a company is abiding by all applicable regulatory requirements, the protocol, SOPs, and GCP any inspection should be issue free, correct? Notwithstanding that idealistic point of view, developing a program of inspection readiness has become a standard practice for the commercial pharmaceutical, biotech and medical device industry, and all medical research centers that engage in clinical trials. Regulators have no problem with such readiness programs in large measure because the presence of such activities demonstrate that companies want to be efficient in processing inspection requests and the deterrent element associated with the potential for inspection is working.

The Fundamentals of Clinical Research: A Universal Guide for Implementing Good Clinical Practice, First Edition. P. Michael Dubinsky and Karen A. Henry.
© 2022 John Wiley & Sons, Inc. Published 2022 by John Wiley & Sons, Inc.
Companion website: www.wiley.com/go/dubinsky/clinicalresearch

34.2   Objectives

This chapter informs the reader about basic approaches that regulatory/competent authorities take in implementing inspection programs as part of their assigned responsibilities. We also describe the ways that sites in particular as well as others subject to regulatory inspection can prepare and ready themselves to process inspections in an efficient and effective manner.

34.3   Scheduling and Conducting GCP Inspections

GCP inspections have been a staple in the inspection programs of many regulatory authorities for some time now and for others GCP inspections are a relatively new undertaking. In the United States, the FDA began their formal GCP inspection programs circa 1978 with the advent of the Bioresearch Monitoring (BiMo) Compliance programs. Those inspection programs served as the gold standard for some time and many still see them as the best model for GCP oversight. In 2001 when the Clinical Trial Directive was published the EU member states began their version of BiMo by establishing a GCP inspection program that has grown considerably since that time and depending upon which member State's inspectors are conducting the work is viewed by many observers as the more rigorous than the FDA. GCP inspections are not specifically required by the US FFDCA but EU Laws do call for such inspections to be conducted as a requirement.

The approach of the inspectorate in terms of scheduling the GCP inspection work differs in some regards and is very similar in others. For example most GCP inspections are announced or scheduled because the inspectorate wants the location to have appropriate key staff available for interviews and records readily available for review. In the EU this preannouncement includes a request for a documentation set which inspectors will review prior to conducting the work. The strategy for the inspectional assessment of a trial overall also differs in that some inspectorates inspect a sponsor first then based on findings there, decide on the nature and scope of the visits to sites. Others approach the overall inspection process by starting at the epicenter of trial activity – the investigational site. Before going further however a brief review of the reasons which prompt regulators to schedule GCP inspections is appropriate.

GCP inspections are scheduled when:

1) A clinical trial authorization has been issued and subjects are being enrolled.
2) A marketing application has been received for review by a regulatory authority.
3) A regulator decides that there is rationale (a cause) for conducting an inspection before, during or after a trial is initiated.

Reasons 1 and 2 above represent the primary reasons for scheduling a GCP inspection and reason 3 can be subdivided further into reasons such as:

a) A complaint is received about the manner in which a trial is being conducted. Complaints can be initiated by subjects, company staff, observers, in sum anyone with some awareness of the trial activity.
b) The sponsor alerts the regulator to some untoward activity about the trial as required by regulation, e.g. serious unexpected adverse reaction(s), significant noncompliance by a site investigator or a serious breach of GCP requirements.
c) The regulator determines that due to the nature of a trial or trials, e.g. a set of trials enrolling infants (vulnerable population), additional inspectional oversight is appropriate.

With regard to trial sites the reasons for inspecting a specific site may go a bit deeper and draw on application data which shows high numbers of subjects enrolled; too many or too few experience reports; data points that seems too perfect to be real; or the site has an already tarnished track record of compliance.

When initially contacting trial sponsors some regulators request that certain documentation be submitted prior to date of the inspection. Active protocols, SOPs and personnel training records might be among the documents request for pre-inspection review.

Most inspections follow a pattern of: (i) introductory meeting when inspectors outline the objective of their inspection before; (ii) proceeding to actual inspection of physical spaces, interview of staff who performed the trial work and in-depth review of documents (hard copy and digital) which document the work performed, i.e. the trial master file. Inspectors usually have a reasonable target timetable to accomplish the inspection work which they will share at the outset. However, that timetable can easily expand if significant findings emerge and additional time is needed. (iii) Inspectional findings are initially reported to the location staff either in writing (e.g. FDA-483) or verbally as general comments. Official feedback is always in writing which includes details as to how best to respond. Most regulatory authorities have written program instructions for their inspectors (Note: for US FDA they are investigators) which are available online. The online information explaining why, how, and who conducts GCP inspection is part of the reference materials provided with this text.

34.4 Inspection Readiness – Preparation, Hosting, and Follow-up

Inspections can occur at any time therefore being inspection ready is important. Anxiety and nervousness often prevail among staff during inspections. That is in part because regulatory inspectors are viewed by some as the police. Keeping in perspective that inspectors/investigators are evidence gatherers and that there are sanctions and penalties imposed for serious violations, being prepared to explain how a trial was conducted according to GCP, the regulations, the protocol and all applicable best practices takes some training and experience. Effectively communicating to an inspector that GCP was implemented can be learned. Inspection readiness includes:

1) Establishing an Inspection Readiness Team and Program – Sites usually receive sponsor support
2) Developing notification/communication procedures to keep staff informed
3) Drafting SOPs and training against them
4) Appointing a Central Inspection Coordinator
5) Defining roles for a readiness team, e.g. host, scribe, subject matter experts.
6) Understanding the dos and don'ts of the inspection process

Details of each of these steps would take a separate text but a synopsis of key practical aspects are:

i) At the initial meeting, as well as the closing meeting, ensure that top management is part of receiving the inspector/inspection team. Inspectors take their work seriously, demonstrate that you do too.
ii) Establish the working venues for inspection tasks such as document review. It should have phone and internet capability and not be in the path of day to day work at the location.
iii) Copying of documents is an inspectional inevitability. Have a plan for providing copies and ensure exact duplicates are retained at the company.
iv) Train staff in interview etiquette such as: be truthful, ask for clarification if unsure of a question, avoid speculation or guessing, only answer questions in your purview, only answer the question you are asked.
v) Things not to do, include: (i) Divulging information about personnel matters except for qualifications, training, job descriptions; (ii) modifying documents; (iii) discussing internal audits; (iv) allowing inspector unescorted access to work areas, and (v) debating what constitutes compliance with the inspector.
vi) Be certain that the company's policies on photographs, recordings and document signing are clear and understood by all staff.
vii) After the inspection is completed arrange meetings with staff and management to discuss observations and frame out draft responses; develop statements of correction and plan to provide written response to the regulator.

This has been a very brief outline of the inspection readiness process. You are encouraged to seek additional insight from other resources and references so that when the inspector(s) do knock your location is prepared.

34.5 Summary

Regulatory inspections will occur and can occur at any time. Therefore the most effective preparation is to conduct the trial in conformance with the key indices – Regulations, protocol, SOPs, and GCP. However, even full compliance with all the requirements is not a guarantee that an inspection will go without a glitch. Honing inspection etiquette skills, treating the inspection process with the respect it deserves and avoiding misunderstandings and miscommunications all aid in making an inspection a productive experience.

Knowledge Check Questions

1) Regulators wait until they receive a complaint before scheduling an inspection of a trial site. True _____ or False _____
2) The US FDA conducts GCP inspections because it is mandated under the FFDCA. Yes ___ or No____
3) Most GCP inspections are scheduled/announced because: (select best response)
   a) The inspectors are on a tight schedule ___
   b) Clinical trial staff seem to always be on vacation ___
   c) The presence of key staff and availability of records is important ___
   d) The prevailing laws on GCP inspections require it ___
4) Receipt of a major marketing application e.g. NDA, is a primary motivator for scheduling GCP inspections. Correct ___ or incorrect ____
5) GCP inspectors always find discrepancies because that is their job. True ___ or False ___
6) Inspection readiness includes the following steps (select all that fit):
   a) Creating a strategic plan that is coordinated by the Company CEO and approved by the Board of directors._____
   b) Selecting a central coordinator who serves as the point of contact for all inspections matters. ___
   c) Training staff in how to best follow interview etiquette with an inspector.___
   d) Selecting a location for the inspectors to occupy and work from including internet access. ____
   e) Obtaining a certification from the National Inspection Readiness training academy ___
7) The best preparation for a GCP regulatory inspection is to conduct the trial in conformance with GCP, regulations, the protocol and SOPs. Correct ___ or Incorrect ___

References for All Chapters

American Society of Health-System Pharmacists (1998). Guidelines on clinical drug research. https://www.ashp.org/-/media/assets/policy-guidelines/docs/guidelines/clinical-drug-research.ashx?la=en&hash=8973560F661752ABFE1F66EC65D7DD6D4EC03b2503 (accessed 17 December 2019).

ANSI WEBSTORE (2011). *Clinical Investigation of Medical Devices for Human Subjects: Good Clinical Practice*. International Standards Organization http://webstore.ansi.org/RecordDetail.aspx?sku=ISO%2014155:2011&source=google&adgroup=iso11&gclid=CO6fhuXkx70CFU5rfgodQGwA9Q (accessed 27 November 2019). ISO 14155:2011.

Authenticated U.S. Government Information (2008). Federal Register/Vol. 73, No. 82/Monday, April 28, 2008/Rules and regulations, human subject protection; foreign clinical studies not conducted under an investigational new drug application, final rule. https://www.govinfo.gov/content/pkg/FR-2008-04-28/pdf/E8-9200.pdf (accessed 27 November 2019).

Azvolinsky, A. (2017). Repurposing existing drugs for new indications. 1 January 2017. https://www.the-scientist.com/features/repurposingexistingdrugsfornew-indications32285?archived_content=9BmGYHLCH6vLGNdd9YzYFAqV8S3Xw3L5 (accessed 27 January 2020).

Bargaje, C. (2011). Good documentation practice in clinical research. *Perspectives in Clinical Research* 2 (2): 59–63. https://www.ncbi.nlm.nih.gov/pmc/articles/PMC3121265/?report=printable (accessed 27 January 2020).

Centers for Disease Control and Prevention. U.S. Public Health Service Syphilis Study at Tuskegee. http://www.cdc.gov/tuskegee/timeline.htm (accessed 27 November 2019).

The Fundamentals of Clinical Research: A Universal Guide for Implementing Good Clinical Practice, First Edition. P. Michael Dubinsky and Karen A. Henry.
© 2022 John Wiley & Sons, Inc. Published 2022 by John Wiley & Sons, Inc.
Companion website: www.wiley.com/go/dubinsky/clinicalresearch

Clinical Trials Transformation Initiative Recommendations (2015). Quality by design. https://www.ctti-clinicaltrials.org/sites/www.ctti-clinicaltrials.org/files/CTTI%252 0Quality%2520by%2520Design%2520Recommendations_FINAL_1JUN15.pdf (accessed 25 May 2021).

EMA (2012). Reflection paper on laboratories that test clinical trial samples. http://www.ema.europa.eu/docs/en_GB/document_library/Regulatory_and_procedural_guideline/2012/05/WC500127124.pdf (accessed 27 January 2020).

EMA (2018). Scientific guidelines. http://www.ema.europa.eu/ema/index.jsp?curl=pages/regulation/general/general_content_000043.jsp&mid=WC0b01ac05800240cb (accessed 27 January 2020).

EMA (2020). Good clinical practice Q&A, GCP matters. https://www.ema.europa.eu/en/human-regulatory/research-development/compliance/good-clinical-practice/qa-good-clinical-practice-gcp#gcp-matters-section (accessed 1 June 2020).

European Commission. Directive 2001/20/EC, clinical trials. https://ec.europa.eu/health/human-use/clinical-trials/directive_en (accessed 27 November 2019).

European Commission (2014a). Regulation (EU) No 536/2014 of the European Parliament and of the Council of 16 April 2014 on clinical trials on medicinal products for human use, and repealing Directive 2001/20/EC. https://ec.europa.eu/health//sites/health/files/files/eudralex/vol-1/reg_2014_536/reg_2014_536_en.pdf (accessed 27 January 2020).

European Commission (2014b). Regulation (EU) No. 536/2014 of the European Parliament and the Council (16 April 2014). Clinical trials of medicinal products for humans for human use. *Official Journal of the European Union* L158: 1–76. https://ec.europa.eu/health/human-use/clinical-trials/regulation_en (accessed 19 February 2019).

European Commission (2014c). Regulation (EU) No 536/2014 of the European Parliament and of the Council of 16 April 2014 on clinical trials on medicinal products for human use, and repealing Directive 2001/20/ECEU Regulation 536, Article 58 - Archiving of the clinical trial master file. https://ec.europa.eu/health/sites/health/files/files/eudralex/vol-1/reg_2014_536/reg_2014_536_en.pdf (accessed 6 April 2020).

European Communities (2001). Directive 2001/83/EC of the European Parliament and of the Council (6 November 2001) on the community code relating to medicinal products for human use. *Official Journal-European Communities Legislation L*, 44(Part 311): 67–128. https://eur-lex.europa.eu/LexUriServ/LexUriServ.do?uri=OJ:L:2001:311:0067:0128:en:PDF (accessed 19 February 2019).

GPO (2004). Federal Register, 32467, Vol. 69, No. 112, Thursday, June 10, 2004 human subject protection; foreign clinical studies not conducted under an investigational new drug application – proposed rule. http://www.gpo.gov/fdsys/pkg/FR-2004-06-10/pdf/04-13063.pdf (accessed 27 November 2019).

Grady, C. (2015). Institutional review boards, purpose and challenges, commentary, chest, November 2015 (1148–1155). https://www.ncbi.nlm.nih.gov/pmc/articles/PMC4631034/pdf/chest_148_5_1148.pdf (accessed 28 May 2020).

International Council for Harmonisation of Technical Requirements for Pharmaceuticals for Human Use (ICH). http://www.ich.org/ (accessed 27 November 2019).

International Council for Harmonisation of Technical Requirements for Pharmaceuticals for Human Use (ICH). https://www.ich.org/home.html (accessed 27 January 2020).

International Council for Harmonisation of Technical Requirements for Pharmaceuticals for Human Use (ICH) (1994). Guideline for Clinical Safety Data Management: Definitions and Standards for Expedited Reporting E2A (1994) Current Step 4 version dated 27 October 1994. https://www.ich.org/page/efficacy-guidelines.

International Council for Harmonisation of Technical Requirements for Pharmaceuticals for Human Use (ICH) (1995). Guideline for Structure and Content of Clinical Study Reports E3 (1995). Current Step 4 version dated 30 November 1995. https://www.ich.org/page/efficacy-guidelines.

International Council for Harmonisation of Technical Requirements for Pharmaceuticals for Human Use (ICH) (2012). Implementation Working Group ICH E3 Guideline: Structure and Content of Clinical Study Reports Questions & Answers (R1) Current version dated 6 July 2012. https://www.ich.org/page/efficacy-guidelines.

International Council for Harmonisation of Technical Requirements for Pharmaceuticals for Human Use (ICH) (2016). Integrated Addendum to ICH E6(R1):Guideline for Good Clinical Practice, E6(R2) (2016). Current Step 4 version dated 9 November 2016. https://www.ich.org/page/efficacy-guidelines.

International Conference on Harmonisation of Technical Requirements for Registration of Pharmaceuticals for Human Use (ICH) (1997). Harmonised Tripartite Guideline: General Considerations for Clinical Trials E8 (1997). Current Step 4 version dated 17 July 1997. https://www.ich.org/page/efficacy-guidelines (accessed 19 July 2021).

International Conference on Harmonisation of Technical Requirements for Registration of Pharmaceuticals for Human Use (ICH) (1998). Harmonised Tripartite Guideline: Statistical Principles for Clinical Trials, E9 (1998). Current Step 4 version dated 5 February 1998. https://www.ich.org/page/efficacy-guidelines (accessed 19 July 2021).

ISO 14155:2011 (2011). *Clinical Investigation of Medical Devices for Human Subjects: Good Clinical Practice*. International Organization for Standardization. https://www.iso.org/standard/45557.html (accessed 27 January 2020).

ISO 9001:2015 (2015). *Quality Management Systems – Requirements*. Geneva, Switzerland: International Organization for Standardization.

Janssen, W.F. (1981). Story of the laws behind the labels, Part 1. The 1906 Food and Drugs Act. https://wayback.archive-it.org/7993/20170111191530/http://www.fda.gov/AboutFDA/WhatWeDo/History/Overviews/ucm056044.htm (accessed 27 November 2019).

Merriam-Webster's. Learner's dictionary. http://www.merriam-webster.com/dictionary/protocol.

NIH (1908a). National Research Act – Office of NIH history. https://history.nih.gov/research/downloads/PL93-348.pdf (accessed 27 November 2019).

NIH (1908b). A short history of the National Institutes of Health, p. 3. http://history.nih.gov/exhibits/history/docs/page_03.html (accessed 11 November 2019).

Penn Medicine (2020). What is an Academic Medical Center. https://www.pennmedicine.org/about/benefits-of-an-academic-medical-center (accessed 27 January 2020).

United States Department of Health and Human Services Food and Drug Administration. Title 21, Chapter I, Subchapter D, Part 316.20. https://www.ecfr.gov/cgi-bin/retrieveECFR?gp=&SID=718f6fcbc20f2755bd1f5a980eb5eecd&mc=true&n=sp21.5.316.c&r=SUBPART&ty=HTML#se21.5.316_12.

United States Department of Health and Human Services Food and Drug Administration (2015). Guidance for industry considerations for the design of early-phase clinical trials of cellular and gene therapy products, Center for Biologics Evaluation and Research June 2015. https://www.fda.gov/downloads/BiologicsBloodVaccines/GuidanceComplianceRegulatoryInformation/Guidances/CellularandGeneTherapy/UCM564952.pdf.

United States Food and Drug Administration (1999). Guidance for Industry, Submission of Abbreviated Reports and Synopses in Support of Marketing Applications, U.S. Department of Health and Human Services, Food and Drug Administration, Center for Drug Evaluation and Research (CDER), Center for Biologics Evaluation and Research (CBER), August 1999, Clinical. https://www.fda.gov/media/71125/download.

United States Food and Drug Administration (2000). Good guidance practices/Guidance documents FDA Regs at 21 CFR 10.115. http://www.accessdata.fda.gov/scripts/cdrh/cfdocs/cfcfr/CFRSearch.cfm?fr=10.115 (accessed 27 January 2020).

United States Food and Drug Administration (2002). Code of Federal Regulations Title 21 CFR 56.115 (b). https://www.accessdata.fda.gov/scripts/cdrh/cfdocs/cfcfr/CFRSearch.cfm?fr=56.115 (accessed 6 April 2020).

United States Food and Drug Administration (2008a). Guidance for industry: CGMP for Phase I investigational drugs. https://www.fda.gov/downloads/Drugs/GuidanceComplianceRegulatoryInformation/Guidances/UCM070273.pdf (accessed 17 December 2019).

United States Food and Drug Administration (2008b). Program 7348.811, chapter 48, Bioresearch Monitoring: Clinical Investigators and Sponsor-Investigators. https://www.fda.gov/media/75927/download (accessed 16 August 2021).

United States Food and Drug Administration (2012a). Consumer updates, Kefauver-Harris Amendments Revolutionized Drug Development. http://www.fda.gov/ForConsumers/ConsumerUpdates/ucm322856.htm (accessed 27 November 2019).

United States Food and Drug Administration (2012b). History of drug regulation in the United States, 1906–2006, p. 6. wayback.archive-it.org/7993/20170114041745/http://www.fda.gov/downloads/AboutFDA/WhatWeDo/History/ProductRegulation/PromotingSafeandEffectiveDrugsfor100Years/UCM114468.pdf (accessed 27 November 2019).

United States Food and Drug Administration (2017). Best practices for communication between IND sponsors and FDA during drug development. https://www.fda.gov/regulatory-information/search-fda-guidance-documents/best-practices-communication-between-ind-sponsors-and-fda-during-drug-development (accessed 27 January 2020).

United States Food and Drug Administration (2019). Investigators Operations Manual (IOM). Chapter 5 Establishment Inspections – Subchapter 5.3 Evidence Development, Responsible Individuals 5.3.6. https://www.fda.gov/media/76769/download (accessed 21 January 2020).

United States Food and Drug Administration Bioresearch Monitoring (BIMO) (2021). Inspection metrics. https://www.fda.gov/science-research/clinical-trials-and-human-subject-protection/bimo-inspection-metrics (accessed 6 April 2020).

United States Holocaust Memorial Museum. United States Holocaust Memorial Museum Note. https://www.ushmm.org/information/exhibitions/online-exhibitions/special-focus/doctors-trial/nuremberg-code (assessed 27 November 2019).

US Department of Health and Human Services. Office of human research protections, the Belmont report. http://www.hhs.gov/ohrp/humansubjects/guidance/belmont.html (accessed 27 November 2019).

US Government Accountability Office. Federal control of new drug testing is not adequately protecting human test subjects and the public HRD-76-96. Published: 15 July 1976. Publicly released: 15 July 1976. http://www.gao.gov/products/HRD-76-96 (accessed 27 November 2019).

World Health Organization (2002). *Handbook for Good Clinical Research Practice.* World Health Organization. ISBN: ISBN 92 4 159392 X. https://www.who.int/medicines/areas/quality_safety/safety_efficacy/gcp1.pdf.

World Health Organization (2005). *Handbook for Good Clinical Research Practice (GCP): Guidance for Implementation.* World Health Organization. https://apps.who.int/iris/handle/10665/43392 (accessed 13 February 2020).

World Medical Association (2018). WMA Declaration of Helsinki – ethical principles for medical research involving human subjects. https://www.wma.net/policies-post/wma-declaration-of-helsinki-ethical-principles-for-medical-research-involving-human-subjects/ (accessed 27 November 2019).

Index

The Fundamentals of Clinical Research: A Universal Guide for Implementing Good Clinical Practice,
First Edition. P. Michael Dubinsky and Karen A. Henry.
© 2022 John Wiley & Sons, Inc. Published 2022 by John Wiley & Sons, Inc.
Companion website: www.wiley.com/go/dubinsky/clinicalresearch

CPSIA information can be obtained
at www.ICGtesting.com
Printed in the USA
BVHW052331170123
655609BV00002B/57